The Psychotherapy of Schizophrenia

The Psychotherapy of Schizophrenia

EDITED BY

JOHN S. STRAUSS
MALCOLM BOWERS
T. WAYNE DOWNEY
STEPHEN FLECK
STANLEY JACKSON
AND IRA LEVINE

Yale University School of Medicine
New Haven, Connecticut

PLENUM MEDICAL BOOK COMPANY
New York and London

Library of Congress Cataloging in Publication Data

Main entry under title:

The Psychotherapy of schizophrenia.

Includes index.
1. Schizophrenia—Addresses, essays, lectures.   I. Strauss, John S.   [DNLM: 1.
Schizophrenia—Therapy—Congresses.   2. Psychotherapy—Congresses.   WM203
P9744 1979]
RC514.C58   616.89'8206   80-16524
ISBN 0-306-40497-4

© 1980 Plenum Publishing Corporation
227 West 17th Street, New York, N.Y. 10011

Plenum Medical Book Company is an imprint of Plenum Publishing Corporation

Printed in the United States of America

Contributors

YRJÖ ALANEN, M.D. • Professor of Psychiatry, University of Turku, Finland

SIDNEY J. BLATT, PH.D. • Professor of Psychology and Psychiatry, Yale University

MALCOLM B. BOWERS, JR., M.D. • Professor of Psychiatry, Yale University School of Medicine; Chief of Psychiatry, Yale-New Haven Hospital

C. BROOKS BRENNEIS, PH.D. • Clinical Faculty, Department of Psychology and Psychiatry, University of Wisconsin

EUGENE B. BRODY, M.D. • Professor of Psychiatry and Human Behavior, University of Maryland at Baltimore; Formerly Chairman, Department of Psychiatry

HILDE BRUCH, M.D. • Professor Emeritus of Psychiatry, Baylor College of Medicine

WILLIAM T. CARPENTER, JR., M.D. • Director, Maryland Psychiatric Research Center; Professor of Psychiatry, University of Maryland School of Medicine

JOHN P. DOCHERTY, M.D. • Director of Education, Yale Psychiatric Institute

T. WAYNE DOWNEY, M.D. • Associate Clinical Professor of Pediatrics and Psychiatry, Yale Child Study Center

STEPHEN FLECK, M.D. • Professor of Psychiatry and Public Health and Deputy Chairman, Department of Psychiatry, Yale University School of Medicine

MICHAEL J. GOLDSTEIN, PH.D. • Professor of Psychology, University of California at Los Angeles

BEVERLY GOMES-SCHWARTZ, PH.D. • Assistant Psychologist, McLean Hospital, Blemont, Massachusetts; Instructor in Psychiatry, Harvard Medical School

DAVID GREENFELD, M.D. • Assistant Clinical Professor, Department of Psychiatry, Yale University

DOUGLAS W. HEINRICHS, M.D. • Department of Psychiatry, University of Maryland

JUHANI LAAKSO, M.D. • Department of Psychiatry, University of Turku, Finland

ROBERT P. LIBERMAN, M.D. • Professor of Psychiatry, University of California at Los Angeles, School of Medicine; Director, Mental Health Clinical Research Center for the study of Schizophrenia

PHILIP R. A. MAY, M.D. • Director, Health Service Research and Development Laboratory, Brentwood V.A. Hospital, Los Angeles, California

GORDON L. PAUL, PH.D. • Department of Psychology, University of Houston, Houston, Texas; Director, Clinical Research Unit, Adolf Meyer Mental Health Center

VILJO RÄKKÖLÄINEN, M.D. • Department of Psychiatry, University of Turku, Finland

RIITTA RASIMUS, M.D. • Department of Psychiatry, University of Turku, Finland

CLINTON RUST, M.P.A. • Executive Director, Camarillo State Hospital

JEAN G. SCHIMEK, PH.D. • Associate Professor of Psychology, New York University

CLARENCE G. SCHULZ, M.D. • Senior Psychiatrist, The Sheppard and Enoch Pratt Hospital

DANIEL P. SCHWARTZ, M.D. • Medical Director, Austen Riggs Center, Inc.

KAREN S. SNYDER, M.A. • Research Associate, University of California at Los Angeles

ALFRED H. STANTON, M.D. • Professor of Psychiatry, Harvard Medical School; Psychiatrist, McLean Hospital

HELM STIERLIN, M.D. • Division of Psychoanalysis and Family Therapy, University of Heidelberg, Germany

JOHN S. STRAUSS, M.D. • Professor of Psychiatry, Yale University School of Medicine

A. HUSSAIN TUMA, PH.D. • Acting Chief, Clinical Research Branch, National Institute of Mental Health

CHRISTINE E. VAUGHN, PH.D. • Associate Research Psychologist, University of California at Los Angeles

CHARLES J. WALLACE, PH.D. • Associate Director, Mental Health Clinical Research Center, University of California at Los Angeles

OTTO A. WILL, JR., M.D. • Clinical Director, Adolescent and Young Adult Inpatient Service, Mt. Zion Hospital, San Francisco, California

LYMAN C. WYNNE, M.D., PH.D. • Professor of Psychiatry, University of Rochester School of Medicine and Dentistry

Preface

This volume is dedicated to Theodore Lidz and Ruth W. Lidz, as was the conference on the Psychotherapy of Schizophrenia held on April 9 and 10, 1979, at which the materials here published were presented. This 1979 symposium replicated in some respects the one held at Yale University thirty years earlier, at a time when psychotherapy with schizophrenic patients was viewed with much optimism and enthusiasm. Ruth and Ted Lidz contributed to this earlier symposium also, emphasizing in their paper the intense mother–patient bond as a therapeutic issue.

Since then, considerable strides have been made in the treatment of schizophrenic patients. The introduction of psychopharmacologic agents, the development of family therapy, and more sophisticated methods in community-based care for such patients, all have had important impacts. Psychotherapy with schizophrenics as such has remained a rather limited practice, partly because it is difficult and demanding of therapists' time and personal investment, and partly because documenting its effectiveness on a statistically or epidemiologically valid plane has eluded us.

In fact, the use of psychotherapy for treating schizophrenic patients is one of the more controversial issues in psychiatry. Two factors besides questions of efficacy contribute to this controversy. First, psychotherapy as a treatment often gets confused with strongly held convictions about etiological questions. Second, the value of psychotherapy for learning about schizophrenia as well as treating it may be at stake. Many view psychotherapeutic exploration of the subjective experiences of schizophrenia as practically unique in providing valuable information for combining with objective data which by themselves consider only one aspect of an ongoing process and life. These and other issues are discussed in this volume.

Brought together here are critics and defenders, all with knowledge of practice and methodology, but with various orientations and interpretations of both. For the practitioner and the investigator, we believe that the papers and discussions in this volume will help to clarify how practice and research can be improved, suggest areas where opposing views can produce a synthesis in which certain disagreements cease to make sense, and highlight continuing differences of opinion that at some point will have to be resolved.

Despite the considerable progress over the three decades which the volume reflects, much remains to be discovered. The importance of subjective and objective data in research and treatment, and the apparent need for multilevel approaches for understanding schizophrenic patients, make this a complex field. However, the strengths and weaknesses of current views, and the directions for future research and treatment, are becoming clearer. We believe that this volume will help in this process.

JOHN S. STRAUSS
MALCOLM BOWERS
T. WAYNE DOWNEY
STEPHEN FLECK
STANLEY JACKSON
IRA LEVINE

Yale University
School of Medicine

Contents

I RATIONALE FOR THE PSYCHOTHERAPY OF SCHIZOPHRENIA

1 PSYCHOTHERAPY IN SCHIZOPHRENIA: HISTORICAL CONSIDERATIONS 3

  Hilde Bruch, M.D.

2 ON THE CENTRAL TASK OF PSYCHOTHERAPY: PSYCHOANALYTIC AND
  FAMILY PERSPECTIVES 13

  Helm Stierlin, M.D.

3 SOCIAL AND FAMILY FACTORS IN THE COURSE OF SCHIZOPHRENIA:
  TOWARD AN INTERPERSONAL PROBLEM-SOLVING THERAPY FOR
  SCHIZOPHRENICS AND THEIR FAMILIES 21

  Robert Paul Liberman, M.D.; Charles J. Wallace, Ph.D.; Christine E.
  Vaughn, Ph.D.; Karen S. Snyder, M.A.; and Clinton Rust, M.P.A.

4 SOME OBSERVATIONS ON THE NATURE AND VALUE OF PSYCHOTHERAPY
  WITH SCHIZOPHRENIC PATIENTS...................................... 55

  Stephen Fleck, M.D.

5 DISCUSSION: RATIONALE FOR THE PSYCHOTHERAPY OF SCHIZOPHRENIA 65

  Eugene B. Brody, M.D.

6 GENERAL DISCUSSION.. 71

II RESEARCH

7   FAMILY THERAPY DURING THE AFTERCARE TREATMENT OF ACUTE
    SCHIZOPHRENIA   77

    Michael J. Goldstein, Ph.D.

8   PSYCHOTHERAPY OF SCHIZOPHRENIA: CAN WE MAKE IT WORK?   91

    Philip R. A. May, M.D.

9   THE NATURE OF THE PSYCHOTIC EXPERIENCE AND ITS IMPLICATIONS FOR
    THE THERAPEUTIC PROCESS   101

    Sidney J. Blatt, Ph.D.; Jean G. Schimek, Ph.D.; and
        C. Brooks Brenneis, Ph.D.

10 PROBLEMS INHERENT IN THE STUDY OF PSYCHOTHERAPY OF PSYCHOSES:
    CONCLUSIONS FROM A COMMUNITY PSYCHIATRIC ACTION RESEARCH STUDY.   115

    Yrjö O. Alanen, Viljo Räkköläinen, Juhani Laakso, and Riita Rasimus

11 INSIGHT AND SELF-OBSERVATION: THEIR ROLE IN THE ANALYSIS OF THE
    ETIOLOGY OF ILLNESS   131

    Alfred H. Stanton, M.D.

12 DISCUSSION   145

    A. Hussain Tuma, Ph.D.

13 GENERAL DISCUSSION..   151

III THE PRACTICE OF PSYCHOTHERAPY WITH SCHIZOPHRENICS

14 COMMENTS ON THE "ELEMENTS" OF SCHIZOPHRENIA, PSYCHOTHERAPY,
    AND THE SCHIZOPHRENIC PERSON.....................................   157

    Otto Allen Will, Jr., M.D.

15 COMPREHENSIVE PSYCHOSOCIAL TREATMENT: BEYOND TRADITIONAL
    PSYCHOTHERAPY   167

    Gordon L. Paul, Ph.D.

16 ALL-OR-NONE PHENOMENA IN THE PSYCHOTHERAPY OF SEVERE
    DISORDERS   181

    Clarence G. Schulz, M.D.

17 PARADOXICAL INTERVENTIONS: LEVERAGE FOR THERAPEUTIC CHANGE IN
    INDIVIDUAL AND FAMILY SYSTEMS 191

    Lyman C. Wynne, M.D., Ph.D.

18 DISCUSSION: THE PRACTICE OF PSYCHOTHERAPY WITH SCHIZOPHRENICS 203

    Daniel P. Schwartz, M.D.

19 GENERAL DISCUSSION.. 209

IV NEW DIRECTIONS

20 THE DEVELOPING GUIDELINES TO THE PSYCHOTHERAPY OF
    SCHIZOPHRENIA 217

    Theodore Lidz, M.D.

21 MEDICATION AND PSYCHOTHERAPY IN OUTPATIENTS VULNERABLE TO
    PSYCHOSIS 227

    Malcolm Baker Bowers, Jr., M.D. and David George Greenfeld, M.D.

22 THE ROLE FOR PSYCHODYNAMIC PSYCHIATRY IN THE TREATMENT OF
    SCHIZOPHRENIC PATIENTS 239

    William T. Carpenter, Jr., M.D. and Douglas W. Heinrichs, M.D.

23 THE QUALITY OF OUTCOME FROM PSYCHOTHERAPY OF SCHIZOPHRENIA 257

    John G. Gunderson, M.D. and Beverly Gomes-Schwartz, Ph.D.

24 TOWARD COMPREHENSIVE UNDERSTANDING AND TREATMENT OF
    SCHIZOPHRENIA 277

    *John S. Strauss, M.D.; John P. Docherty, M.D.; and
    T. Wayne Downey, M.D.*

25 DISCUSSION: NEW DIRECTIONS....................................... 287

    Morris B. Parloff, Ph.D.

26 GENERAL DISCUSSION... 293

    INDEX 297

Acknowledgments

The editors wish to extend special thanks to the following organizations that contributed to the support of the Psychotherapy of Schizophrenia conference and thus made this volume possible: The Center for Studies of Schizophrenia and the Psychotherapy and Behavioral Intervention Section, both from the Clinical Research Branch of the National Institute of Mental Health; Hoffman-LaRoche, Inc.; Sandoz Pharmaceuticals; E. R. Squibb and Sons, Inc., The Warner/Chilcott Co.

Part I

Rationale for the Psychotherapy of Schizophrenia

Psychotherapy in Schizophrenia

Historical Considerations

HILDE BRUCH

The treatment a mentally ill person receives depends to a large extent on the therapist's theoretical conceptions about the nature of the illness. In schizophrenia, there has been a continuous controversy around the question of whether its origin was of a psychological or an organic nature. Kraepelin, who in 1890 had reported that a series of mental disease pictures had a common course, namely termination in a special kind of mental weakness, attributed the illness to some underlying organic, assumedly inherited predisposition. People suffering from this illness (to which he gave the name Dementia Praecox) were considered not accessible to treatment, and their communication was labeled meaningless and not understandable. The abnormal behavior and the disturbed symbolic processes of these patients seemed to him an expression of some organic abnormality, probably of the brain.

In 1917, at the inauguration of The German Research Institute for Psychiatry, he reviewed the progress in psychiatry during the past hundred years, and related various practices to the philosophical concepts of their

HILDE BRUCH • Department of Psychiatry, Baylor College of Medicine, Houston, Texas 77030.

age, to the theoretical assumptions of the scientific speciality, and to rationalizations of the continuation of deep-rooted prejudices.[1-3] As long as the insane were conceived of as violent and dangerous, they were kept in chains, to protect their fellow citizens and wardens. Later on, the explanation was that restraints would pacify and relax them, and thus aid in their recovery. Similar contradictory justifications were given for the use of the lash. In nineteenth-century concepts, the psychiatrist was viewed as needing the power and psychic ability to subdue a patient, tame him, and arouse fear in him. Kraepelin was particularly critical of proponents of psychic theories, according to which insanity was the outcome of personal guilt and sin; therapy was directed at making patients atone for this through suffering, including food and sleep deprivation. Kraepelin took pride in having removed the concept of mental illness from the domain of sinfulness, and having made it a medical condition instead. He did not acknowledge the newer psychological approaches, and the names of his outstanding contemporaries, Bleuler, Freud, and Meyer, are not mentioned. Only the search for organic causes was considered scientifically respectable.

Bleuler proposed the name "schizophrenia" for this disease group, because he saw the elementary disturbance in the lacking unity of subjective experiences, in fragmentation and splitting of thinking, feelings, and will. He also drew attention to the motivational and affective significance of the secondary symptomatology. He considered as the primary symptom a peculiar loosening of the associational link in thinking, and felt that this was the manifestation of a hypothetical morbid process. Meyer, a competent neurologist and neuropathologist, denied the usefulness of any classification according to speculative assumptions that cerebral or glandular lesions or dysfunctions were the cause of the mental disturbance and of the resulting failure in life adjustment. Throughout his teaching, he maintained that schizophrenics needed to, and could, be understood in terms of their life experiences. Bleuler and Meyer disagreed with Kraepelin's basically pessimistic view that the vast majority of patients were forever lost and practically incurable.

This atmosphere of fateful pessimism pervaded the teaching of psychiatry in German medical schools during the 1920s. When I was graduated in 1928, I was offered an assistantship at the Freiburg Psychiatric Clinic, which I declined with the explanation: "I don't want to spend the rest of my life with museum pieces." Nothing in the teaching had suggested that these patients might change or were capable of response. Rosenfeld experienced something similar as a medical student in Germany, and then encountered the same attitude in England a few years later.[4] When he had positive results by talking with hospitalized schizophrenics, his colleagues attributed this to "remission," because relating them to human interaction would imply a psychogenic basis, which at that time (mid-1930s) was not acceptable in England.

My interest in psychiatry reawakened after coming to the United States in 1934. I met several people actively engaged in therapeutic work with schizophrenics, and I distinctly remember my amazed reaction, "But nobody can talk with them!" When I became a resident at the Phipps Clinic of the Johns Hopkins Hospital in the early 1940s, it required a reevaluation of everything I had learned. I didn't quite begin from scratch, because my work with obese children had made me aware of the importance of psychological experiences and the disturbed patterns of family interaction for the disturbances in their symptoms and personality.[5] Several of these severely disturbed fat children later became manifestly schizophrenic.

Under the leadership of Adolf Meyer, the Phipps Clinic had a long tradition of an individualistic approach to schizophrenics. Many different physicians and training centers have taken part in the application of psychological understanding to the treatment of psychotics, and have approached the task from different angles and with various techniques. Outstanding are the names of two psychoanalysts (Harry Stack Sullivan and Frieda Fromm-Reichmann) for their innovative therapeutic work with schizophrenics; they were associated with two private hospitals (Chestnut Lodge Sanitarium, and Sheppard and Pratt Hospital) in the Washington/Baltimore area. I shall refer chiefly to their work, which was organized around the concept of interpersonal relations and communication.[6,7]

Psychoanalysis played an important role in this whole development. Psychoanalysis has provided psychiatry with a genetic, dynamic, and interpretative point of view, and with a treatment method. Freud had at first expressed the opinion that, with proper modification, his approach might be used in the treatment of psychosis; but then he felt that the schizophrenics' narcissism would prevent the development of a therapeutically valid transference relationship, and make them inaccessible to psychoanalytic treatment. Some analysts were not discouraged by this pessimism, and modified the classical analytic approach to fit the needs of schizophrenics. The modification extended in many ways the range and application of psychoanalytic thinking. The first work was done at a time when the basic analytic teaching was that of id psychology. In the work with schizophrenics, the importance of disturbances in ego functions came into the foreground, and much of what is now called object-relationship theory can be traced to these early reevaluations.

Lengthy and sometimes heated debates dealt with the question of whether the modified approach could be properly called *psychoanalysis*. In 1931, Sullivan reported on his, by then already extensive, experiences in a paper called "The Modified Psychoanalytic Treatment of Schizophrenia."[8] He mentioned that his approach was intimately related to the psychoanalytic method of Sigmund Freud, but added that "no argument will be offered to the propriety of the use of psychoanalysis in reference to definite variations from Dr. Freud's technique. The choice of a word must be made a matter of personal opinion." In 1939, he presented a comprehensive formulation of his own theoretical deductions as "Conceptions of Modern Psychiatry."[9] On the other hand, Fromm-Reichmann consistently referred to her method as "psychoanalytically oriented psychotherapy."[10]

In spite of differences in various approaches, they share certain general assumptions. One prerequisite for successful psychotherapy with schizophrenics is that the psychiatrist have respect for the patient in his plight, and be able to visualize the bewildered and frightened schizophrenic as a functioning human being. He needs to be able to see meaning in the distorted verbalizations, bizarre behavior, and fluctuating attitudes, and thus establish a meaningful therapeutic relationship. Thus the patient experiences new modes of interpersonal relatedness, and can come to a new understanding of his own development, and of what has miscarried. The underlying assumption is that the schizophrenic illness is the outcome of disturbed interpersonal experiences, which have resulted in aberrant symbolic processes, with distortions in perception, meaning, and logic, and that this can be corrected, to a certain extent, so that the patient can learn to function more independently, with more realistic awareness of his own self, and with greater capacity for participation in the enjoyment of life.

HUMAN DEVELOPMENT AND FAMILY INTERACTION

Psychoanalysis has recognized the enormous significance of early experiences for personality development, which was conceived of as determined by the psychosexual maturation. The important traumatic experiences occurred presumably during the narcissistic and oral-sadistic phase. Early therapists would refer in general terms to the initial traumatic warp and early thwarting experiences which had exposed the later schizophrenic to unbearable frustration. Stressful experiences later in life would force the patient to regress to the earlier fixations, the original period of schizophrenogenic traumatization. All this was based on reconstructions from the patients' accounts, not on direct observation.

Sullivan departed from the psychosexual model of the theory of instincts. He conceived of personality development as originating in the infant's interaction with the significant adults, whereby the child was conceived of as vulnerable to anxiety-arousing situations.[11] Though he is much more specific and realistic in his reconstructions, he did not carry out direct observation of the families of his patients.

In retrospect, it appears paradoxical that psychoanalysis, with its great emphasis on early development, avoided direct studies of the family. When my own work on childhood obesity led to the study of the family frame, I discovered to my surprise that no psychiatric family studies had been published before 1940.[5] After World War II, a great interest developed in the study of the family, in particular those with children who later became schizophrenic. During the 1940s it was established that abnormal psychological exposure was a frequent occurrence, not merely an assumption based on reconstruction from the few patients who had been studied in intensive psychotherapy. Such survey studies revealed a high frequency of broken homes and of parental rejection in the background of schizophrenic patients. The emphasis was nearly exclusively on the detrimental influence of the mother, and terms like "schizophrenogenic mother" were used as if they conveyed specific meaning. Such grossly abnormal circumstances make it difficult to differentiate the emotional traumatization from the consequences of severe social and economic deprivation. Subsequent studies were carried out on socially intact families, permitting the recognition of more subtle facets of abnormal psychological interaction.

In the study of childhood schizophrenia, it was found that families who had a child in residential treatment differed significantly from control families of comparable social standing with relatively normal children.[12] Those who rated low in "overall adequacy" had schizophrenic children, though with great variability between different families.

In the study of the family background of adult schizophrenics, Lidz and his co-workers at Yale observed that, in spite of the great individual variations, two patterns of interaction could be recognized in these families.[13] In one group, the "schismatic family," there is an open split, with violent fighting between the parents, forcing the children to align themselves with one parent, usually with the one of the opposite sex, against the other. In the other group, the "skewed family," one parent appears seriously disturbed, but the other parent goes along to the extent that a real "*folie à deux* or *à famille*" develops. The child grows up in a disturbed environment that is not reality-oriented. Wynne and his co-workers, working at the National Institute of Mental Health (NIMH), focused on a pattern that they called "pseudo mutuality" to illuminate the disturbing forces in a family that, on first contact, might give the impression of harmonious functioning.[14]

As more details about the disturbed interactions accumulated, a clearer delineation of underlying questions began around the mid-fifties, with increasing efforts to define the factors which interfered with a child's growing into a distinct individual, with needs and impulses clearly differentiated from those of his parents. Psychiatric thinking had been fascinated for a long time by the notion of a specific trauma in maldevelopment. The importance of repetitive patterns in basic learning situations had been neglected. The question shifted from what had gone wrong to what had failed to go right. As family studies progressed, questions were raised about the basic functions of the family that had been taken for granted as inherent in the human state. Increasingly, the importance of *deficits* in acquiring the fundamental aspects of mental functioning, such as learning the meaning of language and behavior clues, were recognized as the background of ultimate maladaptation.[15,16]

STYLE OF COMMUNICATION

The schizophrenic's speech and thinking, which have been described as primitive, prelogical, and unrealistic, have been the object of much speculation. Reality checks, or "consensual validation," to use Sullivan's expression, seem to be lacking. What at first had been called "transmission of irrationality" was studied in increasing detail to illuminate how these disturbances would result in the thinking disorder characteristic of the schizophrenic illness.

In 1956, a group of scientists at Stanford University offered a communicational theory of the origin of the schizophrenic's thinking disorder.[17] They started with the observation that schizophrenic language is rich in metaphors, but that they are "unlabeled," and common metaphors are interpreted in a literal way, in contrast to the use of metaphors in normal speech. They related this to the fact of the later patient's finding himself trapped over and over again in impossible contradictions without the possibility of escape, while at the same time helplessly dependent on the other person who caused the situation. They called the conditions under which this occurs "double bind" situations, which are related to the disturbed patterns of family interaction. The conclusion was drawn that the schizophrenic's inability to discriminate between different levels of abstraction was related to the fact that, as a child, he had been consistently exposed to situations which would have been dangerous if he had perceived them correctly and reacted spontaneously to what was occurring. The novel aspect of this contribution was the way it established a relationship between disturbances in emotional experiences and in language and thought development.

Since this formulation of the "double bind" more than 20 years ago, extensive work has been carried out by other investigators. I refer here only to Wynne and Singer's work on disturbed style of communication.[18] In verbal interaction, parents of schizophrenics tend to wander away from the task at hand; they may disqualify or blur ideas and fail to achieve closure, producing disturbances of language acquistion and/or usage in the vulnerable child. Lidz has focused on the relationship between the parents' and the patient's egocentricity, resulting in the egocentric overinclusiveness characteristic of schizophrenic thinking.[19] These new findings are the outcome of intensive work with schizophrenics and their families, and they offer new guidelines for more effective therapy.

Not only thought processes and speech patterns are disturbed in schizophrenics. Other characteristic features, such as marked feelings of passivity, lack of autonomy, a sense of being controlled by others, indecisiveness, diffuse self-awareness, and so forth, can also be considered as the outcome of disturbed developmental experiences.[20] If confirmation and reinforcement of child-initiated clues are lacking, inaccurate, or contradictory, the infant will be deprived of a learning experience essential for separating self and non-self. He will grow up perplexed and unable to differentiate clearly between alterations in his biological field and emotional reactions, and will be defective in recognizing whether experiences and sensations originate in him or in the environment. Not having developed the essential basis for effective living, he will be the eternal stranger, alienated from the world, frightened by its incomprehensible tasks and demands.

THERAPEUTIC RELATIONSHIP

Since schizophrenics are often withdrawn, hostile, and suspicious, it had been assumed that they were unable to establish a durable relationship to another person. Actual experiences showed that schizophrenics were not only capable of forming human attachment, but that their dependence on the therapist was very intense, but apt to change rapidly from love to hate. The early work was done before effective psychotropic drugs were available, and often on patients whose deteriorated state was a sad monument to neglect and other harmful experiences. Work with such patients required what appears to us now as superhuman patience. The positive heritage from this period is the confidence that even a hostile and mute patient can again be brought into rapport. Although drugs have an ameliorating effect on the most disturbing and destructive symptoms, they do not improve or correct the underlying symbolic deficits, inadequate life experiences, and unrealistic expectations from the therapeutic relationship. Used properly, they are a great adjunct to psychotherapy, and allow previously inaccessible patients to engage more easily in a helpful therapeutic relationship.

When, during the pre-drug period, psychoanalysis was first applied to schizophrenics, the emphasis was on the extraordinary fragility of their reactions. Fromm-Reichmann wrote in 1939:[10]

> Whenever the analyst fails the patient—it will be a severe disappointment
> and the repetition of the chain of frustrations the schizophrenic has pre-

viously endured.—I believe (his unpredictable reaction) to be due to the inevitable errors in the analyst's approach to the schizophrenic.

Fifteen years later, in 1954, she stated:

We no longer treat the patients with the utter caution of bygone days. They are sensitive but not frail. If we approach them too cautiously—we contribute to their low self evaluation, instead of helping them to develop a healthy attitude toward themselves and others.[21]

In the same lecture, she pointed out that the patient had been deprived of valid guidance during childhood, and that it was the therapist's task to supply the needed education in realistic living—a modern-sounding concept.

Recognition of the developmental aspects of the disturbed utterances is of help in understanding the meaning of the bizarre, often incoherent or contradictory communication during the psychotic phase which might be cut short through drugs. It is important for the therapist to be familiar with the psychotic preoccupations of his patient, because they often contain important clues to his chief difficulties and conflicts. In working with this material, it is important not to get lost in symbolic fantasies, but to use them to help a patient to come to a new and clearer understanding of the confusing realities of his life. Often a patient who appears oriented and coherent will continue to communicate in the schizophrenic mode, or relapse into it when he feels threatened in his tenuous security operations, or by thus far unresolved conflicts. It is the therapist's task to recognize the tangible realities that need to be dealt with.

Sullivan expressed quite early (1931) the opinion that a psychiatrist's theoretical attitude was related to his effectiveness as a therapist.[8] He observed that the passive, mirrorlike attitude of the classical psychoanalyst was not conducive to producing a favorable outcome in schizophrenia. He conceived of the role of the psychiatrist as that of a "participant observer." He considered the unanalyzed psychiatrist as having a rigid system of taboos that might make the schizophrenic fearful of him, but that the recently analyzed psychiatrist might superimpose his theoretical convictions, and not recognize a patient's most urgent problems.

Amazingly similar are the findings of Whitehorn and Betz's study at the Phipps Clinic, published in 1954, about the differences in success in treating schizophrenics of different therapists.[22] The highest improvement rate was associated with a tactical pattern of "active personal participation," with the therapist showing initiative in a sympathetic inquiry, challenging the patient's self-deprecatory attitude, and with realistic limits as to what is acceptable in the patient's behavior. Passive permissiveness, or efforts to give a patient insight through interpretation, appear to have much less therapeutic value.

Since these early evaluations, much has been learned about the origin and nature of schizophrenic development, and we are on much more definite grounds in reconstructing with the patient the vicissitudes of his background. Much of the basic orientation has remained the same. Important in all dealings with schizophrenics is unambiguous speech and complete honesty. During his childhood, there has been such an enormous element of dishonesty and distortion about the realities of life, that a schizophrenic learns, even before his breakdown, denial of reality, pretense, and self-deceit as the only way of life. Psychotherapy represents a new experience, where he learns to discriminate between real and simulated behavior, and also to express without distortion and denial what he perceives and hears. The therapist must not give the impression of omniscience or secret knowledge, or imply to the patient the hope of a magic resolution to his problems. There is need for willingness to consider or to admit error, and also to admit the possibility of having slighted the patient, or having been annoyed.

One of the most important tools of a therapist is his openness and curiosity, the honest desire to find out what really has happened, with no implication of knowing it ahead of time. This demands discriminating alertness in recognizing inherent, often minute, contradictions. Treatment proceeds as a series of temporary and tenuous hypotheses that are put to the test of collaborative scrutiny in each treatment session. Knowing realistic details of a patient's background is of help in this effort of unraveling the distortions in his development. It demands that the therapist bring him back at every point to the tangible situation he endured and still faces. He learns also that he is not altogether bad and hateful, and that it is not all his fault, but that he has been confronted with insoluble problems and confusing reality situations which were not of his making, which he could not master as a child. Eventually, he will also learn about his part in continuing this make-believe life from which he finally withdrew into the psychotic world.

As treatment progresses, there will occur a gradual decrease in the sense of utter helplessness that has made the patient feel terrorized by unknown forces impinging upon him from any event or human contact, to which he had responded with mistrust, depression, and withdrawal, or with outbursts of uncontrolled rage and hostility. Recovery, in this orientation, is conceived of, not as an all-or-nothing "cure," or as a resolution of "the schizophrenic core," but as a broadening of the area of effective living through developing new tools of self-orientation.

Even with this clearer awareness of what we are doing, psychotherapy with a schizophrenic continues to be painfully slow work. But, in spite of its inherent difficulties, this work provides great satisfaction in terms of our own human values and a feeling of personal growth.

REFERENCES

1. Kraepelin E: *Hundert Jahre Psychiatrie: Ein Beitrag zur Geschichte menschlicher Gesittung*. Berlin, Julius Springer, 1918.

2. Kraepelin E: *One Hundred Years of Psychiatry*. (W. Baskin trans). New York, Philosophical Library Inc, 1962.

3. Bruch H: 100 years of psychiatry (Kraepelin)—50 years later. *Arch Gen Psychiatry* **21**:257–261, 1969.

4. Rosenfeld HA: Personal experiences in treating psychotic patients, in Frank KA (ed): *The Human Dimension in Psychoanalytic Practice*. New York, Grune & Stratton, 1977, p 29–48.

5. Bruch H: Obesity in childhood: V. The family frame of obese children (with G Touraine). *Psychosom Med* **2**:141–206, 1940.

6. Bruch H: Studies in schizophrenia. *Acta Psychiatr et Neurol Scand Suppl* **130**:34, Munksgaard, Copenhagen, 1959.

7. Bruch H: A historical perspective of psychotherapy in schizophrenia, in Fann WE, Karacan I, Pokorny AD et al (eds). *Phenomenology and Treatment of Schizophrenia*. New York, Spectrum Publications Inc. 1978, pp 311–324.

8. Sullivan HS: The modified psychoanalytic treatment of schizophrenia. *Am J Psychiatry* **88**:519–540, 1931.

9. Sullivan HS: *Conceptions of Modern Psychiatry* (1939). New York, WW Norton & Co, 1953.

10. Fromm-Reichmann F: Transference problems in schizophrenics. *Psychoanal Q* **8**:413–426, 1939.

11. Sullivan HS: *The Interpersonal Theory of Psychiatry*. New York, WW Norton & Co, 1953.

12. Behrens ML, Goldfarb W: A study of patterns of interaction of families of schizophrenic children in residential treatment. *Am J Orthopsychiatry* **28**:300–312, 1958.

13. Lidz T, Cornelison A, Fleck S, et al: The intrafamilial environment of schizophrenic patients. II. Marital schism and marital skew. *Am J Psychiatry* **114**:241–248, 1957.

14. Wynne LC, Ryckoff IM, Day J, et al: Pseudo-mutuality in the family relations of schizophrenics. *Psychiatry* **21**:205–220, 1958.

15. Lidz T, Cornelison A, Terry, D, et al: Intrafamilial environment of the schizophrenic patient: VI. The transmission of irrationality.. *Arch Neurol Psychiatry* **70**:305–316, 1958.

16. Lidz T: *The Family and Human Adaptation*. New York, International Universities Press, 1963.

17. Bateson G, Jackson D, Haley J, et al: Toward a theory of schizophrenia. *Behav Sci* **1**:251–264, 1956.

18. Singer MT, Wynne LC: Principles for scoring communication defects and deviances in parents of schizophrenics: Rorschach and TAT scoring manuals. *Psychiatry* **29**:260–288, 1966.

19. Lidz T: *The Origin and Treatment of Schizophrenic Disorders*. New York, Basic Books, 1973.

20. Bruch H: Psychotherapy with schizophrenics, in Kolb LC, Kallmann FJ, & Polatin P (eds). *International Psychiatry Clinics*. Boston, Little Brown & Co, 1964, pp 863–896.

21. Fromm-Reichmann F: Psychotherapy of schizophrenia. *Am J Psychiatry* **111**:410–419, 1954.

22. Whitehorn JC, Betz BJ: A study of psychotherapeutic relationships between physicians and schizophrenic patients. *Am J Psychiatry* **111**:321–331, 1954.

Chapter 2

On the Central Task of Psychotherapy

Psychoanalytic and Family Perspectives

HELM STIERLIN

FROM THE SEDUCTION THEORY TO THE OEDIPUS COMPLEX

On September 21, 1897, Freud revoked the seduction theory of neuroses. This signaled the most severe crisis in his life and career. Till then, he had believed and publicly asserted that his patients' neuroses could be traced to seductive, traumatizing parents or parent substitutes. Now he thought otherwise. This amounted, so he said, to the "*Sturz aller Werte*," the collapse of all values. He was "certain," he wrote in a letter to Wilhelm Fliess,[1] "that in the unconscious there exists no marker of reality so that one cannot distinguish between truth and affect-laden fiction." And, if this is so, he felt forced to conclude, our search for external traumatizing agents through a psychoanalysis must remain futile.

But out of such a collapse of all values there grew Freud's major theoretical achievements, grew his seminal work on dreams, and grew, in particular, the discovery, or, perhaps better, installment, of the Oedipus Complex.

HELM STIERLIN • Division of Psychoanalysis and Family Therapy, University of Heidelberg, 6900 Heidelberg 1, Germany.

"I have also found in myself," Freud[2] wrote in a subsequent letter, "love [*Verliebtheit*] for my mother and rivalry toward my father, and hold these now to be a recurrent event of early childhood." Accordingly, Freud viewed the Greek myth of Oedipus as giving

> voice to a compulsion [*Zwang*] which everybody recognizes because he has felt it in himself. Each listener was once tentatively and in his fantasy such an Oedipus, and vis-à-vis this dream fulfillment, transformed into reality, he turns away in horror with all that force of repression which separates his infantile from his present condition.

Thus, the Oedipus theory reversed the seduction theory, or, perhaps more correctly, reversed the roles and accountabilities of parents and children: Father and mother figured no longer as active seducers. Rather, they were cast as passive objects of the child's wishes. In this manner, the interactional scenario was—to apply the language of present day communicational theory—newly punctuated, interpersonal causality was newly defined, and blame and exculpation (by implication) newly fixed.

This punctuation, however, did not inhere in the original Oedipal myth; it resulted from Freud's special perception, if not truncation, of that myth. For the Oedipal myth, as commonly transmitted, starts with the actions of Oedipus' father Laios, legendary king of Thebes: Laios lived with his queen Iokaste in a childless marriage. Questioning the Delphic Oracle, he learned a son would be born to him, yet also this son would kill him, because Zeus had heard the curse of King Pelops. As a youngster, Laios had been this king's guest, and had then abducted and seduced Chrysippos, Pelops' beautiful son. (Various Greek sources hold Laios to be the inventor of pederasty, the homosexual love of young boys.) Conscious of his guilt, Laios believed the Oracle, and for a long time separated from Iokaste. When a son was finally born, the parents had him thrown into the wild mountains of Kithairon, his ankles pierced and tied. (Hence his name Oedipus, "swollen foot.") Miraculously, he was saved by a shepherd, and eventually grew up at the court of King Polybos of Corinth. He left this court when the Oracle prophesized that he would kill his father and marry his mother—which he then, after all, did do, in the manner which Sophocles' play unravels.

What, then, caused Freud to turn from the seduction theory to the Oedipal theory? Till today, this question has remained largely unanswered, since Freud's own explanations, as given to Fliess and others, appear contradictory and unconvincing. Here I cannot document this in detail, and must therefore refer the reader to the careful exposition and discussion of this subject by Marianne Krüll,[3,4] a historian and sociologist at Bonn, Germany.

However, Krüll not only critically examines Freud's reasoning, she also presents some answers of her own—thanks to a painstaking research effort carried out over many years, and as yet published only in German. This research led her, among other things, to visit Freiberg, Freud's home town in Moravia, in order to unearth and utilize heretofore unknown documents, to immerse herself in Freud's parents' and especially his father's socio-cultural background, and to reread and frequently reinterpret Freud's and his biographers' writings, particularly Freud's extant dreams and letters. Her main conclusion: Freud abandoned the seduction theory when he, in his self-analysis, came close to discerning seductive, traumatizing, if you wish perverse behavior in his own parents. Krüll even offers the—admittedly dar-ing, but by her, well-supported—thesis that little Sigmund witnessed, and came close to remembering, sexual activities between his mother and her stepson, Philipp. (Freud's father, Jacob, a traveling cloth merchant, was then in his early forties. Freud's mother, Amalie, was almost twenty years younger than his father, and of approximately the same age as Freud's half brothers by the father's first marriage, Philipp and Emanuel. The Freud family lived, then, in a very crammed and small one-room apartment, and the father was often away.)

If we follow Krüll's evidence and arguments—and I, personally, am ready to follow her—there emerges this final conclusion: in revoking the seduction theory, Freud tried to exonerate his own—as well as his neurotic patients'—parents: he now saw the neurotic or psychotic drama spawned *not* by traceable parental behaviors, but by the patient's own compelling drives and fantasies. And the Oedipal theory legitimized such view. It showed such drives and fantasies to be not only compelling, but also ubiqui-tous; showed them, as it were, to derive from a law of human nature. Thus, Freud made the Oedipus Complex not only the bedrock of analytic theory, he also made it a part of what I recently termed our "relational reality."[5,6]

RELATIONAL REALITY

This relational reality could also be called "soft" reality, in juxtaposi-tion to "hard" reality. Hard reality includes what we usually mean by ma-terial reality, i.e., concrete and easily visualizable reality. Relational or soft reality, in contrast, is less easily visualizable, and is more dependent on (i.e., sustained and created by) our interpersonal perceptions, interpretations, and fantasies. In choosing the term "relational reality," I took as my guide Gregory Bateson,[7] who considered the shaping and understanding of his relationships as man's most central and pervasive endeavor. The term "rela-tionship" here covers my relations to myself (i.e., to my inner life, my needs, my body) as well as to others, their inner lives, their expectations, their bodies, as well as to given social institutions. Much more than hard reality, this relational reality appears man- and culture-made, appears sub-ject to historical change, and hence subject to changing conceptual vantage points which shape our assignment of interpersonal causality and agency, while giving coherence and meaning to our actions and motivations.

Seen this way, Freud's Oedipal theory contributed to the shaping of Western man's present-day relational reality: he provided a map, a framework, by which man's relations to himself, to his inner life, as well as to his significant others, could be traced, and by which interpersonal causality and agency could be discovered as well as assigned. Yet Freud created also a setting—the psychoanalytic situation—in which this map could be utilized effectively. Subsequently, map and setting came ever more to fit each other. In an expanding circular process, the observations made in the setting helped to refine the map, and such refinement in turn confirmed the setting.

MODERN FAMILY THEORY AND FREUD'S SEDUCTION THEORY

If we now look at modern family theory and therapy, as spearheaded by Lidz and others,[8] we find it to affect man's relational reality no less importantly than did Freud. We find, too, an expanding circular process between charting a map and use of a new setting, between theory building and refinement of therapy. And we find, further, that this process has—almost!—led us back to the point from which Freud took off in 1897—the seduction theory of neuroses: or, more correctly, has led us back to the question with which Freud then grappled.

However, to fully grasp that question, a semantic correction seems in order: the term "seduction" appears too narrow to describe what is essential here. For at issue is not only sexual seduction, but what Webster's dictionary lists as additional meanings of "to seduce"—"to persuade to disobedience or disloyalty," and "to lead astray" (which in German is rendered "*irreführen*"). In brief, at issue are the many ways in which parents may mislead and/or fail their children. Particularly the research with "schizo-present" families, as carried out by Lidz and his team over the past decades, has made us realize how fatefully the parents' actions and omissions may bear on their children's lives, as when they are unempathic, steep these children in irrationality, overtax them with impossible missions, or exploit them in one way or another. But also, this research has taught us to see these parents as children of their parents, who pass on to their children, or take these children to account for, what was done to them, the parents, by *their* parents. Thus, new perplexing issues were raised as to how interpersonal causality should be defined, and blame and exculpation be fixed—the very issues with which the original Oedipal myth (the pre-Freudian myth, as it were) confronts us.

At the same time, this research has alerted us to those powerful family forces of loyalty, legacy, and delegation that may fatefully shape and distort one's relational reality—as they did in the case of Freud himself. If we trust Krüll's evidence and conclusions, Freud skewed his search for truth when deepest loyalties and legacies, i.e., the defense of his father's and family's honor, were at stake. This is the same Freud[9] who could be so ruthlessly honest with himself as to publicly own up to his death wishes toward his son when the latter served as a soldier in World War I. The research of the last decades on "schizo-present" families showed these families very frequently to be both divided in their loyalties, and deadlocked in bitter and destructive blaming. Such families also were caught up in faulty accounting, and in shared distortions of their relational reality—manifestations and consequences of a faulty epistemology and cognition—of misperceptions, of falsely and too rigidly employed categorizations, of restrictive inner schemata, of erroneous inferences, and inaccurate generalizations, which often are collusively maintained.

Finally, it showed them to be typically caught up in a deadly power struggle, or, in Bateson's words, a symmetrical escalation,[10] in which each party tries to manipulate (rather than negotiate) the relational reality through strategies which lead nowhere. These strategies we have come to know as mystification, as the disqualification of meaning, as the imperceptible shifting of one's focus of attention, the subtle undercutting of the other's statements, the disclaiming of agency, and hence of responsibility, for one's actions and statements. By its very nature, such a power struggle—or, perhaps more correctly, struggle for the power of the stronger reality—can neither be won nor lost. Rather, it locks the agonists into a malignant clinch.[11] And this clinch becomes then ever more difficult to break.

PSYCHOTHERAPY AS FACILITATION OF THE FAMILY-WIDE DIALOGUE

What lessons for therapy may we derive from this research? I see, above everything else, *one* lesson: that therapy should facilitate the in-life, family-wide dialogue, or, to put it differently, that the facilitation of such dialogue should be viewed as the central therapeutic task. This task corresponds with the basic rule of family therapy which Boszormenyi-Nagy and Sparks[12], in contradistinction to the basic rule of psychoanalysis, formulated as follows: try, as much as possible, to talk about those things which till now you could not discuss—for example, ominous family secrets, painful disillusionments, unmourned losses, injustices committed and loyalties betrayed. It is, then, through such a dialogue that a mutually accepted relational reality can be negotiated, consensual validation reached, rights and obligations ascertained, accounts settled, and, hopefully, eventual reconciliation achieved. Viewed in this way, such a dialogue can be said to "heal," as the root meanings of the common Germanic adjective "*heil*" are "healthy and sound," as well as "whole, intact, and saved." A healing through dialogue, accordingly, connotes achievement not only of physical and mental health, but also of integration, reunion, and salvation.

However, to facilitate and carry through such a dialogue may be hard. Freud's very example shows that it may be easier to undergo a lengthy analysis, and thereby own up to—even excessively—one's conflicts and dark sides, than to seek and risk an in-life dialogue with one's family which may stir deepest anxiety and guilt—not only in oneself, but also (and this makes it so difficult) in one's parents and closest relatives.

The task becomes even harder with many schizo-present families whose members, as we noted, are stalemated in bitterest conflict, yet are also—actually or seemingly—unable to confront each other, or to achieve reconciliation or reunion. Here, those who need the dialogue most, are least able or willing to engage in it, and are also least able and willing to let the therapist facilitate it.

To the therapist, committed to facilitate a dialogue, this represents, then, a real dilemma and "Grenzsituation." In my view, it requires the therapist first of all to break the malignant stalemate or clinch, so as to create and then sustain the conditions under which the family-wide dialogue can unfold. To understand what this implies, we return once more to the metaphor of the boxing match. In the boxing ring, it is the referee who usually ends the clinch. To separate the opponents' deadlock, he must often intervene actively and energetically, indeed, he must sometimes quite literally throw his weight in. By such a heavy active intervention, he sets the deadlocked fight in motion again, and creates the space necessary for the interplay of the different individualities, strategies, motivations, etc., which was absent as long as the clinch held.

The family therapist must, I believe, intervene in just such an active way in the case of malign stalemate, interposing the weight of his personality and authority to break the deadlock and create the free space in which the contenders can unfold their individually differentiated values and motives. Of course, the therapeutic situation is incomparably more complex than the boxing ring, and the therapist has a commensurately greater repertoire of possibilities for intervention. The therapist's weight and authority can be best expressed as "the stronger person's reality," a concept I introduced in 1959.[13] The stronger person's reality comes into play in all relationships which develop extreme dependencies, and, consequently, accompanying hopes and expectations directed at the family therapist increase as the relationship between the patient and his family becomes deadlocked and irresolvable. Frequently, the nearer the patient and his family come to being at the end of their tether, the more likely is it that the therapist will, almost automatically, seem to be a potential savior. However, he is not only a potential savior, but also a potential judge—someone with the power to deepen the fear and insecurity of patients already burdened with fear, insecurity, shame, and guilt. The art of the therapist lies then in his ability in what Selvini et al[14] called "positive connotation," the giving of positive meaning: the therapist must avoid any tendency to censure, to frighten, or arouse guilt however subtle or well-concealed: instead, he must as far as possible show approval. Both—the active interpolation of the "stronger reality" of the therapist, and the total avoidance of fear and guilt arousal—create, then, the optimal basis for breaking up the malign stalemate, clinch, and power struggle. It is then possible, for example, to initiate the unlocking strategy known as "paradoxical intervention" or "prescription." As part of such an intervention, the therapist also approves the behavior of the index patient, despite its causing crises and suffering, and he thereby paradoxically mobilizes the wills of both the index patient and of the other members of the family to end such behavior. I do not have space here to discuss how and why this happens, but refer those interested to the relevant literature, which already numbers close to 100 titles,[15] as well as to Dr. Wynne's chapter in this volume.[16] The assertion must suffice, that such an unlocking of the power struggle gives all the participants the chance to make a new start in their mutual individuation and separation—to begin a true dialogue, in which they can own up to their own ambivalences, in which they see others as persons in their own right.

Often, such breaking of the malign stalemate will amount to a reopening of a dialogue which derailed a long time ago when the dependent, trusting child turned to his parents, the persons with the stronger reality, both for safe anchorage and for a share in the making of their common relational reality—yet, along with these parents, became entrapped. Now the paradoxical intervention may serve as the key that springs open the trap—and thereby frees all family members for further growth, individuation, and new forms of relatedness.[13,15]

CONCLUDING REMARKS

But, finally, a word of caution: even though I view the facilitation of the family-wide dialogue as the central therapeutic task, it is not the only task. Many patients—and particularly those labeled as schizophrenics—will need further help in overcoming the lack of skills, lack of experiences, the cognitive distortions, even defects, etc., which are the consequences of their deprivations and the uneven developments suffered during their long family-wide developmental and relational stagnation. Many therapeutic endeavors on the individual, group, milieu, and social levels, as presented elsewhere in this volume, will be helpful here. And yet—so I am inclined to think—they will only be helpful in so far as they subserve such dialogue.

REFERENCES

1. Freud S: *Aus den Anfängen der Psychoanalyse 1887–1902. Briefe an Wilhelm Fliess.* Frankfurt, S Fischer, 1950, pp 186–188, rev ed, 1975.
2. Freud S: *Aus den Anfängen der Psychoanalyse 1887–1902. Briefe an Wilhelm Fliess.* Frankfurt, S Fischer, 1950, p 193.
3. Krüll M: *Sigmund Freud und sein Vater.* München, CH Beck, 1979.
4. Krüll M: Freuds Absage an die Verführungstheorie im Lichte seiner eigenen Familiendynamik. *Familiendynamik* 2:102–129, 1978.
5. Stierlin H: *Delegation und Familie.* Frankfurt, Suhrkamp, 1978.
6. Stierlin H, et al: *Das erste Familiengespräch* (rev ed). Stuttgart, Klett, 1979. English edition: *The First Interview with the Family*, New York, Brunner/Mazel, 1980.
7. Bateson G: *Steps to an Ecology of Mind.* New York, Ballantine Books Inc, 1972.
8. Lidz T, Fleck S, Cornelison A: *Schizophrenia and the Family.* New York, International Universities Press, 1965.
9. Freud S: *Die Traumdeutung.* Leipzig & Vienna, F Deuticke, 1900.
10. Bateson G: Bali: *The Value System of a Study State. Steps to an Ecology of Mind.* New York, Ballantine Books, Inc, 1972, 107–127.
11. Stierlin H: Status der Gegenseitigkeit: die fünfte Perspektive des Heidelberger familiendynamischen Konzeptes. *Familiendynamik* 4:106–116, 1979.
12. Boszormenyi-Nagy I, Spark G: *Invisible Loyalties: Reciprocity in Intergenerational Family Therapy.* Hagerstown, Md., Harper & Row Publishers Inc, 1975.
13. Stierlin H: The adaptation to the stronger person's reality in Stierlin H: *Psychoanalysis and Family Therapy.* New York, Jason Aronson, 1978, pp
14. Selvini-Palazzoli M, Boscolo L, Cecchin G, et al: *Paradox and Counterparadox.* New York, Jason Aronson, 1978.
15. Weeks G, L'Abate L: A bibliography of paradoxical methods in psychotherapy of family systems. *Fam Process* 17:85–98, 1978.
16. Wynne LC: Paradoxical system intervention: Leverage for therapeutic change in families and individual schizophrenics. Presented at the Yale Symposium on Psychotherapy of Schizophrenia, April 10, 1979.

Chapter 3

Social and Family Factors in the Course of Schizophrenia

Toward an Interpersonal Problem-Solving Therapy for Schizophrenics and Their Families

ROBERT PAUL LIBERMAN,
CHARLES J. WALLACE, CHRISTINE E. VAUGHN,
KAREN S. SNYDER, and CLINTON RUST

With the current enthusiasm for biological mechanisms in the understanding and treatment of schizophrenia, a bystander may wonder why there is a clamor for psychotherapeutic approaches to this major psychiatric disorder. After all, doesn't research on genetics, dopamine, and endorphins promise early breakthroughs in deciphering the pathogenesis of schizophrenia? Haven't the neuroleptic drugs shown that schizophrenia is a biological illness that should be treated with somatic methods? Hasn't the value of psychotherapy—whether conducted by seasoned analysts, enthusiastic residents, or optimistic social workers—been shown to be limited, at best, for the great proportion of individuals suffering from schizophrenia? Although these questions may seem naive, dead and buried to those who are committed, through training and experience, to a psychotherapeutic

ROBERT PAUL LIBERMAN, CHARLES J. WALLACE, CHRISTINE E. VAUGHN, KAREN S. SYNDER, and CLINTON RUST • Mental Health Clinical Research Center for the Study of Schizophrenia, Carmarillo State Hospital, Camarillo, California and UCLA School of Medicine, Los Angeles, California 90024. Research Supported by NIMH Grant No. MH 30911 awarded by the Clinical Research Branch. The authors are grateful for the support of NIMH staff: Morris Parloff, Hussain Tuma, Loren Mosher, Samuel Keith, and Joseph Autry III.

approach with schizophrenic patients, they are very much alive in the minds of many rank-and-file psychiatrists, residents-in-training, and health planners, who are the architects of our future national medical insurance programs. Thus, it is important to address the rationale for psychosocial treatment in schizophrenia, and to offer a clear and convincing strategy for its clinical use.

LIMITATIONS OF NEUROLEPTIC DRUGS IN THE TREATMENT OF SCHIZOPHRENIA

Despite hopes and expectations, neuroleptic drugs have not provided a wholly satisfactory treatment for schizophrenia. Antipsychotic medication has not stopped the "revolving door" pattern of discharge and readmission in psychiatric facilities. Relapse and rehospitalization rates for schizophrenic patients released to the community indicate that 50–60% of patients cannot sustain community adaptation for two years.[1,2] Follow-up studies indicate that 34% of schizophrenic patients discharged are readmitted within the first year. There has been a 30% rise in the annual rate of readmission of schizophrenic persons to state and county hospitals in recent years. One recent study of all consecutive admissions of schizophrenics to a typical community mental health center found that 45% were readmitted within six months of discharge.[3] Three to five years after discharge, only 25–35% of patients have not required readmission.[4] Thus, though drug treatment ameliorates acute symptomatology and relieves much suffering, it does not prevent relapse and rehospitalization. Patterns of recidivism can be even more disturbing than sustained chronicity, and have led to widespread demoralization of patients, families, and treatment personnel. This demoralization, in itself, has an adverse impact upon therapeutic efforts.

Neuroleptic drugs cannot be counted upon as the final solution to schizophrenia for another reason. Almost all clinical trials of neuroleptics find that 15–25% of schizophrenic patients do as well on placebos. Although we cannot yet identify those characteristics which predict good response in the absence of drug therapy, it is suspected that the premorbid social competence of the individual, and the family's emotional climate, may be important factors—factors we shall return to later. Also important in promoting good clinical response without drugs is the quality of the therapeutic milieu. In a triple-blind, well-controlled study, maintenance phenothiazines failed to contribute to the responsiveness of hard-core, chronic psychotics when they were treated in active milieu or behavior therapy programs.[5] Similarly, in a series of single-subject studies—in which frequent, repeated measures were taken on highly specific and focal target symptoms of schizophrenia—contingencies of reinforcement were found to be more potent than medication in producing certain types of behavioral change.[6]

Two other related factors limit the applicability of neuroleptic drug therapy, and point to the need for effective psychosocial interventions—side effects, and noncompliance. Side effects of neuroleptics, especially akinesia, akathisia, and the extrapyramidal syndrome, contribute significantly to the patient's reluctance to adhere reliably to a medication regimen.[7] Even among those who take their medication reliably, 48% relapse within two years.[8] Extrapolations from these data suggest that, by five years, almost all patients taking neuroleptic medication will relapse.[9] Thus, neuroleptic drugs retard, but do not prevent, relapse. Neither do drugs teach life and coping skills, nor improve the quality of an individual's life, except indirectly, through removal of symptoms. Most schizophrenic patients need to learn or relearn social and personal skills for surviving in the community. After this litany of limitations of drug therapy, we can move to more positive rationales for the development of psychosocial or psychotherapeutic interventions for schizophrenia.

FAMILY FACTORS IN SCHIZOPHRENIC RELAPSE

A series of studies over the past two decades, begun at the Medical Research Council's Social Psychiatry Unit at the Institute of Psychiatry in London, and now continuing in studies supported by the WHO and NIMH located in Denmark, India, and the United States, have highlighted the importance of the effect of the emotional climate in the family on the course of schizophrenic illness in a family member. Evidence has accumulated which points to the interpersonal processes within the family as among the most powerful predictors of relapse in a person having an established schizophrenic illness. The English studies were begun in response to the changing patterns of mental health care for schizophrenics in the 1950s which resulted in increased rates of discharges, followed by increased rates of readmissions. With the focus of research interest turned into the community for answers to the problem of relapse, George Brown, Ph.D., and his colleagues studied the possible influence of family relationships on the course of schizophrenia. This was stimulated by the early finding that schizophrenic patients who returned to parents or spouses relapsed more often than those discharged to hostels or apartments.[9] Several years were spent devising a standardized method for assessing the quality of the emotional relationship between a schizophrenic patient and his or her key relatives.[10,11] The successful development of an interview format—the Camberwell Family Interview—led to a series of studies, each of which concluded that *the best single predictor of symptomatic relapse in the nine months*

after discharge from hospital was the level of emotion expressed by a rela-
tive toward the patient during a standardized interview at the time of the
patient's hospitalization.[12-14]

Evaluating Expressed Emotion

The Camberwell Family Interview is conducted by a trained inter-
viewer/rater with a single family member in a comfortable setting, usually
the family home. The abbreviated version of the interview lasts about 1½
hours. It is semistructured, and elicits the relative's report of interactions
between the patient and family members, as well as commentary on the
patient's behavior during the three months prior to admission. Circumstances surrounding the decision to hospitalize, acting out, frequency of
quarrels, social isolation, and symptoms shown by the patient are covered.
Of even greater importance for the subsequent ratings of "expressed emotion" are the *feelings* and *attitudes* of the relative toward the patient, and
the patient's relationship with others in the family. Feelings are expressed
spontaneously, or in reponse to probes, during the detailed questioning
about family activities and the development of the patient's disorder. In
measuring the relative's "expressed emotion," the interviewer/rater
evaluates nonverbal elements as well as the semantic verbal content of the
relative's responses. Emphasis is placed on vocal aspects of speech—tone,
pitch, intensity, rapidity, and fluency—in rating the various scales reflecting
emotional qualities.

The scales developed by Brown and his colleagues included warmth,
hostility, positive comments, critical comments, and emotional overinvolvement. Each scale is operationalized with detailed referents and many examples. With sufficient training and supervision, interviewer/raters can reach
acceptably high levels of reliability in scoring these scales. It should be
noted, however, that training ordinarily requires a two-week full-time work-
shop, followed by two to three months of reliability checks on ratings of
tape-recorded interviews.

The two scales which have turned out to be most predictive of relapse
are critical comments, and emotional overinvolvement. The number of
critical comments made by the relative about the patient are rated on how
the relative speaks of the patient. Tone of voice, or clear and umambiguous
statements of resentment, disapproval, or dislike of something the patient
has said or done contribute to the identification of a critical comment. For
example, if a relative reported that the patient, just prior to admission,
"spent all of him time lying around the house," a critical comment would be
rated only if the relative's tone of voice was disapproving, sarcastic, or
angry. On the other hand, if the relative added, "he spent all his time lying

around the house because he's just plain lazy," the accusation of laziness, even without a disapproving tone of voice, would qualify the comment as a criticism.

Emotional overinvolvement is a global rating of the relative's expressions of overconcern, overprotectiveness, or excessive solicitude toward the patient. The rating is based both on the relative's responses to the interview, and on interactions reported by the relative with the patient. Extreme worry or anxiety by the relative about the patient is also coded as overinvolvement. This category can reflect the kind of relationship often referred to as symbiotic or schizophrenogenic by American psychiatrists. It is important to point out that most relatives from the English studies *do not* show excessive criticism or marked emotional overinvolvement. Those that do are frequently not abnormal or strikingly deviant in light of the extremely asocial, impaired, and symptomatic nature of their ill family member.

Expressed Emotion and Relapse

The most recent of the London studies suggests that patients returning to families that are high on expressing criticism and emotional overinvolvement relapse four times as often as those returning to families that are low in these categories of "expressed emotion." A family member qualified for the designation of high on "expressed emotion" if he or she made six or more critical comments during the interview, or was rated at four or higher on a six-point scale of emotional overinvolvement. Fifty-one percent of patients returning to homes where a family member was high on "expressed emotion" relapsed during the nine months after discharge, whereas only 13 percent relapsed who returned to low "expressed emotion" families.[14] The diagnosis of schizophrenia and clinical determinations of relapse were made on the basis of the Present State Examination.[15]

High "expressed emotion" (EE) did not explain all of the variance, since almost 50% of those from high EE homes did not relapse. Thus, secondary analyses were conducted to determine which other factors were contributing to clinical outcome. Two factors were found which appeared to exert an important protective influence on patients in high EE homes: regular adherence to phenothiazine medication, and reduced contact with highly critical or overinvolved family members. Figure 1 shows the way in which (1) the use of antipsychotic medication; and (2) less than 35 hours per week of face-to-face contact, protect schizophrenic individuals from relapse in families. Patients living with family members high on EE who spend much time with their relatives and are not protected by maintenance-drug therapy have a very poor prognosis, with 92% of them relapsing. Relapse

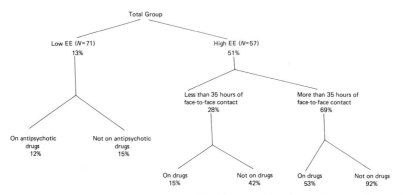

FIGURE 1.   Nine-month relapse rates of 128 schizophrenic patients who were living with relatives rated high and low on "expressed emotion" (EE). Data are drawn from two separate studies carried out a decade apart in London (Brown, Birley, Wing, 1972; Vaughn, Leff, 1976).

rates drop if one of the two protective factors is operating. Prognosis is best of all—and is equivalent to that of patients returning to low EE households—for those who have both protective factors operating.

Replications of these English studies are ongoing at the Mental Health Clinical Research Center (MHCRC) for the Study of Schizophrenia at Camarillo/UCLA; the University of Rochester; the University of Pittsburgh; and the University of Chicago/Illinois State Psychiatric Institute. Preliminary findings at Camarillo/UCLA suggest that patients returning to high EE families do indeed frequently relapse; however, there seems to be a much greater proportion of families high on EE in California than in England. In London, 45% of the families were high on EE, whereas, with two-thirds of the sample collected, the Los Angeles study at Camarillo/UCLA is finding 75% of the families high on EE.

Implications for Clinical Intervention

Of significance in the studies on EE is the fact that a vulnerable target group can now be identified as at high risk for relapse. The group at highest risk are unmarried males living at home with parents who are high on EE. More importantly, independent of chronicity, this vulnerable group can be identified at the time of hospital admission through the administration of a standardized interview. What types of clinical interventions, then, can be utilized with this highly vulnerable group? The evidence from moderating variables on relapse rates suggests that clinicians should aim to provide maintenance antipsychotic drugs for these patients, and to reduce the amount of face-to-face contact between them and their relatives after discharge.

Although special procedures, such as long-acting antipsychotic drug preparations and reinforcement methods,[16] may improve the sustained use of medication, side effects and noncompliance limit the success of this therapeutic avenue. Reducing the amount of face-to-face contact is easier said than done. Many of the high EE families and their schizophrenic member are "glued" together through years of mutual dependency and gratifications. One approach developed by the PACT (Program for Assertive Community Training) project in Madison, Wisconsin,[17] employs "constructive separation" between patient and family. This community-based program, as a continuum of acceptance, requires adherence to specific guidelines which regulate interactions between patients and families via phone, visits, and correspondence. However, as a compensation for the loss of family ties, the PACT staff provide 24-hour, round-the-clock, personal support and crisis intervention. Few agencies working with schizophrenics can offer that degree of support and contact.

Two other approaches, which are being evaluated at the Camarillo/UCLA MHCRC for the Study of Schizophrenia, involve (1) reducing EE in relatives through a specific type of behavioral family therapy; and (2) strengthening the social and communication skills of the schizophrenic patient through a training program aimed at enabling the patient to cope better with high EE from family members, or to leave the family and become more autonomous.

SOCIAL COMPETENCE AND SCHIZOPHRENIC RELAPSE

If one subscribes to the currently popular diathesis—stress theory of schizophrenia, it is necessary to take a closer look at the process by which environmental stressors like high EE, operating on a vulnerable individual, actually produce breakdowns in social and personal functioning, and symptomatic exacerbation or relapse. While it is likely that neuroleptic medication reduces a schizophrenic individual's vulnerability to relapse, and protects the person from the stressful impact of life events and high EE,[14,18] *why* do such individuals succumb to stressors that others take in stride or are able to manage? One possibility is that schizophrenic symptoms—whatever their biological mechanisms—become manifest when a person is overwhelmed by situational challenges and problems that he or she does not have the interpersonal resources to cope with or solve.

From this vantage point, an increase or reappearance of symptoms in a person vulnerable to schizophrenia is an outcome of the balance or interaction between the amount of life stressors and the problem-solving skills of the individual.[19] Either *too much environmental change or stressor*—such as a harshly critical relative with whom the schizophrenic individual is emotionally overinvolved—or *too little in the way of coping and problem-solving skills*—such as a person who always responds to new situations with social withdrawal—can lead to symptomatic flare-ups. This model of symptom formation is equally applicable to other psychiatric and medical disorders; for example, if a person's diathesis is for peptic ulcers or hypertension, excessive stressors or deficient problem-solving ability can lead to the symptoms of a person's particular susceptibility. The significance of this two-way model of symptom formation lies in the emphasis given to the active role of the patient's coping skills in modulating vulnerability to relapse. What is the evidence for the thesis that deficiencies in problem solving might contribute to the process of relapse in schizophrenia?

Correlations between social inadequacy, which presumably indexes low interpersonal problem-solving ability, and symptomatic outcome/rehospitalization have been recognized for many years.[20-22] Many studies have shown that, the higher the person's social level of adjustment prior to developing schizophrenic symptoms and requiring hospitalization, the better will be his or her post-hospital outcome.[23] The Phillips Premorbid Scale and its derivatives generally measure heterosexual adjustment, and the range and depth of personal relationships from childhood to the patient's index hospitalization. Studies utilizing premorbid-adjustment ratings show associations with global ratings of improvement and indices of rehospitalization.[24] For example Farina et al[25] followed female patients for a minimum of five years, and selected two groups markedly different in outcome. One group was considered in remission if each patient spent less than six months in the initial hospitalization, and had no rehospitalizations over five years. The other group was considered deteriorated if each patient spent more than six months in the hospital, and had one or more readmissions in five years. Individuals with higher premorbid levels of adjustment from the Phillips Scale were more likely to be in the remitted group to a statistically significant degree. Vaillant[26] found that nonschizoid premorbid adjustment was an important prognostic factor in differentiating 51 remitting schizophrenics from 128 unimproved patients over a follow-up interval that averaged ten years. Qualifying somewhat the importance of premorbid social adjustment was Vaillant's additional finding that this variable did not discriminate the 20 remitting patients who had a history of frequent relapses from the remaining 31 who sustained their remissions.

In a well-executed study, Gittelman-Klein and Klein[27] investigated the relationship of childhood and adolescent social adjustment with two-year outcomes of 86 schizophrenics. Ratings were made of withdrawal, peer relationships, social interests, and dating and sexual activity. Outcome was defined in terms of a six-point global scale, plus the number of rehospitalizations and the amount of time spent in a psychiatric hospital during the follow-up period. Results indicated that each of the items reflecting premorbid adjustment significantly correlated with the three measures of outcome—correlation coefficients ranged from 0.27 to 0.55.

Although the data from studies using premorbid social adjustment scales are based on retrospective and global ratings of interpersonal competence, a body of more direct and prospective evidence has recently developed, showing that schizophrenic persons have major deficiencies in discrete social skills. For example, patients have been found to generate fewer response alternatives to interpersonal problems.[28]

Spivack and his colleagues have identified six cognitive problem-solving skills: problem recognition, means–ends thinking, alternative thinking, causal thinking, perspective taking, and consequential thinking. In a series of studies, these investigators have found that psychiatric patients generate fewer means to achieve a goal than do normals; and these means are generally less relevant that those generated by normals.[29-31] Within a group of 190 psychiatric patients, many of whom were schizophrenic, poorer problem-solving skills were associated with (1) high scores on the Sc and Pa scales of the MMPI; (2) lower scores on the Goldberg Index; and (3) poorer premorbid competence as measured by the Phillips Scale.

Social performance in role-play situations, or spontaneously enacted with confederates in natural situations, has been measured by direct recording of discrete behaviors presumed to be important elements of social skill. Schizophrenic individuals, as compared to normal controls, have been found to exhibit less eye contact, greater response latency, more dysfluencies, and less appropriate affect.[23] A more direct test of problem-solving ability in schizophrenics was carried out by Wallace and his associates[32] at the Mental Health Clinical Research Center for the Study of Schizophrenia at Camarillo/UCLA. Interpersonal problem-solving skills were conceptualized as including (1) accurate perception of relevant interpersonal and situational cues; and (2) flexible processing of these cues for generating a set of response alternatives and understanding their potential consequences. Twelve schizophrenic inpatients and 12 hospital employees viewed six videotaped problem situations, and then responded to a series of questions designed to assess their social perception and processing skills. The results indicated that the schizophrenic patients had inferior social-perceptive and processing abilities. Interestingly, when pretraining was offered which structured ways for dealing with the situations, the schizophrenics improved their responses, and the normals showed some impairment. This would suggest that normals, having an established way of solving problems, were disrupted by the provision of a new structure; on the other hand, schizophrenics, bereft of cognitive problem-solving skills, were aided by the prestructuring.

In summary, failure to adjust to family and community living, and a reappearance or worsening of psychotic symptomatology in schizophrenics, may be associated with their deficits in social skills and interpersonal problem solving. These deficits may derive from (1) a primary failure to have ever learned social competence (as in the case of the poor premorbid, process schizophrenic); or (2) a loss of performance capability because of excessive environmental stressors leading to affective arousal and cognitive disorganization (as when high EE leads to relapse), or disuse (as through institutionalization). Contributory evidence for this hypothesis comes from current longitudinal studies of children at risk for developing schizophrenia. Investigators have found that these children demonstrate signs of inappropriate social behavior or withdrawal as early as the initial primary school grades. It would be reasonable to assume that, if schizophrenic individuals could have their social problem-solving skills buttressed by an effective therapy procedure, then they might be more resistant to relapses provoked by environmental stressors or life changes. It is this assumption which guides our current work, which aims to develop a comprehensive problem-solving therapy for schizophrenics and their relatives. Our strategy for reducing relapse is to strengthen the social and problem-solving skills of schizophrenics through direct training, and to improve the emotional climate within the family through a therapy that teaches communication skills.

SOCIAL SKILLS TRAINING

Social skills training is a behavior-therapy approach which attempts to increase patients' performance competence in critical life situations. Skill training emphasizes the positive, educational aspects of treatment. It assumes that each individual always does the best he can, given the person's biological endowment, cognitive limitations, and previous social learning experiences. When an individual's "best effort" fails to meet interpersonal needs and goals, it is an indication of a situation-specific deficit in the individual's repertoire. This deficit may arise from a diathesis for process-type schizophrenia, from lack of experience, or from extreme amounts of social stressors (e.g., criticism and/or overinvolvement from a close family member). Whatever the source of the person's deficits of skills, therapists should be able to help the person overcome or partially compensate for the deficits through systematic training in more effective response alternatives.

The objective of training is to strengthen patients' ability to cope with a wide variety of interpersonal situations. Implementation of training is based upon the situationally specific aspects of instrumental and social-emotional encounters between people; thus, the training can take place *in vivo* with the people actually involved with the patient's real-life problems; or it can take place via role-playing. Detailed descriptions of the training process are available,[33-38] the following provides a capsule summary of a prototypical session.

First, the patient is asked to role-play an interpersonal situation, either with the trainer or with a fellow patient. At the conclusion of the role-play, the trainer reviews the patient's performance, reinforces correct behaviors, and provides instructions to use certain other behaviors that will presumably result in a more socially skilled performance. The focus of training is usually the topography of the patient's performance; that is, *nonverbal behaviors*, such as eye contact, speech fluency, voice intonation and volume, facial expression, response duration and latency, posture, and gestures; and *verbal content*, such as requesting changes in the behavior of the other person, expressions of appropriate affect, asking questions, making self-disclosures, and offering compliments.

The situation is role-played again, and the cycle is repeated until the performance meets a criterion specified by the trainer in concert with the patient. Videotaping may be used to aid the review process; modeling and coaching may also be used to demonstrate and prompt more effective behaviors. Thus, many of the principles known to facilitate social learning—instructions, goal setting, modeling, prompting, positive reinforcement, shaping change through successive approximations—are packaged in the training approach. Table I lists the steps in social skills training, and Figures 2 and 3 illustrate trainers working with patients in a role-played situation. It is important to emphasize the directiveness, specificity, and active nature of the therapy process, as these characteristics sharply demarcate this type of behavior therapy from more conventional psychotherapies which rely on indirect discussion of problems and feelings.

Social skills training, like other psychotherapies, must be firmly rooted in a warm, trusting, and empathic therapeutic alliance to be effective. The alliance is further cemented by the problem-solving, trial-and-error nature of the training process, and by the partnership between patient and therapist in defining problems, selecting goals, and actively working together on solutions. An important phase of social skills training is the generalization of in-session improvements to the real world. Generalization, or transfer of therapeutic gains, is promoted by a number of procedures:

1. Giving "homework assignments" to carry out in the real world what was practiced in the training session.

2. Gradually fading the frequency of the sessions with "booster sessions" scheduled as needed.

3. Using multiple therapists and other patients in the role playing, so that the learning will not become stimulus bound to a single therapist.

4. Teaching the patient to use self-instructions and self-reinforcement outside of the training situation.

5. Simulating the natural environment in the therapeutic role playing by bringing in props and role players who resemble the significant others in the patient's life.

6. Choosing scenes for the role playing that are relevant for problem solving in those interpersonal encounters that occur in critical life situations and that mediate successful family and community adjustment.

7. Working with family members and other community-based individuals, such as the patient's social network, who can reinforce the patient's progress.

SOCIAL SKILLS TRAINING FOR SCHIZOPHRENICS

We were encouraged to commit our MHCRC's resources to a long-term program of studies on social skills training by findings from both single subject and group studies which indicated that schizophrenic patients favorably responded to specific training of the behavioral elements of

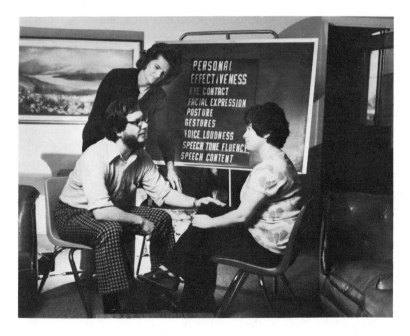

FIGURE 2. Therapist (standing) prompting patient to touch his partner in role-playing a scene in social skills training.

TABLE I.   Outline of the Training Procedure for Social Skills Training Using Role Playing and Behavioral Rehearsal to Simulate Real-Life Situations

1.	Specify the interpersonal problem by asking:
	What affect or communication is lacking or not being appropriately expressed?
	With whom does the patient want and need to improve social contact?
	Where and when does the problem occur?
2.	Formulate a scene which simulates or recapitulates the features of the problem situation.
3.	Observe while the patient and surrogate role players rehearse the scene and, during this "dry run," position yourself close to the action.
4.	Identify the assets, deficits, and excesses in the patient's performance during the "dry run," and give constructive feedback.
5.	Give instructions and prompts to initiate changes in behavior.
6.	Use models to demonstrate more adaptive expressive skills.
7.	Focus on all dimensions of social competence:
	Topical content and semantic choice of words and phrases
	Nonverbal components
	Timing and reciprocity
	Perceptual and discrimination skills
8.	Give positive feedback to reinforce progress, or even effort, as the patient again rehearses the scene in a "rerun."
9.	Shape behavioral changes in small increments, start where the patient is and don't expect too much improvement at any one time.
10.	Generalize the changes over settings, responses, and time, by:
	Repeated practice and overlearning
	Specific, attainable, and functional "homework assignment"
	Positive feedback for successful transfer of skills to real life
	Training in self-instructions and self-reinforcement
	Fading the structure and frequency of the training

interpersonal competence. Wallace and his colleagues at the Camarillo/UCLA MHCRC have published a thorough and critical review of these studies,[32] which will be only summarized here.

Single-Subject Studies

Hersen, Bellack, Eisler, and their colleagues have conducted several studies using single subject designs that clearly demonstrate the effectiveness of training on the topographical elements of social skills in chronic psychiatric patients.[36-38] An experiment conducted with two verbally abusive psychotic patients exemplifies the single-subject approach.[39] The patients were trained to increase their rates of eye contact and assertive requests, and to decrease their rates of irrelevant, hostile, and inappropriate comments. Training consisted of instructions, modeling, behavioral rehearsal, and feedback. A total of 14 role-played interpersonal situations were used

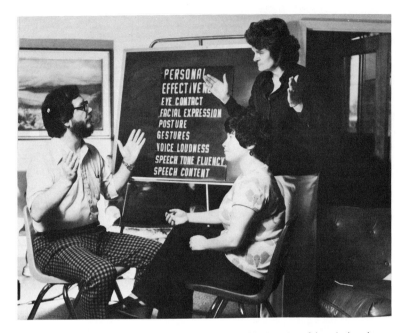

FIGURE 3. Therapist coaching a patient, through the use of hand signals, to lean forward while speaking in a role-played scene in social skills training.

for each patient; seven were used during training, and seven were used to assess the generalization of training to novel situations. Generalization to a confederate other than the trainer, as well as to situations spontaneously enacted on the patients' ward, was also assessed. After three baseline sessions, in which the 14 situations were simply role-played and the patients' responses assessed, training was applied to the first patient while the other patient continued in the assessment-only condition. After three more sessions, the second patient also received training.

The results indicated that each patient's behaviors changed only as the training was applied, suggesting that training was the effective element in the change. The results also showed that training generalized to different confederates, and to both the seven novel situations and the patients' interactions on the ward. These results have been replicated in other, similar, single-subject studies conducted by Hersen and his colleagues. In addition, several of their studies have indicated that treatment gains, as measured by improvements in discrete verbal and nonverbal assertive behaviors, were maintained for as long as six months after training ended.[40,41] Matson and Stephans[42] found that training not only improved the social skills of four aggressive patients, but also increased nurses' ratings of the patients' cooperativeness and interpersonal appropriateness. While gains, including reductions in fighting and arguing, were maintained over a 12-week follow-up period, once the follow-up checks were discontinued, the patients' appropriate behavior rapidly deteriorated to prebaseline levels.

Using a multiple baseline design with three relapsing schizophrenics diagnosed by the Present State Examination, Liberman and his colleagues[43] sequentially applied social skills training to each of three problem areas—in-hospital situations with staff and other patients; family interactions; and social and vocational interactions in the community. Training was provided during 11 sessions per week, 30 hours per week for eight weeks. Outcomes were assessed by the patients' ability to complete homework assignments in each of the three problem areas, with verification coming from the targets of the assignments. During the first two weeks, before training was begun, baseline assessments were made of homework completion, with the patients simply being urged to do as many of the assignments as they could. Training was then applied to interactions in the hospital during weeks 3 to 6; to in-hospital plus family interactions during weeks 7 and 8; and, finally, to all three arenas of interaction during weeks 9 and 10.

The results are presented in Figure 4, and indicate that completion of homework assignments did not increase until training was applied to each specific interpersonal arena, suggesting that the training was the causally effective variable in the homework completion. Furthermore, generalized improvements were found in a variety of other outcome measures—a naturalistic, mildly stressful conversational encounter with confederates; ratings of conversational skills on the ward by nursing staff; the Behavioral Assertiveness Test; MMPI; and the Whitaker Index of Schizophrenic Thinking.

Group Comparison Studies

The studies that have evaluated the effects of social skills training by means of group comparisons are difficult to summarize, since many different training methods and many different outcome measures have been used. Nevertheless, certain trends have emerged from the literature. Improvements were noted in six of seven studies that used self-reported assessments of competence and comfort by patients in interpersonal situations. In eight studies that have evaluated the effects of training on the topographic features of social skills, improvement was noted which persisted for as long as 24 months after-treatment. Two studies, both utilizing outpatients and self-reported ratings, found no improvements beyond those found in control groups. When the effects of training have been evaluated in situations dissimilar in format from the training sessions, the results have been less promising. Only one study has unequivocally documented generalized improvement in a new situation. Goldsmith and McFall[44] found that in a mildly stressful, five-minute conversation with a stranger, trained

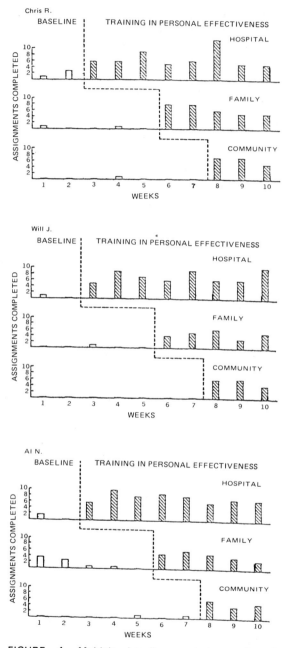

FIGURE 4. Multiple baseline analysis, replicated across three patients, of the impact of training in personal effectiveness (social skills) on completion of homework assignments in three interpersonal spheres—hospital, family, and community interactions.

patients were rated significantly higher in skill and comfort than either assessment-only or "pseudotherapy" patients; in addition, the trained patients successfully completed more interpersonal tasks in the conversation with the confederate than did patients in the control groups.

In an elegantly controlled study covering six years, Paul and Lentz[45] randomly assigned chronic, refractory psychotic patients to three intramural regional hospital programs—a traditional, continued treatment service, a milieu-therapy program, and a social learning/token economy program. In the latter two programs, staff were kept constant by rotation across wards. Criteria for release from the hospital were standardized for all three programs. Once discharged, patients were followed for 18 months in the community, with active aftercare consultation.

Impressive and clear-cut results were found favoring the social learning approach. Over 90% of patients treated in the token economy remained continuously in the community at the time of the 18-month follow-up. Some had been in the community for over five years. Over 70% of the residents treated by milieu therapy had achieved significant releases with continuing community stay, compared to fewer than 50% of hospital patients. The patients' level of functioning in the community decreased during the first six months out, followed by increases over the last year of follow-up. The social learning program emerged as effective on an absolute level (e.g., over a third of the patients were functioning at a level indistinguishable from normals), and significantly more effective than either the traditional hospital program or the milieu-therapy program. The social learning program improved the level of functioning more, achieved greater numbers of significant institutional releases, maintained community stay, and, in economic terms, was the most cost-effective program to operate as well.

With these encouraging studies as a background, we began a clinical trial of social skills training with chronic, relapsing schizophrenic young males who come from families high on EE—a group that can be considered vulnerable to environmental stressors and to future relapses. In addition to social skills training, a behavioral, multiple family group therapy is being offered to the patients and their relatives, in an effort to reduce the levels of EE within the family system. A randomly selected comparison group receives equally intensive "holistic health therapy" and insight-oriented family therapy.

THE CAMARILLO/UCLA MHCRC TRAINING
PROGRAM FOR RELAPSING SCHIZOPHRENICS

The Mental Health Clinical Research Center (MHCRC) for the Study of Schizophrenia is a multidisciplinary program for psychosocial research into the causes and treatment of schizophrenia. Supported by a research grant from the National Institute of Mental Health, the MHCRC is jointly sponsored by the UCLA Department of Psychiatry, and Camarillo State Hospital. As one of its primary objectives, the MHCRC is developing and evaluating a social skills training program for chronic, relapsing schizophrenics and their relatives.

The schizophrenic patients selected for the treatment program are currently hospitalized males who are considered to be at high risk for relapse. Patients between 18 and 50 are selected if their diagnosis of schizophrenia is verified by the administration of the Present State Examination (PSE). The PSE, which elicits specific symptoms of schizophrenia through a standard interview, is an internationally accepted instrument for cross-cultural research on schizophrenia. The criteria for diagnosing schizophrenia with the PSE are similar to those used by the World Health Organization, the proposed Third Edition of the American Psychiatric Association's *Diagnostic and Statistical Manual* (DSM-III), and the NIMH Research Diagnostic Criteria.

If the PSE is positive for schizophrenia, a trained interviewer from the MHCRC staff meets with the patient's family for about two hours to administer the Camberwell Family Interview. This interview assesses the relatives' level of negative expressed emotion, as defined by critical comments about the patient and/or emotional overinvolvement with the patient. Patients are accepted into the study it they:

1. Have a diagnosis of schizophrenia confirmed by the PSE, with first rank symptoms during the past month.

2. Have lived for at least one of the three months preceding their current hospitalization with a relative(s) who is determined to be high on EE by the Camberwell Family Interview.

3. Had the onset of illness before age 40.

4. Were not hospitalized cumulatively for more than one year in the past five.

5. Have no organic brain syndrome.

A cohort of patients is selected every three months, and transferred to the Clinical Research Unit at Camarillo State Hospital. The CRU is a 12-bed, coed unit, that is richly staffed with nurses and technicians who are trained to make special observations and interventions within a consistent behavior-therapy milieu. The unit has a multilevel credit system, which provides credits for prosocial behavior in self-care, interpersonal and daily living skills that can be exchanged for privileges, snacks, cigarettes, and small luxuries. The milieu of the CRU has been described in detail in another publication.[46]

Patients are admitted in groups of six to the Clinical Research Unit for ten weeks of treatment; they are randomly assigned to either social skills training or holistic health therapy. The holistic health therapy emphasizes coping with the stressors that have often precipitated past psychotic episodes; it includes yoga, jogging, and meditation, plus instructions in correct nutrition and in redefining schizophrenia as a growth experience. Because this chapter focuses on social skills training, the holistic therapy program—which has been effective in reducing symptoms of patients participating in the first three cohorts of patients—will not be described further. The two treatments are equated for time spent in therapy, and for the effects of different therapist characteristics. Therapists rotate between the two treatments on a daily basis, so that, at the end of ten weeks, they have spent an equal amount of time with both groups. The ten-week inpatient treatment program has several components, that are systematically evaluated to establish their utility in the treatment of hospitalized schizophrenic patients.

Social Skills Training

The techniques of the social skills training program, developed by Charles Wallace, Connie Nelson, David Lukoff and Chris Ferris, include as the core element a daily two-hour role-playing session. In these five-day-per-week sessions, the patient learns to solve interpersonal problems that are deemed important for effective functioning in the social arenas of the hospital, his family, peers and the community.[32,47] The sessions are led by two co-therapists, who work with a group of three patients. The hospital and community problems have been standardized, and include such areas as interacting with other patients, nursing staff, apartment managers, human service agency officials, and residential care staff. The family scenes are individualized for each patient, based on reports of problematic situations, and on the family members' responses to the Camberwell Family Interview.

The format of the training sessions emphasizes the cognitive factors that are involved in effective social performance and problem solving. The interpersonal communication process has been broken down into three separate phases, each characterized by a component of effective problem-solving:

1. Receiving Skills—the ability to attend to and accurately perceive problem situations and cues.
2. Processing Skills—the ability to interpret interpersonal cues, to generate possible alternatives for action, to consider the potential consequences of each alternative, and then to decide on a reasonable course of action.
3. Sending Skills—the ability to deliver effectively a social response, using verbal and nonverbal expressiveness.

During the role playing of the situation, the patient must initiate the interaction or respond to a trainer who takes the role of the significant other (e.g., nurse, parent, agency clerk, friend). The scene is role-played and video-taped; then the patient is asked the following questions, to assess his skill in receiving and processing the information in that social situation:

Receiving Questions	Processing Questions
Who spoke to you?	Name one other alternative
What did _____ say?	you could have used when
What was _____ feeling?	_____ said _____?
What was your short-term goal?	If you were to _____, what would the other feel?
What was your long-term goal?	What could the other do?
	Would you get your short-term goal?
	Would you get your long-term goal?
	Would you use that alternative and why?

A set of 14 active behavioral alternatives or response options has been developed that appears to fit most person-to-person, instrumental scenes. Each scene has a recommended alternative that is suggested to the patient if he does not spontaneously select one of the potentially effective alternatives. The alternatives include:

Compromising
Terminating rudely
Terminating politely
Ignoring criticism
Getting angry
Repeating your request
Asking for assistance
Highlighting the importance of your need
Complying with the other's request
Refusing to comply with the other's request
Explaining your position
Asking for more information
Coming back later (e.g., ask for an appointment)
Acknowledging the other's position and . . . (use one of the above)

An incorrect or inappropriate answer at any point in this process results in a training procedure designed to highlight the relevant cues and immediately elicit and reinforce the correct answer.

In learning sending skills, the patient views the videotape playback of his performance, and gives a self-evaluation of his performance in response to questions from the therapist:

> How was your eye contact?
> How was your voice volume?
> How was your fluency?
> How was your posture?
> How was your facial expression?
> How were your gestures?

If ineffective responses are shown, the patient rehearses the scene again with coaching and modeling as necessary. Patients rotate in their responding to questions and prompts, and take turns in being the protagonist in a training scene.

Training in Cognitive Skills

During the last five weeks of the program, the emphasis switches from scenes in which instrumental needs are obtained to more complex friendship and dating situations. Using a graduated approach, appropriate social skills are introduced, beginning with the initiation of a conversation, and ending with the termination of a completed conversation. Approximately five weeks are spent shaping complete conversational skills. The major skills emphasized are: identifying potential topic areas in the other person's response, using verbal and nonverbal listening skills, deciding when it is your turn to talk, deciding what level of self-disclosure is appropriate for the situation, changing the topic, and terminating the conversation. These conversational skills are taught using instructions, modeling, role playing, feedback, and reinforcement, with the addition of several discrimination exercises.

The receiving, processing, and sending questions are modified to conform with the goal of initiating and maintaining satisfactory social relationships. In the early sessions of the peer and friendship module, relatively few questions are utilized. More questions are added to the therapy process as additional conversational skills are acquired. The final two weeks of therapy consist of simulated practicing of conversations with friends and dates. At the end of each role-play, the following questions are asked:

Receiving Questions	Processing Questions
Who spoke to you?	What was your short-term goal?
What was the main topic of conversation?	What was your long-term goal?
What was the other person feeling?	

The initiating statement of the role-play is then replayed on the video equipment, and the following questions are asked of the patient who had done the role playing:

Receiving Questions	Sending Questions
What topic area did you choose?	Did you use an open-ended question?
Can you think of another topic area?	Can you think of an open-ended question you could have used?

The last group of questions are asked intermittently (every 10–15 meters of tape) during the video playback:

Sending Questions

Did you ask a question?
Was it open or closed?

Processing Questions

What level of self-disclosure should you be at?
How can you tell?
Do you want to continue or terminate?
Does the other person want to continue or terminate?
How can you tell?
Is one person doing most of the talking or is it about 50–50?
Is it time to change the topic?

Receiving Questions

What are some possible topic areas to change to?
Has the role player changed the topic?
What topic did he change to?

In addition to these questions, the therapists are instructed to stop the tape at any time, to reinforce the following sending skills: active listening skills, gestures, good open-ended questions, and appropriate laughter.

Community Homework Assignments

While the role-played training sessions are critical for overcoming deficits in skills, poor performance is often a result of motivational deficits. One of the major inadequacies of many social skills training approaches is that they do not arouse adequate levels of motivation for patients to use their newly acquired skills. To have the patients use their newly acquired skills outside of the training sessions, they are given homework assignments. By completing homework assignments outside of the training sessions, the patient obtains "success experiences," and natural, social reinforcement that can help to raise his level of motivation for engaging in social behavior in the future.

Homework assignments require the patients to interact with nursing staff, community agencies, family members, and peers, without the direct supervision of the therapists. Each assignment has a specified "permanent product" that proves that the assignment was carried out by the patient. Patients are asked each day if they have completed any of the assignments, and to turn in the "permanent products" to the therapists. Ample opportunities are provided for the patients to do the assigned tasks. Semiweekly trips into the community allow time for community-based homework assignments, and weekly family therapy sessions, as well as weekend home visits, provide opportunities for family-based homework assignments.

Examples of homework assignments are:

In Hospital

At a patient planning meeting request a special outing.
   Permanent Product: Bring a note from supervising staff member.

In Community

At ice cream store, ask to taste two different flavors before choosing a flavor.
   Permanent Product: Bring ice cream tasting spoons the clerk gives you.

In Family

Call parent and ask that a special item of clothing or personal article be brought for you at next family therapy meeting.
   Permanent Product: Have parent verify call at therapy meeting and bring in the item.

Friendship and Dating

Ask fellow patient to go with you to have coffee in town or see a movie.
   Permanent Product: Have fellow patient verify invitation and bring back a restaurant receipt or ticket stub.

Community Survival Skills

There is considerable evidence suggesting that patients who have experienced frequent, albeit short-term, admissions to institutions are deficient in many of the basic self-care skills necessary for leading satisfying and productive lives in the community. For this reason, one evening each week is devoted to the acquisition of independent living or community survival skills. These basic survival skill areas include grooming, recreation, use of newspapers, telephones, and community agencies, cooking, apartment living, job interviews and vocational planning, transportation, use of laundromats, medical emergencies, Medicaid, first aid, budgeting and money management, and checking accounts.

A variety of training techniques are employed in these sessions, including instruction, open discussion, practice, problem solving, and role playing. The material is, to a large extent, self-paced, and the sessions typically run for about two hours. Criteria indicating competence in each skill area are established prior to the introduction of a new skill area. This necessitates a highly individualized instructional format. The function of this module, then, is to help the patient to make a smooth transition into the community and into the aftercare program.

Family Therapy

The three patients receiving social skills training and their relatives meet weekly during the ten-week hospital period, in a multiple family group. The group has three co-leaders, who jointly direct the demonstrations and discussions, and then work separately with each family during the second half of each two-hour meeting. The first two sessions are spent on discussions of schizophrenia, its causes, course, and treatments. Information is translated to a layperson's level of understanding, with schizophrenia presented as a disorder marked by severe problems in living—working, self-care, socializing, thinking, and feeling. The families are helped to lighten their burdens of guilt, overresponsibility, confusion, and helplessness. The patients are encouraged to grasp the scope of their problems, obtain reasonable hope for modest improvements in coping, and deal with denial. One session is focused on the assertive use of community and psychiatric resources during the posthospitalization period.

The remaining seven sessions are given over to family communication skills, which are described, rationalized, demonstrated, and then rehearsed in the family groups—expressing positive feelings and feedback; making positive requests, active listening skills, expressing negative feelings; and coping with symptoms. The same model of problem solving used with the patients' social skills training is implanted with the families. Each patient and his relatives work with a therapist to (1) pinpoint and specify problems in living; (2) develop several options or alternative responses to deal with the problem; (3) weigh the pros and cons of each alternative, particularly in terms of the potential consequences should it be utilized; (4) choose one alternative that seems reasonable; (5) decide on how to implement the response as a family; (6) provide mutual support in implementation; and (7) reevaluate the problem after the alternative has been used. The family therapy is evaluated by before-after ratings of expressed emotion from Camberwell Family Interviews; a Family Conflict Inventory; and knowledge about schizophrenia and its treatments on a questionnaire.

Aftercare

Aftercare planning is done beginning the first week of hospitalization in a weekly Aftercare Group. The group is organized around various phases of life in the community—income, living arrangements, use of time, continued psychiatric treatment, education, vocational training, and employment. The following questions are used to guide the discussion of each area:

1. What have you had in the past?
2. What do you have now?
3. What will you need when you leave?

From this general discussion, the patient proceeds to specific individual planning and resource development. Each patient also learns to identify "warning signals" of impending relapse, and how to obtain help when such symptoms or experiences occur.

After the patient leaves the hospital, he is followed in the community by a social worker, who provides supportive contact, and conducts periodic research evaluations for nine months. Follow-up contacts are initially frequent when the patient leaves the hospital—twice weekly in person, and once weekly by phone—but are gradually reduced, and faded completely after nine months. By that time, the patient is expected to be connected and involved with appropriate helping resources and agencies in the community.

Evaluation

The effects of the entire package of techniques are evaluated using a multilevel assessment battery. The battery includes patient-reported measures of psychopathology, assertiveness, and social anxiety; role-played tests of social skills in several different types of social situations; behavioral and cognitive tests of interpersonal problem-solving skills; and ratings of psychopathology and general functioning by a psychiatrist, the nursing staff, and the family. All measures are obtained before and after the hospital period of therapy, with ratings of psychopathology made semimonthly by the psychiatrist, and weekly by the nursing staff. The majority of the measures are again administered at 1, 3, 6, 12, 18, and 24 months after hospital discharge, with all measures administered at a follow-up evaluation nine months after treatment. Table II lists the outcome measures used in the research.

TABLE II.   Outcome Measures Used in the Camarillo/UCLA Study on Training Schizophrenic Patients and Their Relatives in Social Skills and Problem-Solving Skills

Names of dependent variable	Frequency of assessment*	Rater
Brief Psychiatric Rating Scale (BPRS)	Biweekly and every follow-up	Psychiatrist
Psychiatric Assessment Scale (PAS)	Biweekly and every follow-up	Psychiatrist
Clinical Global Impressions (CGI)	Biweekly and every follow-up	Psychiatrist
Nurses' Observation Scale for Inpatient Evaluation (NOSIE–30)	Weekly	Nursing Staff
Nurses' Global Impressions (NGI)	Weekly	Nursing Staff
Social Interaction Schedule	Four times daily	Nursing Staff
Tests of Interpersonal Cognitive Problem Solving Skills (MEPS; Options)	Pre and post and 9-month follow-up	Staff
Rathus Assertiveness Schedule	Pre and post and every follow-up	Patient
Social Anxiety and Distress Scale	Pre and post and every follow-up	Patient
Fear of Negative Evaluation Scale	Pre and post and every follow-up	Patient
Minnesota Multiphasic Personality Inventory (MMPI–168)	Pre and post and every follow-up	Patient
Symptom Check List 90 (SCL–90)	Pre and post and every follow-up	Patient
Confederate Test of Social Skills	Pre and post and 9-month follow up	Staff & Patient
Role-Play Test of Social Competence	Pre and post and 9-month follow-up	Staff
Shipley–Hartford IQ Test	Pre and post and 9-month follow-up	Patient
Tennessee Self-Concept Test	Pre and post and 9-month follow-up	Patient
In-therapy process assessments	Daily	Staff
Katz Social Adjustment (KAS)	Pre and 9-month follow-up	Patient & Family
Present State Examination (PSE)	Pre and post and 9-month follow-up	Psychiatrist

* Follow-ups are scheduled at 1, 3, 6, 9, 12, 18, and 24 months post therapy.

DISCUSSION

While the MHCRC treatment program, emphasizing the training of social and family communication skills, appears to address important problems in the pathogenesis of schizophrenic relapse, there are a number of questions which must be answered by empirical results before this psychosocial strategy is viewed as an advance in our therapeutic efforts with schizophrenics. First, *can schizophrenics and their families learn the problem-solving methods to be used in everyday interpersonal relations?* This is a "process" matter, and will be revealed by the evaluation of the patients' and their relatives' demonstrating problem-solving skills during the therapy sessions. Thus far, with half the project completed, it appears that most of the patients and their relatives do learn the skills *while they are being monitored in the sessions.* One qualification is that a schizophrenic patient who is still incoherent, with intrusive hallucinatory and delusional speech, is not able to attend to the social skills training sequence, or to assimilate it. Therefore, a minimum level of restitution of the thought disorder, not yet determined, is likely to be necessary for a patient to learn the methods.

The second question addressed by the research is, "If the schizophrenic patient is able to learn the problem-solving model, and does show improvement in social skills through training, *does this lead to improvement in other behavioral areas, such as psychopathology, social adjustment, social anxiety, self-care skills, cognitive capacities, and affect?* This is a question, then, of response generalization. Thus far, improvements in some areas of psychopathology, affect, and self-care skills have been noted; however, the decisive data have yet to be collected.

Third, the questions of situational and temporal generalization arise. If improvements brought about by the training are seen during the hospital period of intensive treatment, *will they generalize to the home, the workplace, the various community settings in which the patient will live after discharge?* And, if they do generalize to the posthospital situations, *how long will they be maintained?* The follow-up evaluations, to be carried out over a two year period, will tell this story. Brief therapy may start a person on a trajectory of change, but only long-term studies can assess truly durable change. It is to be expected, however, that with much of human behavior being situationally supported and determined, natural reinforcers in the community will have to be mobilized to consolidate the gains made by patients during the intensive phase of treatment.[48] Several learning strategies are being used in the social skills training to enhance generalization across settings and over time:

1.   The training of a cognitive "problem-solving" model, which serves as the core element of the treatment program, may equip a schizophrenic with a "built-in" mechanism to cope with stressful life events.

2.   Use of overlearning; that is, the same problem-solving methods are repeatedly taught, day after day, using different situational problems and challenges.

3.   A variety of therapists are deliberately brought into contact with the patients, so that their learning is not attached or discriminated to any one therapist—this should promote their use of skills learned in therapy with a range of other individuals after discharge.

4.   Communication and problem-solving skills are the primary focus of the family therapy, with the aim to establish a more reinforcing and cohesive support system for the patient after discharge.

5. The aftercare follow-up includes efforts, albeit with limited contact, to prompt and reinforce the patients' use of their social and problem-solving skills.

Despite systematic efforts to promote durability of treatment gains, it may be necessary to engineer more permanent social support networks for the schizophrenic person in the community. On the drawing boards at the Camarillo/UCLA MHCRC are plans to develop *in vivo* training methods for community survival skills, based upon learning technology and the successful support system created by Stein and Test.[17] We may find, in the future, a variety of semipermanent, transitional social support systems which serve to maintain a schizophrenic individual's social and cognitive adaptations, much as artificial limbs and mechanized transport maintain the functioning and mobility of a physically handicapped person. An important ingredient in future efforts at rehabilitation of schizophrenics will be educating toward greater tolerance and receptivity the families, gatekeepers, human service workers, and other citizens who come into everyday contact with schizophrenics. These people, in the community, will need to learn a problem-solving "set" to use in their encounters with a schizophrenic as much as the schizophrenic himself needs to learn problem solving.

The idea that social skills training will be useful for changing the course or outcome for schizophrenic patients is intuitively appealing, because of the social deficits found in patients before and after the onset of their illness. However, the current testing of the effects of social skills training is somewhat akin to "putting the cart before the horse." There is only suggestive evidence that problem-solving skills are related to outcome. Thus, this raises additional questions for the current research—are the social and problem-solving skills being taught in the current MHCRC program related to relapse; and, if they are, will a schizophrenic person who has become more competent in social interaction and problem solving be less likely to suffer a symptomatic relapse?

Our lack of knowledge of the specific details surrounding the phenomena of relapse and remission keep us in the dark about the role of social, communication, and problem-solving skills in the reactions of schizophrenic persons to environmental stressors. We need to know much more about the problems and problem-solving efforts of schizophrenic persons faced by a variety of situations. Patients returning to conjugal homes will surely face a set of problems that are different from those faced by patients who return to a parental home; schizophrenics returning to both of these types of families will not face the same types of problems as are faced by patients returning to small or large residential care facilities. Our current efforts in understanding the nature of social skills are slowed by lack of assessment tools that would allow us to differentiate the type of social skills deficit from among disparate sources, such as perceptual and knowledge deficits, response or repertoire deficits, or motivational and rein-forcement deficits. For example, for those individuals who relapse because of a social problem-solving deficit, did the deficit represent a failure to perceive the situation accurately, a lack of know-how in the situation, an inability to respond effectively, or an environmental contingency that rewarded unskilled and disturbing behavior, and/or that extinguished or punished incipient efforts at a skilled response.

We also need to determine whether ineffective coping and interpersonal problem solving actually leads to affective arousal, cognitive distortions, and symptomatic relapse—or whether social incompetence only incon-veniences the patient and those around him. For example, if symptomatic exacerbation precedes deficits in social skills, then perhaps the best preven-tive strategy would be to provide stress and arousal reduction techniques, such as brief periods of reduced social stimulation and increases in medica-tion. On the other hand, if we can identify social problems and behaviors which are relevant to the process of relapse, then we will be better placed to design an educational curriculum for social skills training that will have a higher probability of efficacy. Obtaining data on these more specific and refined relationships between interpersonal problem solving and the course of schizophrenia must await longitudinal, follow-through research studies.

A start has been made toward an empirically based, therapeutic approach for the psychosocial treatment of schizophrenia. With the opti-mistic assumptions that our schizophrenic patients have the capacity to learn; that their relatives' attitudes and feelings can become more positive; and that conducive environments—both in and out of hospitals—can be designed to override the biologically mediated diathesis toward schizo-phrenia, we can continue to make modest but important progress in helping our schizophrenic patients live more rewarding lives.

SUMMARY

The psychotherapeutic hearth for schizophrenia glows and warms its adherents only in a few academic ivory towers and private psychiatric hos-pitals, while most of American psychiatry is swept by a tide of psychothera-peutic nihilism, in so far as schizophrenia is concerned. In most treatment settings, the question is not whether intensive psychotherapy, or even brief therapy, is of value for schizophrenics, but, rather, whether the schizophrenic patient will have time to brush his teeth and take a shower before being discharged through the hospital's "revolving door" with fluphenazine in his butt, a prescription in his hand, and an appointment to see a well-meaning but harassed aftercare worker two or three weeks later. This is the current practice and professional reality that must be confronted by those who are developing, evaluating, and justifying psychosocial approaches for the treatment of schizophrenia.

Despite their widespread and accepted usage, neuroleptic drugs leave much to be desired as a satisfactory treatment for schizophrenia. Drug therapy has delayed but not solved the problem of recurrent relapse in schizophrenia; has led to a decrease in census, but an increase in read-missions to mental hospitals; has been accompanied by a host of unpleasant and sometimes irreversible side effects; has had its full efficacy limited by a staggering noncompliance rate; and does not enable the schizophrenic person to learn those social and life skills necessary for survival and satisfy-ing functioning in the community. While medication undoubtedly reduces symptomatology and facilitates interpersonal contact, more is needed for a comprehensive treatment of the person with schizophrenia.

Two sources of data have accumulated over the past 20 years, pointing to the potential value of a combined social skills training and family therapy approach to the treatment of schizophrenia. A wide variety of studies has suggested that the level of social competence attained by a person before a psychotic episode has a major impact on the individual's adjustment in the future. The prognosis for a schizophrenic's later work and social function-ing improves to the extent that the individual had close peer and heterosocial/heterosexual relationships, and successful school and work performances, before falling ill. A second source of data indicates that the emotional climate of a family has a definite, predictable effect on the course of the schizophrenic illness of a family member. In fact, ratings of certain emotions and attitudes expressed by key family members are powerful pre-dictors of relapse in persons having an established schizophrenic illness.

A family's attitudes and feelings toward a schizophrenic member, evaluated with the semistructured, standardized Camberwell Family Inter-view, classify a patient as being from a home high or low on two aspects of "expressed emotion"—excessive criticism, and emotional overinvolvement. Results of three replicated follow-up studies indicate that patients with rela-tives high on "expressed emotion" relapse at a rate four times greater than patients with relatives low on "expressed emotion."

These sources of data led to a convergence on a psychosocial treatment strategy for schizophrenics and their family members that aims:

!. To strengthen the social competence and interpersonal skills of relapsing schizophrenics, enabling them to obtain their social, family, and daily living needs.

2. To improve the quality of familial relations, reducing overinvolve-ment and critical attitudes while increasing cohesion and communication clarity within the family.

At the Camarillo/UCLA Mental Health Clinical Research Center for the Study of Schizophrenia, a comprehensive psychosocial treatment strategy, together with neuroleptic medication as needed, is being developed and evaluated. The strategy utilizes social skills training in groups for schizophrenic patients, and a multifamily therapy for the patients and their relatives.

Social skills training is designed to teach patients effectively to solve the interpersonal problems that are part and parcel of daily living. Effective solving of interpersonal problems is hypothesized to consist of accurate *receiving* of situational information, flexible *processing* of the information in order to generate a set of alternatives and their likely consequences, and effective *sending* of an appropriately chosen alternative. The training techniques are designed to improve patients' receiving, processing, and sending skills, in the context of standardized instrumental and friendship/peer heterosocial situations.

The family therapy, conducted one evening a week for two hours, begins with two sessions of mental health education. During these sessions, the patients and relatives are helped to ventilate their past frustrating and painful experiences with schizophrenia, and to understand, in concrete and personal terms, the nature, course, and treatments for schizophrenia. The remaining sessions are devoted to systematic training of communication skills and problem-solving methods.

The social skills training and family therapy are intensive, with patients receiving 30 hours per week of treatment over a ten-week inpatient period. This regimen is being compared with an equally intensive approach, offered by the same therapists, consisting of meditation, yoga, jogging, art therapy, and stress-reduction methods. Patients are randomly assigned to these two treatment conditions, and will be followed for symptomatic, social, occupational, and community adjustment for nine months. It is hoped that this developing line of research will produce an evolution of increasingly effective psychosocial interventions, that will reduce the rate of relapse and improve the quality of life among schizophrenic persons.

ACKNOWLEDGMENT

The work reported in this paper is the outcome of an interdisciplinary team effort by the staff of the Camarillo/UCLA Mental Health Clinical Research Center for the Study of Schizophrenia. The authors acknowledge the central importance of the following colleagues in making this work possible: Robert Aitchison, Dorothy Argabrite, Rick Brickey, Patricia Brown, Karen Burke, Gene Couture, Ian Falloon, Chris Ferris, William Freeman, Susan Hodge, Arvis James, Simon Jones, Cecilia Kwolek, Portia Loughman, David Lukoff, Barringer Marshall, Jr., Pauline Martin, Jose Martinez-Diaz, F. Ann McElroy, Joan Moore, Connie Nelson, Dennis

O'Bosky, Tim Oliver, Jenny Payne, Sandra L. Rappe, Bob Riley, Julie Strand, and Mark Terranova.

REFERENCES

1. Mosher LR: Madness in the community. *Attitude* **1**:2–21, 1971.
2. Talbot JA: Stop the revolving door: A study of recidivism to a state hospital. *Psychiatr Q* **48**:159–167, 1974.
3. Evans JR, Goldstein MJ, Rodnick EH: Premorbid adjustment, paranoid status, and patterns of response to phenothiazine in acute schizophrenia. *Schizophr Bull* **3**:24–37, 1973.
4. Kohen W, Paul GL: Current trends and recommended changes in extended-care placement of mental patients: The Illinois system as a case in point. *Schizophr Bull* **2**:575–594, 1976.
5. Paul GL, Tobias LL, Holly BL: Maintenance psychotropic drugs in the presence of active treatment programs. *Arch Gen Psychiatry* **27**:106–115, 1972.
6. Liberman RP: Behavior therapy for schizophrenia, in West LJ, Flinn D (eds): *Treatment of Schizophrenia*. New York, Grune & Stratton, 1976, p 175.
7. Van Putten T: Why do schizophrenic patients refuse to take their drugs? *Arch Gen Psychiatry* **31**:67–72, 1974.
8. Hogarty GE, Goldberg SC, Schooler NR: Drug and sociotherapy in the aftercare of schizophrenic patients: II. Two-year relapse rates. *Arch Gen Psychiatry* **31**:603–608, 1974.
9. Brown GW, Carstairs GM, Topping G: Post-hospital adjustment of chronic mental patients. *Lancet* **2**:685–689, 1958.
10. Brown GW, Rutter M: The measurement of family activities and relationships: A methodological study. *Human Relations* **19**:241–263, 1966.
11. Rutter M, Brown GW: The reliability and validity of measures of family life and relationship in families containing a psychiatric patient. *So Psychiatry* **1**:38–53, 1966.
12. Brown GW, Monck EM, Carstairs GM, et al: Influence of family life on the course of schizophrenic illness. *Br J Prev So Med* **16**:55–68, 1962.
13. Brown G, Birley JLT, Wing JK: Influence of family life on the course of schizophrenia. *Br J Psychiatry* **121**:241–258, 1972.
14. Vaughn CE, Leff JP: The influence of family and social factors on the course of psychiatric illness: A comparison of schizophrenic and depressed neurotic patients. *Br J Psychiatry* **129**:125–137, 1976.
15. Wing JK, Cooper JE, Sartorius N: *The Measurement and Classification of Psychiatric Symptoms*. London, Cambridge University Press, 1974.
16. Liberman RP, Davis J: Drugs and behavior analysis, in Hersen M, Eisler R, Miller PM (eds): *Progress in Behavior Modification*. New York, Academic Press, 1975, p 307.
17. Stein LI, Test MA (eds): *Alternatives to Mental Hospital Treatment*. New York, Plenum Publishing Co, 1978.
18. Leff JP, Hirsch SR, Gaind R, et al: Life events and maintenance therapy in schizophrenic relapse. *Br J Psychiatry* **123**:659–660, 1973.
19. Zubin J, Spring B: Vulnerability: A new view of schizophrenia. *J Abnorm Psychol* **86**:103–126, 1977.
20. Zigler E, Phillips L: Social competence and outcome in psychiatric disorder. *J Abnorm Soc Psychol* **63**:264–271, 1961.
21. Levine J, Zigler E: The essential-reactive distinction in alcoholism. *J Abnorm Psychol* **81**:242–249, 1973.
22. Strauss JS, Carpenter WT: The prediction of outcome in schizophrenia. II. Relationships between predictor and outcome variables. *Arch Gen Psychiatry* **31**:37–42, 1974.

23. Hersen M, Bellack AS: Social skills training for chronic psychiatric patients: Rationale, research findings, and future directions. *Compr Psychiatry* **17**:559–580, 1976.

24. Kokes RF, Strauss JS, Klorman R: Premorbid adjustment in schizophrenia: Concepts, measures and implications: II. Measuring premorbid adjustment: The instruments and their development. *Schizophr Bull* **3**:186–213, 1977.

25. Farina A, Garmezy N, Zalusky M, et al: Premorbid behavior and prognosis in female schizophrenic patients. *J Consult Psychol* **26**:56–60, 1962.

26. Vaillant GE: A 10-year follow up of remitting schizophrenics. *Schizophr Bull* **4**:78–85, 1978.

27. Gittleman-Klein R, Klein DF: Premorbid social adjustment and prognosis in schizophrenia. *J Psychiatr Res* **7**:35–53, 1969.

28. Platt JJ, Spivack G: Problem-solving thinking of psychiatric patients. *J Consult Clin Psychol* **39**:148–151, 1972.

29. Platt JJ, Siegel JM, Spivack G: Do psychiatric patients and normals see the same solutions as effective in solving interpersonal problems? *J Consult Clin Psychol* **43**:297, 1975.

30. Spivack G, Platt JJ, Shure MB: *The Problem-Solving Approach to Adjustment.* San Francisco, Jossey-Bass, 1976.

31. Platt JJ, Siegel J: MMPI characteristics of good and poor social problem-solvers among psychiatric patients. *J Psychol* **94**:245–251, 1976.

32. Wallace CJ, Nelson CJ, Liberman RP, et al: A review and critique of social skills training with schizophrenic patients. *Schizophr Bull,* **6**:42–63, 1980.

33. Liberman RP, King LW, DeRisi WJ, et al: *Personal Effectiveness: Guiding People to Assert Themselves and Improve their Social Skills.* Champaign, Ill, Research Press, 1975.

34. Goldstein AA: *Structured Learning Therapy.* New York, Academic Press, 1973.

35. Trower P, Bryant B, Argyle M, et al: *Social Skills and Mental Health.* Pittsburgh, University of Pittsburgh Press, 1978.

36. Hersen M, Bellack AS: A multiple baseline analysis of social skills training in chronic schizophrenics. *J Appl Behav Anal* **9**:239–245, 1976.

37. Hersen M, Turner SM, Edelstein BA, et al: Effect of phenothiazine and social skills training in chronic schizophrenics. *J Clin Psychol* **31**:588–594, 1975.

38. Williams MT, Turner SW, Watts JG, et al: Group social skills training for chronic psychiatric patients. *Eur J Behav Anal Mod* **1**:223–229, 1977.

39. Frederikson LW, Jenkins JO, Foy DW, et al: Social skills training to modify abusive verbal outbursts in adults. *J Appl Behav Anal* **9**:117–127, 1976.

40. Foy DW, Eisler RM, Pinkston S: Modeled assertion in a case of explosive rages. *J Behav Ther Exp Psychiatry* **6**:135–137, 1975.

41. Bellack AS, Hersen M, Turner SM: Generalization effects of social skills training with chronic schizophrenics: An experimental analysis. *Behav Res Ther* **14**:391–398, 1976.

42. Matson JL, Stephans RM: Increasing appropriate behavior of explosive chronic psychiatric patients with a social skills training package. *Behav Mod* **2**:61–77, 1978.

43. Liberman RP, Lillie F, Falloon I, et al: Social skills training for relapsing schizophrenics: An experimental analysis. Unpublished manuscript, 1978. Available from the first author at the Mental Health Clinical Research Center for the Study of Schizophrenia, Box A, Camarillo, CA 93010.

44. Goldsmith JB, McFall RM: Development and evaluation of an interpersonal skills training program for psychiatric inpatients. *J Abnorm Psychol* **84**:51–58, 1975.

45. Paul GL, Lentz RJ: *Psychosocial Treatment of Chronic Mental Patients: Milieu vs. Social-Learning Programs.* Cambridge, Harvard University Press, 1977.

46. Liberman RP, Wallace C, Teigen J, et al: Behavioral interventions with psychotics, in Calhoun KS, Adams HE, Mitchell EM (eds): *Innovative Treatment Methods in Psychopathology.* New York, Wiley, 1974, p 323.

47. Wallace CJ: Assessment of interpersonal problem-solving skills in chronic schizophrenics. Paper presented at the Annual Meeting of the American Psychological Association, Toronto, September 1978.
48. Liberman RP, McCann M, Wallace CJ: Generalization of behaviour therapy with psychotics. *Br J Psychiatry* **129**:490–496, 1976.

Chapter 4

Some Observations on the Nature and Value of Psychotherapy with Schizophrenic Patients

STEPHEN FLECK

Medical practitioners, meaning physicians during the scientific era as much as during the prescientific millennia, have always drawn inferences from more or less impressionistic therapeutic effects upon the nature of causation or etiology. Equally often, an etiological theory, once formulated, has led to therapeutic prescription, or even, in the case of schizophrenia, to therapeutic nihilism. The history of the treatment of schizophrenics is replete with enthusiastic therapeutic endeavors, sometimes based on very erroneous premises, such as the alleged mutual exclusion of epilepsy and schizophrenia, which led to convulsive treatments, therapies which then led to other etiological credos.[1-4] Psychotherapy, effective as it can be with schizophrenics, is no exception to such *post hoc propter hoc* etiological hypothesizing. We know that the pathogenic mechanisms in psychological development and in familial behaviors which we can identify during psychotherapeutic work are basic, but we do not know if they are the only, *sine qua non* etiological factors. They, or some chromosomal aberration, may or may not be the first level in a spiral of abnormalities, but this is as

STEPHEN FLECK • Department of Psychiatry, School of Medicine, Yale University, New Haven, Connecticut 06519.

uncertain as is the position or role of abnormal dopamine activity in such a developmental spiral culminating in schizophrenic manifestations.

What is overridingly important is that chemical measures affect certain symptoms and behaviors in particular, often those that can prohibit the patient's even sitting for any length of time; but that, with or without medication, schizophrenics can also be treated psychologically, and that all of them, especially young ones, require psychosocial treatments, psychoeducational guidance, and rehabilitation or even habilitation.

In contrast to these relatively technical measures, dyadic psychotherapy is primarily the use of self—all of one's self—on behalf of another person. This includes those aspects of one's person with which one would rather not be acquainted. In psychotherapeutic work with schizophrenics in particular, attention to these more archaic facets within ourselves may be as important as our cognitive selves (i.e., our knowledge of theories or facts about personality development and structure, about the biology of schizophrenia, and the chemistry of neurotransmitter systems).

Using oneself in this total way on behalf of another, specifically a schizophrenic person, is anxiety-provoking as well as unbelievably fatiguing. Yet, without such total investment of oneself, I do not consider the psychotherapy of schizophrenics a valid endeavor, especially for therapy evaluation purposes, notwithstanding that other psychotherapeutic measures, like behavioral techniques, especially in groups, and sociotherapy, are also important, as already indicated. Yet, when colleagues like the late Elvin Semrad, and Otto Will, and others here on the program, speak of psychotherapy of schizophrenics, I believe, indeed, I know, that it is this total psychoemotional involvement of one person with another that most of them have in mind.[5-10] Other writings and discussions of psychotherapy of schizophrenia, including some studies in which some of these same colleagues have participated, like the remarkable research at the Massachusetts Mental Health Center under Grinspoon,[11] or studies done by May[12] on the West Coast, do not conform to the model of therapy as I have defined it.[13] There is currently also a tendency to define psychotherapy negatively (i.e., everything that is not somatic or drug treatment is called psychotherapeutic). Psychotherapy with severely disturbed schizophrenics cannot usually be accomplished in two sessions a week, or incident to dispensing medications, although the frequency of encounters is by and large less important than is the nature of the mutual investment in exploring the difficulties both the patient and the therapist experience in their encounters.[9,10]

A 46-year-old professional married woman, the mother of several children, was referred to me by an older colleague with the mandate to get her back into the hospital. She had been first diagnosed as schizophrenic more than five years before that, and had been hospitalized much of the time since then. She had received insulin and electric shock treatments, and had remitted for only several months at a time. She had been outside the hospital for about a year at the time of referral, and had worked during part of that time effectively in psychotherapy with a colleague, but a month or so before the referral had begun to become psychotic again, which neither she nor her therapist could understand or work out together. She was then seen by still another colleague, who, after a couple of sessions, rejected her, or so she felt, and she was referred to me. Although blatantly psychotic, and a considerable burden to her family at the time, she adamantly refused to return to any hospital—a stand which I could somehow respect, and therefore I proceeded to explore with her how she could manage living at home, and, for the time being at least, come to see me every day. She was willing to see me, but not every day, although she gave in on that point, and we quickly established a working relationship, with subsidence of her overt psychotic symptoms. After two and one-half weeks of this, she failed to keep her appointment, and over the phone refused to return or tell me why she would not return. During a second phone call that same day, she agreed to come and discuss her alleged decision not to continue in treatment with me. When she came, she was sullen and silent. During the previous two sessions, she had expressed wishes to be close to me. Once I focused on these expressions, specifically on her fantasy that she would like to be down at the beach with me skipping along in the sand and holding hands; she suddenly glared at me and said, "Yes, and you put your hand in your pocket." I acknowledged that I might have done so, although I was not aware of it, and that her interpretation that I rejected her wish was correct in that I wished to work with her and could not do so at the beach, skipping along in the sand, holding hands or not. At this she brightened up, and we continued treatment for several years.

I will return to some other facets of this treatment and her story later on, in order to illustrate further how difficult it can be to fathom and encompass the total process and interchanges. The therpist cannot afford to be lax in awareness of himself, his actions, or his own needs and defenses.

Our more systematic understanding of such personal investment and interpersonal engagement began with Freud, who not only taught us about unconscious mechanisms, but discovered and elucidated transference and countertransference. Yet Freud's clinical interpretations, psychological theories, and analysis of transference phenomena remained circumscribed, with a focus on personality development and structure—a focus on defenses (against instinctual drives) in particular; which led him to believe that schizophrenics, whose defenses are not well structured, fail to establish transferences, let alone develop transference neuroses as a focal element in traditional psychoanalysis.[14]

Others, however, accepted the necessity, and found ways to widen the scope of therapeutic relatedness. Among such psychoanalytic pioneers were

Sullivan,[15,16] Fromm-Reichmann,[5] Sechahaye,[8] Simmel,[17] and Hill[7]—all of whom dared tread where Jung, in a sense, gave up, at least to proceed systematically, although he continued treating schizophrenics. Some of us here, including our honorees and the late Elvin Semrad, are a sort of second generation of schizophrenia therapists, disciples of Sullivan and Fromm-Reichmann, and many more here are already third generation. It needs to be understood that psychotherapy with schizophrenics is a limited field, and those who engage in it need one another for mutual reassurance and reaffirmation in this work, which is arduous, lonely, often painful and upsetting, and always uncertain. There is no cookbook, as Otto Will[10] has said.

Some of the most difficult and painful events, sessions with schizophrenic patients and also some severe borderline patients, concern the unspeakable sadness and forlornness these patients can exude, by which the therapist certainly will be affected and may feel engulfed. I say "unspeakable," and mean it quite literally, because this sadness relates to preverbal experiences and a sense of helplessness and hopelessness, which one can observe at least partially in Monica's apathetic turning away, demonstrated so cogently by Engel.[18] Unfortunately, I, for one, have never been able to pinpoint with patients retrospectively just what particular conditions or maternal neglect patterns did occur so early in life. Inconsistency in mothering is very probably one factor, seen later in transformation as the need–fear dilemma described so well by Burnham and his co-workers.[19] The intense need for attachment leads to fearsome overcloseness, which drives the patient to a stance of negativistic mute sullenness, to paranoid constructs, or, worse still, to aggressive action. We can fathom this experience from the data on imperviousness and intrusiveness of many mothers of schizophrenic patients that we and others have gathered. But it is not clear to me what particular interactional elements may be missing in either the mother or the infant, or both, that imprint the infant with this lasting terror of such a forlorn state, often elaborated later on into a sense of worthlessness and unlovability, and also connected with a crucial developmental deficiency or failure in acquiring object constancy. Without the acquisition of object constancy, cognitive development is hampered too, especially in the sense of persistent egocentricity, as pointed out by Lidz.[20]

It is these core problems from which schizophrenic patients suffer which have tremendous implication for the therapeutic process, although I hasten to add that I do not mean to invalidate other important psychodynamic aberrations in personality development and structure. Among these, the deviations leading to and imbedded in faulty linguistic development are particularly important.[21] However, the basic problem of forlornness also constitutes a potent force in the evolution of therapeutic relationships. It makes for the tremendous intensity with which such patients relate and attach themselves to therapists, and for the patient's demandingness and longing for symbiotic union with the therapist, which are as intense as they are unfulfillable. These longings lead in turn to fantasies of dismemberment on the part of the patient, fears of fragmentation of him- or herself or of the therapist when separation occurs or threatens. Such intense relationships between therapist and patient are indeed different from the neurotic patient's transference.[14,22]

I do not need to elaborate on the vicissitudes of trust these patients experience, trusting in a magical way one moment, and finding the therapist totally untrustworthy the next. Furthermore, when patients feel under-attended or insufficiently loved, they also easily resort to distortions and paranoidal constructs. For instance, if a therapist repeats a phrase of the patient's, such as, "I must be defective," the patient may claim it to be the therapist's judgment about the patient by the next day or even within the same hour, leading to agony for the patient, negativistic, incensed distancing in the next hour or beyond it, and perplexity for the therapist.

Serious and dangerous destructive behavior can ensue from such "misunderstandings," the quotes being there because these impasses are not amenable to the usual corrective statements about misunderstandings between people. The patient referred to above, about two and one-half years after the episode described, had such an hour with me, and again I could not discover what had gone awry between us. She let me know only that she felt desperate, and was convinced that I did not give a hoot about her, but gave me no indication what particular event or omission in my hearing or respon-siveness had led to this conviction. By then the patient had returned to her professional work, and there were a number of people we knew in common. My wondering about having received some unwelcome or disturbing information in this way about me was denied. The next hour I saw another patient, but was aware that the first patient had gone to the bathroom, and had not left the suite. This concerned me enough that I interrupted the hour with the second patient, and went to the bathroom, where I found her almost unconscious. She had taken a large amount of barbiturates, and fortunately could be rushed to a nearby hospital, where she was saved by dialysis, recovering completely eventually after more than a day's uncon-sciousness, unresponsiveness, and subsequent pneumonia. Later I found out that this renewed nadir experience occurred after she had learned that we were giving a party that weekend to which she had not been invited (there had never been any social contact). I can add here that this led also to a clarification of the impasse she had reached with the previous therapist, who, indeed, had become very friendly with her, and had included her in social activities, eventually leading to her feeling rejected by him, and result-ing in renewed psychotic disorganization.

We worked for another fifteen months, at which time both of us left town, in different directions. The patient, indeed, did undertake further professional training, and for the past twenty years has been effective in her work, and has established much improved relationships with her children. She also entered more formal analysis with a senior colleague, which went well despite my misgivings and having recommended against this. She has remained well and asymptomatic from a psychiatric standpoint, and, as I said, is functioning superbly in her profession as a teacher. During the first several years, she would touch base with me rather regularly through a phone call or a note, but now this happens only very occasionally. I emphasize this because one of the aspects of psychotherapy with schizophrenics is very important—it never ends completely. Somehow such patients remain attached, and although they no longer need any direct contact for long periods of time, every so often they do need it, and then it may be quite crucial for them. However, it may not occur even once a year. One could conjecture that their capacity for achieving object constancy remains weak, and needs shoring up once in a while.

It is important to emphasize that most follow-up studies of schizophrenics, no matter how they were treated, are "stills" instead of subsequent life histories. The latter are difficult to come by unless the outcome is poor, leading to the familiar data on chronicity and recurrent hospitalizations. Indeed, this is often viewed as the natural history of the "disease," because data on these patients are so readily gathered. Not so with recovered patients, who are usually reticent to make themselves available for meaningful follow-up studies, except for the contacts with their former therapists to which I have referred. But generally, data on patients who do well remain scattered, and epidemiologically unavailable. Meaningful follow-up data constitute the importance of Bleuler's[23] work based on personal contacts spanning 25 years, presenting a very different natural course than one finds in our textbooks.

Unlike recovered addicts, former schizophrenic patients are reticent about declaring themselves. Green,[24] an exception, may be proving the point, but patients who have recovered and are successful in life cannot be reported on without their consent, and may even be readily identifiable by others. Recently I saw a lady 15 years after several years' hospitalization at a sister institution which is also devoted to psychotherapy of schizophrenic patients. Like most of our "graduates" from the Yale Psychiatric Institute, successful or not, she was very negative and resentful about her hospital experiences, and was just then incensed at what she considered the hospital's clumsy and intrusive follow-up research. She, too, had done well since discharge, had weathered surgery for a malignancy, but also had maintained quite regular contact with her therapist through the years. She was referred to me because of her continued need for support, and yet was essentially asymptomatic, was working, and had successfully managed her move to new surroundings.

An ex-patient's single follow-up contact with a stranger, often consisting of completing a schedule of symptoms and behaviors, cannot result in meaningful information about personal growth and change processes which follow years of intimate work in a special relationship between two people. Epidemiological surveys are important to establish indices of cognitive and social functioning.[25] They cannot provide data of how corrective changes came about in a person, any more than anybody can quickly and easily ascertain what relationships or experiences with a significant other, family member, teacher, or friend made for growth and significant change within oneself.

The importance of *effective* psychotherapy with schizophrenics is not in its extent, since obviously not many patients compared to the huge number of schizophrenics in the world can be treated this way. Its importance lies in the fact that it is possible to help some of the most severely psychotic people in this fashion to help themselves and rejoin our world effectively, indicating thereby that there is enough plasticity in both personality malformation and whatever neurochemical systems may be involved to change toward more conventional patterns and interactional responses. Psychotherapy may be a clumsy and costly way to effect changes in the neurochemical substrate, or even in the miscarried development of psychosocial structures and behavior patterns, but it demonstrates that no matter what and how severe the pathology may be, living as a member of the human race can be achieved.

In addition to demonstrating the plasticity of all these structures, treating such patients is a crucial learning experience for psychotherapists. The qualities a therapist must bring to and cultivate for this work encompass, among others, tolerance for ambiguity and anxiety, and tenacity in keeping oneself involved even when fatigued or bored. Furthermore, the theistic ambitions which many of us harbor more likely hinder than help the process. Therapists must evolve a mix of empathetic collaboration and curiosity, of cognitive-interpretive activity and guidance, which will be different with each patient. Some, but not all, psychotherapists must learn how to sit with, respond to, and interact beneficially with these psychotic patients, with and without the help of chemicals, because there is much to be learned in this therapeutic process about the nature of being, and, more important, of becoming human.

This experience is important not only for those of us who become therapists primarily, but also for administrators or leaders of psychiatric institutions and services. Without the experience of living, so to speak, with psychotic patients, program directors will likely not address the needs of these patients effectively and compassionately. Furthermore, it is essential knowledge if we are ever going to prevent this crippling condition. I believe we have made progress in this direction, not so much through psychotherapy *per se*, but by having been led through our psychotherapeutic experiences to family studies.[26] It is possible now in a gross, albeit yet incomplete way, to state what the essential ingredients of familial inputs into human development are, and this is one of the most promising leads to pursue for understanding and eventually preventing schizophrenia as a deficiency disease in psychosocial nurturance and enculturation.[20,27-29]

There is the question of how much it costs to treat a schizophrenic person. It is the wrong question, no matter how insistently our third-party payers or medical-cost watchers ask it. How much does it cost *not* to treat a disturbed person optimally? What price human misery—the patient's, his or her family's, not to mention the price society pays, not only in dollars, but also by living with the guilty knowledge of ignoring the professed principle that we are our brother's or sister's keeper? As long as we believe in and strive toward the idea that the individual counts—that the search for well-being and full development is for everybody, we cannot honestly abrogate or forego the best forms of help we know, inadequate as such knowledge may be.

Schizophrenia or mental ill health in general is not the only medical condition in our professional lives where we fall short in providing adequate care and services, and where our knowledge is only partial; but psychosis happens to be our specialty, and it is our duty to advocate optimal treatment for our patients, and optimal education for our colleagues-to-be. Until we discover differently, psychotherapy with schizophrenics not only offers some patients hope for real life, but also constitutes one of the major research opportunities for the study of this condition, and for the study of humanness and of humanness gone awry.

REFERENCES

1. von Medina L: *Die Konvulsions Therapie der Schizophrenie*. Halle, East Germany, Marhold, 1937.
2. Sakhel M: Zur Methodik der Hypoglykaemie. *Behandling von Psychosem. Wien. Ke. Wochochn* **49**:1278–1288, 1936.
3. Bleuler ME: The long-term course of schizophrenic psychoses, in Wynne LC, Cromwell RL, Matthysse S (eds): *The Nature of Schizophrenia*. New York, John Wiley & Sons, 1978, pp 631–636.
4. Jackson DD: Introduction, in Jackson DD (ed): *The Etiology of Schizophrenia*. New York, Basic Books, 1973.
5. Fromm-Reichmann F: Transference problems in schizophrenics. *Psychoanal Quart*, **8**:412–426, 1939.
6. Gunderson JG: The value of psychotherapy of schizophrenia: A Semrad memorial. *McLean Hosp J*, **3**:131–145, 1978.
7. Hill L: *Psychotherapeutic Intervention in Schizophrenia*. Chicago, University of Chicago Press, 1955.
8. Sechahaye M: *Symbolic Realization*. New York, International Universities Press, 1951.

9. Semrad EV, Menzer D, Mann J, et al: A study of the doctor–patient relationship in psychotherapy of psychotic patients. *Psychiatry* **15:**377–384, 1952.
10. Will OA: The conditions of being therapeutic, in Gunderson JG, Mosher LR (eds): *Psychotherapy of Schizophrenia.* New York, Jason Aronson Inc, 1975, pp 53–66.
11. Grinspoon L, Ewalt J, Shader R: *Schizophrenia: Pharmacotherapy and Psychotherapy.* Baltimore, Williams & Wilkins, Co, 1972.
12. May PRA: *Treatment of Schizophrenia: A Comparative Study of Five Treatment Methods.* New York, Science House, 1968.
13. Fleck S: Schizophrenia, in Conn HF (ed): *Current Therapy: 1978.* Philadelphia, WB Saunders Co, 1978, pp 864–868.
14. Freud S: *Die Psychoanalytische Technik.* Gesammelte Werke Vol XVII. London, Imago Publishing Co Ltd, 1941, pp 97–108.
15. Sullivan HS: Peculiarity of thought in schizophrenia. *Amer J Psychiatry* **82:**21–86, 1925–1926.
16. Sullivan HS: The modified psychoanalytic treatment of schizophrenia. *Amer J Psychiatry* **88:**519–540, 1931–1932.
17. Simmel E; The psychoanalytic sanitorium and the psychoanalytic movement. *Bull Menninger Clin* **1:**133–143, 1937.
18. Engel GL: *Psychological Development in Health and Disease.* Philadelphia, WB Saunders Co, 1962.
19. Burnham D, Gladstone AI, Gibson RW: *Schizophrenia and the Need–Fear Dilemma.* New York, International Universities Press, 1967.
20. Lidz T: *The Origin and Treatment of Schizophrenia Disorders.* New York, Basic Books, 1973.
21. Wynne LC: Communication disorders and the quest for relatedness in families of schizophrenics, in Sager CJ, Kaplan HS (eds): *Progress in Group and Family Therapy.* New York, Bruner/Mazel, 1972, pp 595–615.
22. Lidz RW, Lidz T: The family environment of schizophrenic patients. *Amer J Psychiatry* **106:**332–345, 1949.
23. Bleuler M: *Schizophrenic Disorders: Long-Term Patient and Family Studies.* New Haven, Yale University Press, 1978.
24. Green H: *I Never Promised You a Rose Garden.* New York, Holt Rinehart & Winston, 1964.
25. Brown GW, Birley JLT, Wing JK: Influence of family life on the course of schizophrenic disorders: A replication. *Br J Psychiatry*, **121:**241–258, 1972.
26. Lidz T, Fleck S, Cornelison AR: *Schizophrenia and the Family.* New York, International Universities Press, 1965.
27. Alanen YO: The family in the pathogenesis of schizophrenic and neurotic disorders. *Acta Psychiatr Neurol Sand*, Suppl 189, Vol 24, 1966.
28. Fleck S: The family and psychiatry, in Freedman A, Kaplan H, Sadock B (eds): *Comprehensive Textbook of Psychiatry*, ed 2. Baltimore, Williams & Wilkins, 1975, pp 382–397.
29. Lewis J, Beavers WR, et al: *No Single Thread.* New York, Bruner/Mazel, 1976.

Chapter 5

Discussion: Rationale for the Psychotherapy of Schizophrenia

EUGENE B. BRODY, M.D.

The authors of these four papers are clearly sensitive to close encounters with schizophrenic patients, and, despite the announced theme of the session, this may be one reason why none of them focused exclusively on the rationale for psychotherapy with schizophrenics. I think that most of us who have been in the field believe that the personally involving nature of the therapeutic experience really precludes any need to justify it. The possibility of intensive interaction constitutes its own rationale, because it contains an element of hope; with the prevalence and the devastating character of the disorder, no further justification is required.

The papers suggest that our conclusions about psychotherapy with schizophrenics, and our reasons for believing that it is worthwhile, are based on two kinds of knowledge, or, following President Giamatti's introduction, two kinds of evidence, clinical and scientific. There is a fuzzy line between these two, and I am not imputing particular value to either category. Fleck and Bruch deal mainly with clinical knowlege, gained through the dyadic therapeutic intervention. Helm Stierlin's ideas are also based importantly

EUGENE B. BRODY • Department of Psychiatry, Institute of Psychiatry and Human Behavior, University of Maryland School of Medicine, Baltimore, Maryland 21201.

on clinical knowledge, but that gained through multiple transactions with family members. These three authors have all subscribed to a particular value which has informed their research and therapy, that is, the value of total, unreserved personal commitment to the work over a very long period of time with a single patient.

Liberman's contribution, on the other hand, deals mainly with data obtained through systematic observation following the experimental model. He would rank highest in this morning's papers on some scale of objectivity, positivism, or empiricism. He also referred most directly to the rationale for psychotherapy with schizophrenics in terms of the limited effectiveness of available drug treatments, and the tremendous and demoralizing incidence of recidivism. I was very glad to hear him refer to the revolving door, which has become one of the banes of our current psychiatric civilization.

Drugs may be part of the answer, but, as Liberman points out, they don't constitute its entirety. He differentiates a series of psychosocial approaches, all of which might be understood as education for information processing, and all of which involve relationships with therapists selected on the basis of their personal attributes. So there is a clear linkage between his message and that of the other speakers.

The psychosocial approaches include individual psychotherapy, family therapy, psychotherapy as an adjunct of drug treatment especially to ensure compliance (a horrible word in some respects), and training to improve the patient's adaptive and coping capacities and community survival skills. As Liberman notes, even variations in drug response seem related to the non-specific factor of social competence. The psychosocial treatment methods which he describes are valuable in several ways: preventing initial or later episodes, which implies reducing vulnerability; reducing the frequency and length of episodes, which implies increasing the frequency and speed of remissions; and preventing or reducing the likelihood of relapse. Here work with the familial context is especially important.

Liberman's is a reasoned and significant paper, especially important for its heuristic value. His problem-solving approach provides a framework in which the other contributions, concerned with more specific psy-choanalytically informed psychotherapy, can be understood. But, more than that, he may very well be sorting out deficits and training processes which get to the heart of the perceptual and cognitive disorders of schizophrenia. Maybe, at long last, we are approaching that period to which Otto Will referred some time ago; perhaps, after all, we are developing a cookbook which will allow us to train larger numbers of therapists, who in turn will be able to deal with larger numbers of patients.

Hilde Bruch, too, noted the limited impact of drugs, as well as their usefulness as adjuncts. She differentiates psychotherapy dealing with the person from what she calls education in realistic living, comparable to

Liberman's detailed training. Training and education, again, often deal with general adaptive or coping skills, rather than with something specific to schizophrenia, although that differentiation may be less clear than it once was.

Beyond all this, however, Bruch, from her own vast experience, gives us a very lively sense of the evolution of the psychotherapeutic approach. The slow accumulation which allowed successive generations of therapists to view their patients with increasing optimism was an important social phenomenon. Looking back to earlier periods, she says, "Work with such patients required what appears to us now as superhuman patience." The positive heritage from this period is the confidence that even a hostile and mute patient can again be brought into rapport, and that confidence of course may in itself be an important therapeutic factor.

I take the confidence to be a sufficient rationale for continuing psychotherapeutic work, but she is more specific. She refers to psychotherapy as the only way to "correct underlying symbolic deficits, inadequate life experiences, and unrealistic expectations from the therapeutic relationship." That relationship is understood as a model of other relationships, and learning how to become attached to others is crucial to her concept of psychotherapy for schizophrenics. Psychotherapy seems, to her, rational on the basis of the schizophrenic person's deficits in acquiring the capacity to relate, to discriminate, and to use symbols during development.

Finally, Bruch refers to the person of the therapist, a reflective, self-aware being who requires engagement with others. This work, she says, provides great satisfaction in terms of our own human values and the feeling of personal growth. I would be very much interested in knowing how Liberman's selective criteria for his therapists fit with those that might be arrived at by Hilde Bruch, Stephen Fleck, or Helm Stierlin.

Stephen Fleck begins with an important scientific point. He warns us that the fact of earlier pathogenic family environments and developmental experience does not justify an exclusively psychotherapeutic approach to the here-and-now schizophrenic patient; that is, a psychosocial etiology neither requires a psychosocial treatment, nor does it preclude a biochemical one. What is overridingly important, Fleck says, is that chemical measures affect certain symptoms and behaviors, often those that could prohibit even sitting with the patient for any length of time, but that with or without medication, schizophrenics can also be treated psychologically, and all of them, especially the young ones, require psychosocial treatments, psychosocial guidance, and rehabilitation or habilitation.

But, having made this bow to objectivity, Fleck goes on to express his own very important commitment to the total investment of oneself on behalf of the schizophrenic person. His ultimate rationale for psychotherapy with schizophrenics is pragmatic, and clearly in accord with the value attached to being human, rather than to social survival, or community adjustment as such. I think we all resonate very positively to that.

Fleck says it is possible to help some of the most severely psychotic people in this fashion to help themselves and rejoin our world effectively, indicating thereby that there is enough plasticity to change and return to living as a member of the human race is possible. After this, Steve, like the good professor he is, again became more detached. He noted first that doing psychotherapy with schizophrenics is a crucial learning experience for all therapists, and also for psychiatric administrators and leaders, with which I agree. Second, it represents a major research opportunity for the study of what is essentially and uniquely human, a point of view espoused by Ted Lidz over many years.

Finally, Helm Stierlin's rationale for therapy was never explicitly declared, but was constant, inherent, and forceful. In his own statement of therapeutic commitment, Stierlin, following Lidz's work, emphasizes the family. If schizophrenia is rooted in family distortions of what he calls rational reality, an interesting concept which I would like more fully explicated, it is only "through such a dialogue that a mutually accepted relational reality can be negotiated, consensual validation reached, rights and obligations ascertained, accounts settled, and eventual reconciliation achieved. Healing through dialogue connotes integration, reunion, and salvation."

Clearly no further justification is needed. Those psychosocial approaches to which our other speakers have referred as training or education will only be helpful in Stierlin's view in so far as they subserve such a dialogue.

These four papers have spoken for themselves, and very eloquently. And, of course, and not uniquely, they speak to me. My central concern is the search for meaning in human behavior, and more specifically in human beings. I expect to find clues to meaning in neurochemical structures and processes, and in observed reductionistically arrived-at behaviors. I *expect* to find it there, but so far I have only *experienced* it in relations with and communications with others. In clinical work, therefore, I take the object of knowledge (and this is true for Liberman's work as well as that of the others) to be not the patient or the family, but rather the unit, patient–therapist or family–therapist.

I would like to close by reminding you again that it is possible to regard this symposium as dealing with two kinds of evidence, scientific and clinical. Medical knowledge depends, following Wartofsky, on the activity of intervention in a world reconstructed or transformed in reality by medical practice. What this means is that medical or psychotherapeutic knowledge is knowledge for the sake of some good. It is value bound with immediate consequences for human life. It is not grounded in theory and observation. It is grounded, rather, in theory, practice, and intervention by the clinician. And there is a difference, as Stephen Toulmin has pointed out, between the detached descriptive understanding of an individual's biographer, and the committed prescriptive understanding of his personal advisor. The generality characteristic of biomedical science has to achieve an effective union with the particularity of clinical treatment, and most particularly with the individuality of the relationship between the patient and his personal physician. This last I think represents a central effort of each of this morning's speakers, that is, to achieve an effective union between, on the one hand, the generality of science, and, on the other, the particularity of the clinical relationships with troubled human beings who have responded therapeutically to specifically modulated human intervention.

I believe, also, that our impressions justify the expansion of psychotherapeutic research in this area with the same systematic and careful effort which we devote to biochemical or physical research, and that without the former we will not be able to understand the latter.

Finally, I would like to repeat a theme alluded to in Liberman's reference to the new nihilism. We are without question in an era of exciting new genetic and neurochemical knowledge, much of it, although I am not sure just how much, relevant to schizophrenia. But these advances carry their own hazards for patients and their families. Patients who do not respond to drugs tend to be shunted aside, and many who, ten or fifteen years ago, would have had the opportunity for psychotherapy, no longer have that chance. Beyond that, in many places there are whole new generations of psychiatrists growing up without the knowledge or attitudes gained by the intensive, intimate therapeutic work with these patients. And until that day when we have a definitive, nonpsychological therapy for this disorder—and I personally consider that as likely as being able to teach someone a new language with an injection—we cannot afford to neglect this field of research, education, and therapy.

Chapter 6

General Discussion

QUESTIONS FROM AUDIENCE

QUESTION TO PANEL: To what extent is psychotherapy with schizophrenic patients dependent upon adequate knowledge regarding etiology? Will future etiologic information necessarily change our therapeutic strategies?

DR. BRUCH: I think theoretical knowledge needs to be based on evidence, on factual data, and on assumptions; psychotherapy depends very much on assumptions. If you hold the assumption that schizophrenia is an unchangeable, organic illness, then psychotherapy will not be useful, and will be very ineffective.

DR. STIERLIN: I think our therapeutic efforts with these patients have much to do with our notions as to what causes this condition. If we have the notion that at its basis there is a defect in neurotransmitter mechanisms, then the family does not play a major role. In fact, recently a national magazine quoted one investigator as saying he would be surprised if the family has anything to do with schizophrenia. When you go from the assumption that schizophrenia is a problem in living and education reflecting inappropriate coping mechanisms, learned in the formative periods of life, then it makes sense to try the various techniques which Bob Liberman has detailed here. When you have the basic assumption that the main problem, at least during certain phases, is that the schizophrenic is deadlocked in a terrible stalemate which has gone on for many years, sometimes decades, and that he and his symptoms are needed for the survival of the whole family system, then your primary approach is to break up the system. Anybody who has worked with such systems knows how difficult that is.

I am not as optimistic as Dr. Brody about the possibility of reconciliation—even though it is a favorite word of mine—of these various approaches. But I think we can come closer to such reconciliation when we have notions of stages and phases. Thus, the first task might perhaps consist in breaking up what I have called the "malign clinch." Maybe the schizophrenic patient can manage on his own after this clinch is broken. Or he may reveal the defects and lacks in social skills which involve him in negative cycles. He may then need help with these along the lines Dr. Liberman suggested. What we need is really a complex, multiphasic, multisystems concept of schizophrenia.

DR. FLECK: Well, I'm optimistic about Dr. Brody's punch line living on. The problem is whether you think of schizophrenia as a thing, or whether you think of schizophrenics as persons to be treated. Now, that problem isn't peculiar to schizophrenia. It pertains to pneumonia, and to hyperthyroidism, and any other condition. It was Osler who said, about a century ago, and I think I have the quote verbatim, "It is more important to know what kind of a patient has the illness than what kind of an illness the patient has." As long as we take cognizance that people are ill, and that the schizophrenic person has these particular deficits and difficulties in living and thinking, and interacting and living with him or herself, we can and ought to respond to that, no matter where it comes from.

QUESTION FOR DR. STIERLIN: Could you comment on the well siblings in schizophrenic families? Are they less loyal or do they have a different, healthier means of expressing their loyalty, and are developmental or legacy issues more significant in the well siblings?

DR. STIERLIN: I would like to refer here to the study of Ted Lidz and his group on siblings.* They found that these so-called well siblings are often very restricted. They save themselves psychologically by staying out of that drama of conflict, engulfment, guilt, and self-punishment, into which the schizophrenic member gets drawn. It's my repeated experience that, when we see this drama played, it's the schizophrenic patient who strikes us as the healthiest one, in the sense that, even though he gets engulfed and involved in this drama, he struggles with it. In fact, he takes it upon himself to reveal and act out aspects of the conflict which the parents and the well siblings cannot reveal or act out. Thus, we can say that he is more loyal, more in tune with deep and conflictual legacies, than the "well" sibling. However, this is a generalization. I have also found so-called well siblings who have been very resourceful, very committed to helping the family. This means for the therapist that he must try to find and tap the resources of *all* members. By this I mean, for example, these members' ability and willingness to involve themselves with the others, to make sacrifices, to test out reality, etc. But the strange thing is the therapist most often finds such resources in the so-called schizophrenic patient. That at least is my experience.

QUESTION FOR DR. LIBERMAN: Since the cognitive and perceptual deficits of many schizophrenics reflect a preverbal quality of thinking, how do you facilitate the patient's ability to use a cognitive secondary process, such as insight, to accomplish meaningful change in affective experience?

DR. LIBERMAN: There is great difficulty in training cognitive problem solving and social competence with a person who is *totally* immersed in primary process. However, behavioral methods for teaching people to improve their attentional processes, even in the midst of a flagrant psychotic decompensation, have been developed; but progress in this type of intervention is tedious and slow. We have found, with subacutely psychotic individuals who still have primary process symptoms, such as delusions and hallucinations, that if we can focus their attention sufficiently to follow the steps in our training

* T. Lidz et al, Schizophrenic patients and their siblings. *Psychiatry*, **26**:1–18, 1963.

procedure, the training has a salutary effect on their cognitive organization, as measured in a variety of ways. They are better able to use their abstracting skills, and they show a reduction in their psychopathology. Thus, the very process of our structured approach to training seems to help still symptomatic schizophrenics "internalize" the step-by-step, problem-solving training procedure.

QUESTION FOR DR. BRUCH: Are there differences in family patterns and parent–child interaction which differentiate eating disorders from schizophrenia?

DR. BRUCH: Some of the patients with eating disorders become schizophrenic, but on the whole the families with eating disorders are more structured, less chaotic, than those of schizophrenics. In both conditions, the parents have trouble helping their children develop clear-cut concepts about their bodily existence. Usually in families that produce a fat child or adolescent, the disharmony is more in the open. The anorexic family has a surface harmony; their more subtle problems usually are not expressed in overt fighting. The schizophrenic family impresses me as more seriously disturbed, and with a wider variety of disturbances.

QUESTION FOR PANEL: What seems to be different in treating schizophrenics in contrast to nonschizophrenics?

DR. LIBERMAN: Some of the general dimensions are probably the same in working with all kinds of patients. But getting back to that first question, about how etiological knowledge will shape our future treatment efforts, we hope that the more we find out about interactions between deficits in the individual and stressors in the environment, and how they lead to relapse or remission in schizophrenia, the more specifically we can tailor our therapy programs. For example, when we find out that there are certain types of critical life situations that, given the vulnerability of schizophrenics, lead to a flareup of symptoms or relapse, then we can design therapy procedures that may help schizophrenics to cope better with that kind of situation. The "expressed emotion" studies are interesting in this respect, because they have found that depressed people also relapse much more quickly if they return to families who express high levels of criticism, and overinvolvement. Thus, in some respects, what we're finding out about schizophrenia also holds for other categories of illness. Hopefully, in the future we will have sufficient knowledge about relationships between behavioral deficits and environmental stressors to design programs that will be of specific benefit for schizophrenics; however, I doubt that psychosocial treatments will be ever applicable only to schizophrenics.

DR. BRUCH: I think the difference is one of degree, and depends on the quality of—what shall I call it?—tools of orientation and perception. Probably nobody is one hundred percent perfect in his style of thinking, or always correct and realistic. In a neurotic or nonschizophrenic, you can count on a broader capacity for accurate perceptual and conceptual interpretation of the world. In the schizophrenic, and even in some of the eating disorders, this accuracy occurs only in a narrow range. The main task, certainly the initial task, in treatment is to help a patient develop more reliable tools of orientation and responding.

DR. STIERLIN: This touches again on our notions of etiology. Here we must consider what happens in the family *and* in the person. At the moment, we know less about what happens inside the person than what happens in the family. In families that eventually have or produce—however you want to put it—schizophrenics, certain abnormalities or deviances accumulate. Missions becomes "impossible," legacies clash with each other, while the relational and cognitive tools needed to have confrontations and achieve true reconciliation are lacking. Multiple systems functions are involved. Applying a general systems kind of viewpoint, as with a grid, one could see how many more things have been wrong and gone wrong in 'schizo-present' families than, say, in families with an obese patient, or even an anorexic who is not psychotic. It is possible that with so-and-so many points of abnormality, a certain general kind of serious condition is generated. This need not necessarily be schizophrenia, but at least psychosis, for example. With fewer points, perhaps, the person may be more likely to have a neurotic development. It may also depend on the developmental stage at which the family dysfunction and/or deficiency occurred. This is where the data are pointing. As Hilde already said—nobody escapes from the family unscathed. We all have scars. Some of the things that go on in schizophrenic families go on also in normal families. It's the accumulation of family dysfunction that matters. Our treatment approaches have to take into account these dysfunctions.

DR. BRODY: The question of what treatment for what disorder can be responded to in a variety of ways. It may deal with overall claims which are unexceptionable, such as becoming human, rather than with strategies and tactics. This aim is less central for a neurotic or character-disordered patient. For example, if I work psychotherapeutically with a schizophrenic patient who presents initially with a problem of relating to other people, I may cope with his silences by speaking at some length about myself, often in terms of the generalities of my fantasy life or my background which are similar to those of the patient. And that's very easy, because, as Sullivan and Otto Will and many others have pointed out, we are all much more similar than we are different. What I do in this manner is make of myself, using the Freudian language, a narcissistic object, a person who is available to the patient to relate to. As he becomes capable of relating to me, he may in time generalize, and become able to learn how to relate to other people.

Part II

Research

Chapter 7

Family Therapy during the Aftercare Treatment of Acute Schizophrenia

MICHAEL J. GOLDSTEIN

BACKGROUND

With the last few years, the thrust of the community mental health center movement at the national and local levels has generated a treatment model for acute schizophrenia composed of two phases—a brief inpatient phase, measured in days, followed by an extended period of aftercare in the community. In the old system, relatively complete remission of schizophrenic symptoms was the goal, whereas minimal remission of only the most acute and disorganizing symptoms is the goal of inpatient treatment in the new system. The balance of the recovery process, it is believed, can be more effectively achieved once the patient has been returned to community life.

Although this new model emphasized aftercare in the community, it was far from certain what this meant, particularly for the acute, young, first-admission schizophrenic. A number of key questions still remain to be answered concerning effective modes of treatment in community settings. First, what role should antipsychotic drugs play in the aftercare program?

MICHAEL J. GOLDSTEIN • Department of Psychology, University of California, at Los Angeles, Los Angeles, California 90024.

We know well the impact and significance of these drugs during extended inpatient treatment of schizophrenics.[1] But, given our knowledge of the difficulties involved in continued acceptance by patients of these drugs following discharge, how can they be utilized in community-based treatment of acute schizophrenics, and for how long?

Second, many patients released from community mental health centers still manifest residual symptoms and adjustment difficulties. What models of social therapies are appropriate to deal with the reintegration of such patients into the community, and perhaps prevent future psychotic breakdowns? The issue of psychotherapeutic approaches to schizophrenia has moved to a new arena, and deals with a different stage of the illness. No longer do we ask whether psychotherapy is effective in aiding the patient to reconstitute from psychotic confusion. Now we ask whether, once some partial restitution has been effected, social therapies can play a significant role in the treatment of schizophrenia.[2,3] Can the interacting roles of drugs and social therapies be utilized to maximize the effects of each? The research project described in this paper represents an attempt to attend to these issues.

METHOD

Design of Study

The study conducted with my colleagues, Eliot Rodnick and Phillip May, was carried out at the Ventura (Calif.) Mental Health Center. In this center, schizophrenic patients are released to the community after an average of 14 days' hospitalization. A previous study,[4] on a sample of all consecutive schizophrenic admissions over an 18-month period in that center, found that 45% were readmitted for substantial periods within six months of discharge. Further, the majority of readmissions (31%) occurred within three to four weeks. Two other facts were noted: first, patients simply did not take the oral dose of phenothiazines prescribed on discharge; second, they rarely used the outpatient supportive social therapy that was provided. Therefore, we developed an experimental design that focused on the first six weeks after discharge (a critical period, according to the above data), and then studied the relative significance of depot phenothiazine treatment and crisis-oriented family therapy carried out during that critical period. This study involved almost all first-admission schizophrenics in a county of half a million people. The 2×2 factorial design of the study had two levels of maintenance phenothiazine (high and low dose), and two social therapy conditions (present or absent).

Selection of Patients

All consecutive first and second inpatient admissions to the Ventura Mental Health Center were screened for the presence of schizophrenic symptoms. Independently interviewed by the project psychiatrist and psychologist, each patient was rated on a 5-point scale on the probability that he was schizophrenic.[5] Each patient who passed this initial screening was studied for another two to three days, and then rated on the New Haven Schizophrenia Index.[6] Those who received a score of 4 or higher (a cutting score found by Astrachan et al.[6] to correlate highly with a clinical diagnosis of schizophrenia) were entered into the study. Of the 104 patients selected for the study, 69% were first life-time admissions, and the balance recent second admissions (during the same calendar year). They were young (mean age 23.36 years; SD, 4.21), and predominantly white (79%), with 14% of Hispanic origin, and 7% black. Forty percent had not graduated from high school, 35% were high school graduates, and 25% had some college. Sixty-two percent were single, 15% previously married, and 23% currently married. They were hospitalized only briefly (mean 14.24 days; SD, 5.97) before discharge to the aftercare program.

After a patient was selected, he or she and a relative were interviewed separately, and informed of the nature of the study. Both the patient's and the relative's consent were required for the patient to participate. The patient was informed that he or she could withdraw from the study at any time.

The Phenothiazine Drug Condition

It was decided to compare a relatively high therapeutic dose level of phenothiazine with a therapeutically marginal or lower dose level of the same drug. The original intent was to use orally administered phenothiazines, but this was not feasible because of a low rate of compliance. Accordingly, we shifted to a longer acting injectable phenothiazine, fluphenazine (Prolixin) enanthate, which solved the problem of medication delivery successfully.

Fluphenazine therapy was started within a day after the patients had been admitted to the center. A test dose of 0.25 ml was given; if no sensitivity was noted, the patient was then assigned by a random method to one of two conditions: high or low dose. Originally we had intended that the high dose should be 1.5 ml, and the low dose 0.5 ml, but pilot data suggested that the side effects of the higher dose were too severe; dosages were therefore reduced in the actual experiment to 1 ml for the high-dose condition, and 0.25 ml for the low-dose condition, and were kept fixed throughout the study. (Although we use the term "high dose" for the 1-ml condition, it is clear that, in contrast to other studies using this same drug with acute schizophrenic patients,[7] a more appropriate term would be "moderate dose.") Prophylactic antiparkinsonian medication was provided routinely: benztropine mesylate, 2 mg intramuscularly with each injection of fluphenazine; and trihexyphenidyl, 5 mg/day orally during both the inpatient and aftercare phases of the study. The study period was typically one to two weeks as an inpatient, and a six-week after care period as an out-patient. During the inpatient period, if the treating psychiatrist thought that more medication was needed, he was permitted to administer phenothiazine orally. During the aftercare period, three injections were administered at 14-day intervals, the first on the day of discharge. The study was single blind, as the patient was blind to dose level, but the treating psychiatrist was not. However, all ratings of clinical behavior were carried out by raters blind to drug and family therapy status.

Crisis-Oriented Family Therapy

The social therapy used was family oriented. Here, our original desires or goals were modified by experience. It was our hope, based on other work, that we could move into some kind of relationally oriented family therapy. However, it became obvious that this was not feasible for such disorganized patients. Instead, a crisis-oriented six-session family therapy was devised, directed at the following sequence of objectives: (1) the patient and his family are able to accept the fact that he has had a psychosis; (2) they are willing to identify some of the probable precipitating stresses in his life at the time the psychosis occurred; (3) they attempt to generalize from that to identification of future stresses to which the patient and his family are likely to be vulnerable; and (4) they attempt to do some planning on how to minimize or avoid these future stresses. We find that this concrete form of family therapy can be meaningfully carried out with schizophrenics and their families during this phase of treatment. The primary goal in this therapy is to help the patient and significant others use the events of the psychosis, rather than sealing it over and deflecting attention away from the psychotic episode.

RESULTS

Deliverability and Compliance

Of the 104 patients who agreed to participate in the program, eight withdrew after release from the hospital. Three of these left the area immediately; five remained in the area, but rejected compliance with their assigned treatment program. Thus, 92% participated in the aftercare program. The treatment refusers came from three groups: high-dose therapy (two), low-dose therapy (three), and low-dose no-therapy (three).

Figure 1 presents the rate of relapse within each treatment condition at the end of the six-week controlled trial and at the time of the six-month follow-up contact. During the six-week controlled treatment period, ten patients deteriorated clinically, such that either they had to be rehospitalized, or their medication had to be altered substantially—a relapse rate for treatment accepters of 10.4%. This is substantially less than the 31% rate for the comparable six-week postdischarge period found for a very similar consecutive admission cohort at this same facility.[7] Relapses were ordinarily not the decision of the research team, as they usually involved action by the center's emergency psychiatric team, carried out independently of the project team. In cases where the decision to hospitalize was made by the research staff, a consensus of staff—both blind and nonblind to treatment status—was necessary.

Although this is a small number of relapses to search for differential trends across treatment conditions or patients' attributes, some suggestive findings do appear. These data indicate that there are two extreme groups in the sample, the high-dose therapy group, with not a single relapse, and the low-dose no-therapy group, with 24% relapse. The other two conditions fell between these two, and do not differ significantly. Only the extreme groups differ at a statistically significant level. The trends in the marginal totals for dose level and therapy effects, though suggestive, are not statistically signifi-

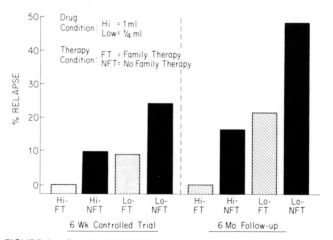

FIGURE 1. Relapse rate within each treatment condition at the end of the six-week controlled trial and at the time of the six-month follow-up contact.

cant for either factor. Thus, despite the small number of relapsing patients, they are concentrated largely in the group with minimal medication and an absence of family-oriented intervention.

The number of breakdowns following the completion of the controlled period parallels the pattern for the first six weeks. There was not a single relapse in the high-dose therapy group, whereas by the six-month point nearly 50% of the low-dose no-therapy group had had some sort of clinical regression. The other two conditions had more breakdowns than the high-dose therapy group, but less than the low-dose no-therapy group. Thus, even though the high-dose therapy patients were no longer receiving therapy, and were no longer rigorously assigned to a maintenance medication condition, they continued to remain outside of a hospital for a six-month period.

If we add together the relapses during the controlled period with those that followed into an overall cumulative six-month relapse figure, a significant drug effect ($p < .01$) and a near significant therapy effect ($p < .10$) are found.

Symptomatic Status at End of Aftercare Period

Patients were rated four times (at admission, at discharge, at six weeks, and at six-month follow-up), using the Brief Psychiatric Rating Scale (BPRS).[8] The rater was a research psychologist who remained blind to drug and therapy status throughout the six-month period. Factor analysis of admission BPRS ratings was carried out to reduce the 16 scales to a smaller set of dimensions. Fourteen of the scales loaded on four factors, *anxious-depression*, *hostility*, *emotional withdrawal*, and *schizophrenic thought*. Data were anlyzed in two ways, with relapsed patients deleted (all completers), and with last contact ratings used to include all starters in the sample.

Family Therapy Effects

The strongest effects are noted when the endpoint ratings for the relapsers are included in the analysis. Significant effects were found for the family therapy variable on: total BPRS score ($p < .01$); *withdrawal* ($p < .02$); and *anxious depression* ($p < .05$), for all patients who began the therapy (all starters). In all instances, there was evidence of less residual psychopathology in the samples that received family therapy.

The magnitude of the therapy effect on *withdrawal* is as significant for all completers as for all starters. Therefore, the impact of the family therapy on *withdrawal* applies to all cases in the sample. The mean scores on the *withdrawal* factor are presented separately below for all starters and all completers:

All Starters ($p < .02$)		All Completers ($p < .03$)	
Therapy	No Therapy	Therapy	No Therapy
2.41	3.65	2.39	3.72

If we examine, for the completers, the individual BPRS scales constituting the *withdrawal* factor, one stands out particularly, *blunted affect* ($p < .005$), in which the therapy cases manifested significantly less flattening of affect at six weeks than the no-therapy cases.

Analyses of BPRS data at the time of six-months follow-up was only significant for the *withdrawal* factor, but only in the group that originally received the high phenothiazine dose. As before, family therapy cases on high dose showed less residual psychopathology than comparable no-therapy cases ($p < .05$). However, the therapy advantage, previously observed with low-dose patients, was no longer observable at six-month follow-up. Note that the sustained effect on the high-dose group persisted long after those patients were systematically receiving the drug. It suggests a prophylactic effect of the adequate dose upon the retention of family therapy effects over the more extended time period.

Further Analyses of the Family Therapy Process

Up to this point, we have been treating the psychotherapeutic intervention as a homogenous process applied equally to all patients. However, we recognize that there is considerable variation in styles of therapy and the ability of patients and therapists to utilize each other's resources.

An analogy may be drawn with a similar issue in pharmaco-therapy, when patients are assigned medication but often fail to comply. Thus, it has been necessary for researchers to devise methods to assure delivery, or at the very least monitor compliance. We felt that a comparable index of the deliverability of a psychotherapeutic intervention would permit a more accurate appraisal of its effects, as well as greater insight into the process of change.

Previously we indicated that the crisis-oriented therapy had relatively specific objectives. Four specific sequential objectives were designated:

1. Acceptance by patient and family that he has had a psychotic episode, and achieving consensus concerning the important precipitating stresses at the time the psychosis occurred.

2. Development of strategies to prevent the occurrence of identified stresses and for coping when stress occurs.

3. Evaluation of progress in implementation of prevention and coping strategies.

4. Anticipatory planning to prevent future stresses and to cope with those which arise.

In this study, therapists rated the extent to which the patient and participating family members achieved each of the four objectives.

A graduate student, Charles King, and myself[9] hypothesized that the greater the number of therapy objectives attained, the greater the sustained benefit by patient and significant others.

Measures

Achievement of Objectives in Therapy. At the completion of therapy, therapists rated each patient on a 5-point scale of the extent to which he was successful in achieving each of the four therapy objectives. The scale included descriptions of typical patient achievements for each point on the scale for each objective. For the purposes of analysis, the four objectives were treated as a Guttman Scale, with the assumption that achievement of a given objective implied achievement of all of the lower objectives. A patient was considered to have achieved an objective if he was rated 3 (moderately successful) or above. The highest objective achieved by each patient became his single score for the achievement of objectives in therapy. These scores range from 0 to 4, distributed as follows: 0, 20.5%; 1, 20.5%; 2, 9%; 3, 9%; 4, 41%. For some analyses, subjects were categorized as "achievers" or "nonachievers" of therapy objectives, employing a median split on highest objective achieved. Thus, subjects who achieved objectives 3 or 4 were classified as "achievers"; those who achieved no higher than objective 2 are referred to as "nonachievers".

Achievers and nonachievers did not differ significantly on the demographic variables of age, marital status, race, education, or father's education. In addition, there was no significant difference between achiever groups in the number of family members participating in therapy sessions.

Ratings of Achievement of Therapy Objectives as a Dependent Variable. First, we examined whether factors observed prior to the initiation of the aftercare family therapy could predict therapists' perceptions of the level of objectives achieved. The variables used were the individual difference measures of sex, premorbid status, paranoid status, Global Assessment Scale, GAS[10] level ratings at admission, and BPRS factor scores at admission and discharge. For the quantitative variables, a median split was used to subdivide groups. In addition, we examined whether assigned drug level (high versus low) was associated with greater success in delivering the therapy model.

None of the individual difference variables or drug levels were found related to therapist ratings of patients' achievement of objectives in therapy.

Next, interactions between individual difference variables and drug level were examined to determine whether the combination of certain patient attributes and assigned drug level could predict the therapists' perceived success in attaining the four levels of therapy objectives.

Hostility and *suspiciousness* are important barriers to the development of therapeutic trust. Therefore, we examined the relationships among ratings on the BPRS factor *hostility*, rated at discharge (the period immediately before the initiation of family therapy), drug level, and the level of therapy objectives attained. For this analysis, patients were classified as high or low on *hostility*, based on a median split. The interaction between drug level and *hostility* at discharge, depicted in Figure 2, was highly significant, $F(1,36) = 9.25, p < .005$. This figure indicates that when a patient showed considerable *hostility*, *suspiciousness*, and *uncooperativeness* at discharge, therapists indicated that they could achieve the majority of their therapy objectives only when the patient was on the *high* dose. However, an inverse effect was noted for patients below the median on BPRS *hostility* at discharge. Attainment of therapy objectives was more likely for patients assigned to the low-dose condition. No other BPRS factor score interacted with drug level in predicting level of therapy objective attained.

Ratings of Achievement of Objectives as a Predictor Variable. After examining some of the variables which affect ratings of patients' achievement of objectives in therapy, we next determined whether the variance in these ratings related to clinical status at six-week and at the six-month follow-up period. For these analyses, patients were divided on the basis of a median split on the Guttman scaling of the ratings of achievement of objectives. Patients below the median achieve no higher than objective 2, and are referred to as "nonachievers." Patients above the median achieved objective 3 or 4, and are referred to as "achievers."

A repeated measure ANOVA using GAS[10] ratings at admission, six weeks, and six months indicates a large improvement for both groups

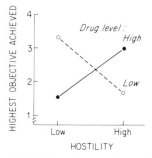

FIGURE 2. Mean ratings of highest objective achieved in therapy. The interaction of drug level and BPRS factor *hostility* rated at time of discharge from inpatient treatment, is illustrated.

$F(1,36)$ for linear trend = 201.5, $p < .005$. However, a significant difference in the slope of the GAS scores was found for achievers and nonachievers of therapy objectives $F(2,42) = 5.10$, $p < .01$. As Figure 3 indicates, patients who were rated as achieving therapy objectives showed greater improvement than patients who did not achieve objectives. GAS scores were also analyzed separately for each period. There were no significant differences between these groups at admission or at the end of the six weeks but patients who achieved therapy objectives were rated significantly higher at six-months follow-up, $F(1,36) = 4.65$, $p < .04$. It appears that the two groups were similar at admission and at the end of treatment. Between the end of the controlled period treatment and the six-month follow-up, patients who were rated as having achieved therapy objectives continued to improve markedly on independent ratings of functioning, whereas patients who did not achieve higher therapy objectives improved little during this period.

Analyses of the BPRS factor ratings at six weeks and six months were conducted in order to identify the specific symptom clusters which contributed to the greater improvement of patients rated as having achieved therapy objectives. Of the four factors, only *thought disorder* revealed clear differences between achievers and nonachievers. There was no difference between these groups at six weeks, but achievers displayed significantly less thought disorder at six months, $F(1,36) = 8.13$, $p < .01$. Figure 4 indicates that patients who were rated as achieving therapy objectives continued to

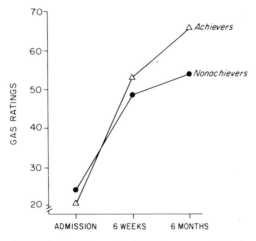

FIGURE 3. Mean Global Assessment Scale (GAS) Ratings. Ratings were made at admission, six weeks, and six months for achievers and nonachievers of therapy objectives.

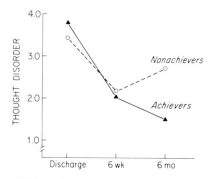

FIGURE 4. Mean *thought disorder*   007
factor scores. The Brief Psychiatric Rating Scale was administered at discharge, six weeks, and six months, for
achievers and nonachievers of therapy
objectives.

show decreases in thought disorder whereas patients who did not achieve therapy objectives displayed a tendency for thought disorder to return to prior levels.

Behavioral Correlates of Therapist Ratings of Objectives. The previous analyses indicated that therapist's perceptions of the degree to which they could deliver the objectives of the crisis-model significantly predicted the longer term course of the patient's disorder, particularly on key symptoms of the schizophrenic process. But, what were therapists reacting to in their ongoing contacts? Evidently, it was something other than classic symptoms of psychopathology. In an effort to get a clearer idea of therapeutic behavior that differentiated achievers from nonachievers, Dennis Schorr, currently a graduate student in psychology at Yale, coded the audiotapes of the therapy sessions. He coded them blind as to therapist rating of objectives.

Schorr's coding system drew from many sources, but most interestingly from the work of Vaughn and Leff[11] on a concept they termed *expressed emotion* (EE), which has been reported to predict relapse in schizophrenics. EE refers to familial attitudes of criticism, hostility, and overinvolvement specifically directed at the identified patient. Schizophrenics returned to high-EE homes have been found to have very high rates of relapse. Schorr developed codes to mirror the EE components of hostility, criticism, and overinvolvement as they might be expressed in actual family interaction in the therapy tapes. Using tapes from the latter part of the six-session crisis-oriented series, he found that higher levels of EE type behaviors were observed in nonachiever-rated family units ($p < .002$). Interestingly, the criticism, hostility, and overinvolvement was as likely to be manifested by the patient as the family member. While this is a gross oversimplification of Schorr's data, it does indicate clearly that there are clear behavioral differences observable between families rated as achievers or nonachievers. The differences observed indicate that, late in the course of therapy, high-EE type behaviors are still occurring in the nonachiever group, providing a link between the Vaughn–Leff literature on relapse and the current intervention study. Currently, we are investigating whether these high-EE behaviors are present in different degrees in early therapy sessions in achievers and nonachievers samples. If they are, then clearly there are systematic differences between these two types of families, which persist throughout six weeks of therapy. If they are not present initially, then it tells us something about possible failures in the application of the crisis model which are potentially correctable.

COMMENT

The present study indicates clearly that both phenothiazine medication and a form of family therapy play a very significant role in decreasing relapse in acute, young schizophrenics after discharge into the community. In the short run, all therapy cases showed less residual symptomotology than cases who did not receive therapy, with the most notable effects on *emotional blunting* and *withdrawal*. Over the longer follow-up period, only the therapy cases who had originally been maintained at the higher dose level sustained their earlier gains. We do not know at this point how this delayed effect was achieved—whether high-dose patients were more likely to follow subsequent treatment recommendations, or whether this is a genuine delayed effect of a short-term intervention remains to be established.

Although all therapy patients showed positive results on *emotional withdrawal*, impact on other components of the core schizophrenic symptoms were dependent upon the degree of therapist success in delivering the full model of the crisis therapy. These data suggest that there may be two levels of therapy effects, nonspecific and specific. Nonspecific effects are the consequence of maintaining a relationship with patient and significant others, but do not require attainment of all therapy objectives. Such a family support system appears to reduce the affective symptoms associated with the postacute phase of a schizophrenic episode such as *emotional withdrawal, blunted affect*, and to a lesser degree *anxiety* and *depression*.

Specific therapy effects, on the other hand, require achievement of discrete therapeutic objectives, such as those identified by the current crisis model. Achievement of these specific objectives is not necessary for improvement in affective symptoms, but is critical for sustained improvement in a core symptom of schizophrenia—*thought disorder*. Signs of the return of thought disorder are evident in cases who did not move beyond step 2 of the crisis model, whereas continued attenuation is noted for those who were rated as attaining steps 3 or 4. If we examine the difference between steps 1 and 2, and 3 and 4, it delineates a shift between a past and future time perspective. Patients who are rated as 3 or 4 can extrapolate from a look at the immediate, crisis-laden past to develop strategies for dealing with future stresses. When that shift in time orientation is noted, there is sustained improvement for the next six months, not only in the affective symptoms, but in thinking as well. These data support the position that, when the schizophrenic individual can integrate the psychotic experience into his life and use this integration in dealing with subsequent life events, a more positive outcome can be anticipated.

REFERENCES

1. May PRA: *Treatment of Schizophrenia*. New York, Science House Inc, 1968.
2. May PRA: The implications of psychopharmacological research for the treatment of schizophrenia, in West L. Flinn D (eds): *Treatment of Schizophrenia: Progress and Prospects*. New York, Grune & Stratton, 1976, pp 61–77.
3. Schooler NR: Antipsychotic drugs and psychological treatment in schizophrenia, in Lipton MA, DiMascio A, Killam KF (eds): *Psychopharmacology: A Generation of Progress*. New York, Raven Press, 1978, pp 1155–1168.
4. Evans JR, Goldstein MJ, Rodnick EH: Premorbid adjustment, paranoid diagnosis and remission in acute schizophrenics treated in a community mental health center. *Arch Gen Psychiatry* **28**:666–672, 1973.
5. Mosher LR, Pollin W, Stabenau JR: Families with identical twins discordant for schizophrenia: Some relationships between identification, thinking styles, psychopathology and dominance-submissiveness. *Br J Psychiatry* **118**:29–42, 1971.
6. Astrachan BM, Harrow D, Adler D, et al: A checklist for the diagnosis of schizophrenia. *Br J Psychiatry* **121**:529–539, 1972.
7. Chien C, Cole JO: Depot phenothiazine treatment in acute psychosis: A sequential comparative clinic study. *Am J Psychiatry* **130**:13–18, 1973.
8. Overall JE, Gorham DR: The brief psychiatric rating scale. *Psychol Rep* **10**:799, 1962.
9. King C, Goldstein MJ: Therapists' ratings of achievement of therapy objectives: An aid to research on psychotherapy with acute schizophrenics. *Schizophr Bull* **5**:118–129, 1979.
10. Endicott J, Spitzer RL, Fleiss JF, et al: The global assessment procedure for measuring the overall severity of psychiatric disturbance. *Arch Gen Psychiatry* **33**:766–771, 1976.
11. Vaughn CE, Leff JP: The measurement of expressed emotion in families of psychiatric patients. *Br J So Clin Psychol* **15**:157–165, 1976.

Chapter 8

Psychotherapy of Schizophrenia

Can We Make It Work?

PHILIP R. A. MAY

A discussion of the future of Psychotherapy Research in Schizophrenia must consider not only the directions that we may want to go, but also the deeper conceptual and social context that may influence these directions and affect the course of the research.

CONTEXT

Apart from certain political and ideological fixed positions that I will refer to later, we have, I believe, reached the point where there is a realistic basis for humble optimism about the future for psychotherapy research in schizophrenia. To a very large extent, the parochial dogmatism and polemics of a decade or two ago have been replaced by a large dose of humility, and we have slowly come to the painful realization that all treatments, physical, psychological, and social, have their inherent limitations,

PHILIP R. A. MAY • Director, Health Services Research and Development Laboratory, Veterans Administration Medical Center, Brentwood and Professor of Psychiatry, Neuropsychiatric Institute, Center for Health Sciences, University of California, Los Angeles, California 90073.

and that there is as yet no universally effective and lasting cure for schizophrenia. Many patients can be helped to regain their premorbid level of functioning, and a good deal can be accomplished in prevention of relapse—but only when things are favorable (i.e., when patient and family are willing and cooperative; when adequate community or private resources are available; and when the providers of care are knowledgeable and experienced in psychological intervention, rehabilitation, social support, and pharmacotherapy). Reordering a pathological personality style is, however, a task of a different order, one that is difficult, if not impossible, to achieve by the methods currently available.

Drugs, for example, may alleviate overt psychotic thinking disorder; improve symptoms, and behavior; and reduce the risk of relapse. They are, therefore, often essential to set the stage for other forms of treatment. But they don't work in all cases, and they sometimes have toxic effects. And, even more important, they can never unravel the tangled bitterness of a lifetime; they cannot show a new way of life; they cannot provide social support; they cannot teach different modes of behavior; and they cannot enlighten a person about new or different sources of pleasure and satisfaction.

In the 1940s and 1950s there was a widespread belief that psychotherapy was the royal, indeed, the only, road to solving the deep and fundamental basic problems of psychosis. Thirty years later, we know that, for hospitalized patients in the acute phase of psychosis, the results are often small compared with the amount of time and effort that it requires,[1] and that the main potential of psychotherapy probably lies in the restitution phase, after the overt psychotic manifestations have subsided and the patient is, literally and figuratively, back in the real world. Just as with drug therapy, psychotherapy and psychotherapists have their limitations. They also have toxic effects—patients can be pushed into suicide and aggression, or into other forms of acting out, and families may be humiliated and split or ignored.

It may be of academic and heuristic value to conceptualize the therapeutic world as divided into psychotherapy, seen as psychological treatment of psychological problems and conducted by therapists from various professions, in contrast to biologic therapy, defined as physicial forms of intervention into physiological processes and administered by physicians.[1] But it is also well to remember that both the givers and the receivers of these therapies are persons who think, feel, behave, remember, metabolize, cycle AMP, release neurotransmitters, and generate electrical currents and potentials, all at the same time. The artificial duality of our concepts is neatly captured by Hoch's statement[2] that

> Psychotherapy itself, is, of course, a procedure which is as organic as the introduction of a drug, but it is not applied to the nervous system. It has to pass through all the filtering and defense mechanisms which shield the

organism against external stimulation whereas drugs are introduced
directly into the organism.

Regrettably, the social dynamics of our treatment system—or perhaps
I should say nonsystem—tend to encourage and perpetuate fragmented
treatment. Agencies and private therapists guard their boundaries jealously,
often to the detriment of a more comprehensive and rational treatment
plan. Indeed, in this respect the patient's internal splitting mirrors—and,
often unwittingly, accentuates—the splitting and lopsided attitudes in the
system. It is rare, for example, to find equal attention being paid to
psychotherapy, occupational rehabilitation, recreational opportunity, social
support, family intervention, and drug therapy.

It would also be unrealistic to assume that the zeitgeist is now all sweet
reason and light. There is still a wide range of ideological rhetoric to hamper
research in this area.

First, the Abolitionists, along with Szasz assert that there is no such
thing as schizophrenia and no such thing as psychotherapy; that they are
brutal fabrications that would disappear like magic if one did away with hospitals, clinics, and treatment professionals; and that "treatment" and
"psychotherapy" therefore are frauds, hoaxed upon an unwilling patient and
ignorant public.

Actually, if you can ignore Szasz's polemics and try not to be put off
by the provocative language, he has a point. But one has to realize that he is
making a political statement, and not a scientific one. There is, in fact, no
evidence that those whom we now call schizophrenic would be better off if
we did it his way. Indeed, I would assign top priority here and now to a
really well-designed and tightly controlled comparison of a good so-called
nonmedical model (as defined by good nonpsychiatrists) with a good
medical model of treatment (as defined by good psychiatrists).

Next come the Legalists who are busily redefining legal rights,
malpractice, and the ground rules for research and everyone's responsibilities, except perhaps their own. The danger is that somewhere in the furor
of their well-meaning efforts, society may lose sight of the patients' needs and
responsibilities, and of the rights and needs and responsibilities of the family
and the community, and of the rights and needs and responsibilities of the
treatment professionals.

It must not be forgotten that a research atmosphere, a spirit of inquiry
and questioning in and of itself, leads to higher standards of care. And even
apart from this secondary gain, society, all of us, have a responsibility to do
what we can to improve the quality of life of present and future generations—and this is what, in the final analysis, research is all about.

Third, are the Alarmists, the anti-professionals and anti-mental health
movers and shakers, whose vigilant hyperscanning leads them to concerns

that therapists may, under the guise of treatment, wittingly or unwittingly be brain-washing, conditioning, programming, and drugging good solid citizens into social and political confirmity. In this respect, it seems to faze them not one whit that there already exist proven, if less scrupulous, methods of coercion and thought control that are far more likely to be used—the press, radio, television, secret police, threats, torture, bribery, and intimidation, for example.

Last, the Professional Nonconformists, for example, along with Laing, believe on the one hand that schizophrenia is a social disease caused by an insensitive and callous oppressive society, and on the other hand that it can become a great growth experience, an inner voyage of discovery. Most of us will agree that this is a hard world, at some times anyway, and that there are many things that should be changed. But we have to live in it. So do our patients—and it is not likely to help them much to blame everything on mother, or on father, or on society. Nor does it seem particularly humane to ignore the pain and suffering of psychosis by polyanna trumpeting about the hypothetical and speculative possibility that every psychosis may supposedly have a silver lining.

It is also well to remember that Freud believed that chemical forms of intervention should play supplemental rather than competing roles in the treatment of psychoses. He wrote:[3]

> The hope of the future here lies in organic chemistry or access to it through endocrinology. The future is still far distant, but one should study analytically every case of psychosis because their knowledge will one day guide the chemical therapy.

Nevertheless, such ideas should not be dismissed lightly. They are important for psychotherapy research, and we disregard them at our peril. It is well to attend to the messages behind the inflated rhetoric. Szasz is right: it is society's prerogative to decide whether or not deviant behavior should be defined as a crime or as an illness or as a social problem and to decide who should be responsible for doing something about it. And it is fair enough to say that we must always watch out for the rights of the individual, and not be too authoritarian or too paternalistic. And it is fair enough to say that we need a lot more tolerance for eccentricity, and that we don't need to rush in and "treat" everyone who acts oddly. But we should never forget that relatives and others in the community have rights and feelings too, and that you can't please everyone all the time.

Nor can one find fault with the (not particularly original) proposition that, if you hve a painful experience, you should try—or be helped to try—to profit from it. If a person falls down and breaks his leg, he can certainly learn from it. He can learn that he should not walk carelessly, or that he should not walk in that particular place. In *The Magic Mountain*, Thomas Mann depicted that one can profit from the experience of tuberculosis. So, if a person becomes psychotic, he should be helped, if possible, to learn something from the content of the psychosis and from the circumstances in which it developed. The UCLA group conducted a study of the efficacy of combining such an approach with drug therapy and found that it was effective.[4]

STRATEGY

Leaving on one side studies that purport to be of theoretical interest only, a sound general strategy for psychotherapy research would be:

1. To develop specific methods (for example, of technic, case selection, etc.). In the development stage, time and cost are not an issue.

2. In a carefully controlled trial, evaluate the use of these methods in the hands of the most expert persons who might be expected to use them. At this point, cost effectiveness is not necessarily an issue.

3. If the trial is successful, develop methods to teach the methods to others.

4. Reevaluate. At this point, cost effectiveness becomes an issue.

5. Finally, study the learning–time–experience curve to identify the optimum cost-effective point for acquiring this particular skill.

I must emphasize the scientific importance of studying the outcome of treatment as given by experts *first*—not last! Many of the past and current problems of psychotherapy research in schizophrenia are attributable to the unhappy fact that in the past the experts taught their methods directly to others, without controlled evaluation.

We don't have an FDA-equivalent to monitor and approve psychological forms of treatment—at least, not yet. But it has been suggested. We need to recognize that, even though it is justifiable to spend large amounts of money and time on research and in developing new methods, in the end we must demonstrate that a treatment is effective *before* it can be considered suitable for teaching to others and for widespread adoption.

TACTICS AND CONTENT

Which directions seem most likely to be profitable for psychotherapy research in schizophrenia, and which should be nominated for instant retirement?

Research Classification and Nomenclature of
Psychotherapy and Psychotherapists

This is needed to promote clear communication among researchers, and between researchers and treating clinicians. We do not need any more "definitions" of psychotherapy. But there should be an agreed, standardized, defined, systematic way to classify for research purposes who does what (or is trying to do what) (or is using which technics), and in what dosage, and for how long. At the very least, such a system would reduce the degree to which gross blunders are made in comparing studies, in interpreting results, in generalizing from one study to another, or from one context to another, and in applying research findings to clinical practice.

The classification system must be wide enough to overlap with and include behavior therapy, milieu therapy, rehabilitation, counselling, and family therapy since some definitions of psychotherapy include much of what might otherwise be classified under these other rubrics.

Research Diagnostic Criteria Versus Research
Classification

In the absence of substantive and widely accepted proof that any particular set of diagnostic criteria has greater validity for the prediction of treatment outcome than another set, I am deeply skeptical of the current bandwagon to include in research studies only those patients who meet cetain rigid and highly exclusive diagnostic criteria.

It is clear that such straightjackets exclude a substantial number of patients for whom good clinicians would agree on diagnosis of schizophrenia. Indeed, such criteria may exclude precisely the kind of patient that might be helped most by psychotherapy.

The objective, therefore, should be to use these diagnostic systems, not as rigid criteria for acceptance into a study, but as instruments to assess and describe the degree to which the patients in this study possess certain characteristics. And, rather than being mesmerized by diagnosis, it might be more helpful to insist on some fairly simple prognostic subclassification. At the very least, it is of prime importance to know how much prior treatment the patients have had and whether we are dealing with good prognosis, fair prognosis, poor prognosis, or chronic treatment failures.

Outcome versus Process

Although fashionable and convenient, the unwise use of a distinction between Outcome and Process studies may impede progress in this field by obscuring two facts: (1) A process is not a process unless it has an outcome, and (2) If a patient–therapist process is truly relevant, the outcome of this process must, sooner or later, be related to a process of clinically meaningful change in the patient.

Studies of the Efficacy of "General Purpose" Psychotherapy

At this point in history, it would seem that studies of the efficacy of what might be characterized as "nonspecific," general purpose, good-for-what-ails-you, relationship psychotherapy are useful only as a baseline control with which to compare some other more "specific" or more "goal-directed" or more "targeted" form of treatment.

Individual Differences

As our statistical technics and design become more sophisticated, studies should examine the characteristics of patients for whom "specific" types of psychotherapy are indicated—and also the characteristics of those who will do well with minimal doses of "general purpose" psychotherapy, and for whom other "specific" psychotherapeutic interventions are not indicated, or offer little or no advantage.

Specific Focused Technics

In the light of previous controlled research and epidemiologic studies, I have no hesitation in proposing that the most fruitful direction at the moment is the development of specific focused technics of psychotherapy aimed at defined and limited problems, the borderland between behavior therapy, psychotherapy, milieu therapy, and family therapy. A major point of treatment strategy should be defining clear goals for each patient. It is particularly important to distinguish between trying to achieve or maintain restitution, and trying to remake the patient. It is also necessary to remember that what is good for one patient may not be good for another; that what helps in the early stages of treatment may not help at all later on; that measures aimed, for example, at getting the patient a job may have no direct effect on grandiose attitudes, or on inappropriate behavior. It is, therefore, essential to define clearly what the goals are, and to plan specific interventions accordingly—and to make appropriate adjustments as treatment progresses.

The "Problems" to be worked on may be defined in social terms (e.g., role performance at work, at home with the family, or elsewhere), or in psychological terms (e.g., concept formation, emotional communication and recognition, cognition or overinclusion), or in psychodynamic terms. The point is that the intervention should be aimed at a specific target, and that outcome must be measured *first* in terms of effect on the target problems, and *secondarily* in terms of generalization to other areas.

Outpatient Therapy

I also have no hesitation in saying that the critical area today is outpatient therapy: how to hold the patient in the community, how to reduce his vulnerability to relapse, how to mitigate the toxic effects of the environment, and how to improve the quality of life for him and his family, and for those who are around him.

Family Therapy and Significant Others

Implicit in the above is the concept that psychotherapy research should not, as in the past, direct itself almost exclusively to the patient. Recent research has underlined the importance of developing strategies to mitigate stresses and burdens and interactions within the family. This is well, but it should not prevent us from seeing that it may be important also to develop therapeutically oriented interventions with others in the community; police and teachers, for example.

Psychotherapy and Drug Therapy

We know that drugs work: there is overwhelming controlled evidence. We also know that the end results of drug treatment still leave much to be desired; that drugs don't work in every case; that they don't do everything; and that they have toxic effects and side effects that may interfere with other treatments.

We would, therefore, be well advised to give up trying to show that drugs are no good or not necessary, and concentrate instead on some of the problems of combining drugs with psychotherapy—compliance, monitoring psychological response, adjusting for optimal dose, investigation of subjective response to drug effect, counteracting side effects by psychological intervention, unconscious resistances to drug therapy within the therapist, etc. Some of the more adventurous might even rise to the challenge of "pharmacopsychotherapy"—developing psychotherapeutic interventions that might potentiate drug effect or reduce side effects by altering drug concentration at target sites.[1]

Toxic Effects

Despite ample evidence to the contrary, it is still common to act and talk as if psychotherapy has no dangers, and that, even if not effective, it is at least entirely innocuous.

A more reasoned approach would be to assume that any treatment will have toxic effects if it is given at the wrong time, in the wrong dose, to the wrong subject, or in a wrong way. This opens the way to research that aims to identify toxic effects more precisely, to examine their etiology and mechanisms, and to develop methods to avoid or to reduce such toxic effects.

Therapist Factors

The most profitable direction in this area would seem to be to focus on therapist activities, perceptions, and feelings that may be related to toxic effects from therapy.

We hear a good deal about "matching" therapists and patients. In a world where most therapist–patient matching is determined by forced assignment, by chance, by geography, or by finances, I can see little practical future for therapist–patient matching studies—except perhaps for difficult cases, or when treatment goes badly.

Therapist Skill, Knowledge and Experience

This can be just another red herring, or it can be an interesting subject for serious, carefully controlled, and well-designed study. As I indicated at the beginning of this paper, experience becomes an issue only after it has been demonstrated that a treatment is effective, and that it can be taught. At that point, the research question becomes "How much teaching and experience are necessary before the treatment is given effectively, and what is the cost-effective point on the learning curve?"

Left-Brain and Right-Brain Therapy

Ours is a verbal society, and so are our therapies. Yet we know only too well that body image is a central issue in early development; that nonverbal interaction precedes verbal; and that at least some schizophrenics pay close attention to what people do, rather than to the words they use.

It is surprising, therefore, that so little attention has been given to the nonverbal aspects of therapy, and to the systematic development of nonverbal psychotherapeutic technics.

In this connection, Myslobodsky and Weiner[1] have made a nice and catchy differentiation between left and right brain therapy. I join them in urging that attention be given to the latter.

CONCLUSION

I have reached the end of my alloted time, but I have nowhere near run out of ideas for future psychotherapy research. This should suffice to demonstrate that the problem with psychotherapy research should never be a lack of ideas. As Blériot said in 1909, before his first cross-channel flight between England and France: "To have an idea is nothing. To build the mechanism is better. To make it work is everything." Our challenge is to make psychotherapy of schizophrenia work.

REFERENCES

1. Myslobodsky MS, Weiner M: Clincal psychology in the chemical environment. *Pscychol Rep* **43**:247–276, 1978.
2. Hoch P: Aims and limitations of psychotherapy, in Nolan DC, Strahl, L, Strahl, M (eds): *The Complete Psychiatrist*. Albany, State University of New York Press, 1968, p 237.
3. Freud S: Letter to Marie Bonaparte Jan 15, 1930 in Jones E (ed): *The Life and Work of Sigmund Freud*. New York, Basic Books, 1957, vol 3, p 449.
4. Goldstein J, Rodnick EH, Evans JR, et al: Drug and family therapy in the aftercare of acute schizophrenics. *Arch Gen Psychiatry* **35**:1169–1177, 1978.

Chapter 9

The Nature of the Psychotic Experience and Its Implications for the Therapeutic Process

SIDNEY J. BLATT, JEAN G. SCHIMEK,
and C. BROOKS BRENNEIS

Effective psychotherapy with schizophrenic patients requires an extensive understanding of the nature of the psychotic process. In our research, we have tried to gain some understanding of the psychotic experience by studying how psychotic patients think about people, and how they interact. We have attempted to investigate the concept of the object (or object representations) in psychosis. In this paper we shall summarize briefly our research findings about the nature of the object world in psychosis and consider in detail the implications of these findings for understanding the psychotic experience and the therapeutic process with schizophrenic patients.

In a number of different disciplines, there have been recent and important discoveries about the nature of cognitive schemata and the development of the representation of self and of others, and their role in

SIDNEY J. BLATT • Department of Psychiatry, Yale University, 25 Park Street, New Haven, Connecticut 06519.   JEAN G. SCHIMEK • Department of Psychology, New York University, New York, New York 10003.   C. BROOKS BRENNEIS • Department of Psychology and Psychiatry, University of Wisconsin, Madison, Wisconsin 53706.

personality organization. Developmental psychologists (e.g., Piaget,[1] Werner,[2] Werner and Kaplan,[3] Decarie[4]) and developmental psychoanalysts (e.g., Anna Freud,[5] Wolff,[6] Jacobson,[7] Mahler,[8] Fraiberg[9]) have made major contributions to the understanding of the complex cognitive, affective, and interpersonal factors inherent in the development of the representation of the object world. In our research on object representation, we have found that the Rorschach and the manifest content of dreams can provide reliable data for investigating the representation of the self and of others. We conducted an extensive analysis of the human response on the Rorschach based on Heinz Werner's developmental concepts of differentiation, articulation, and integration, and have found some unexpected and exciting results which may have important implications for the therapeutic process. These findings, which we have presented in detail in an earlier report,[10] have recently been replicated on data gathered independently at the University of Rochester.[11]

In comparison to a matched normal control sample, a group of seriously disturbed adolescent and young adult inpatients had a significantly greater number of human responses at lower developmental levels; that is, responses of quasi-human and distorted figures engaged in unmotivated, incongruent, passive, and malevolent activity. What was surprising was that these responses at lower developmental levels in patients were often accurately perceived $(F+)$—that is, the responses conformed to the configurations of the inkblot. What was even more surprising and unexpected was the fact that inaccurately perceived $(F-)$ human responses of psychotic patients, responses that did not conform to the configuration of the inkblot, were often at higher developmental levels than in normals. Inaccurately perceived human responses of patients were often more articulated, differentiated and integrated. Psychotic patients had a significantly greater number of developmentally more advanced responses, responses that were undistorted, intact, functionally articulated, integrated, and benevolent, than did normals, but only on inaccurately perceived responses.[10] When patients were in contact with conventional reality, they functioned at lower developmental levels than normals. But when patients gave idiosyncratic interpretations of reality, they functioned at higher developmental levels than normals.

In an attempt to understand these findings further, we examined in detail the human responses of patients that were inaccurately perceived, but at developmentally more advanced levels. These responses did not occur on any particular Rorschach card, but the content of the responses was almost always positive and tended to be grandiose and mythical, such as figures of Napoleon, Lincoln, a soldier from a Friml opera, a princess, the Little King, a Martian, and a knight. Many of these responses seemed to be preformed images, that were internally determined and elaborated with little contact with the external stimulus. But they were well-articulated, organized and integrated. They stood in sharp contrast to the accurately perceived responses of patients that were at developmentally lower levels of organization.

These data indicate that the capacity to perceive reality adequately does not necessarily aid psychotic patients to organize their experiences more effectively and to function at higher developmental levels. Quite to the contrary, it seems that in psychotic patients, contact with reality, at least in a conventional sense, brings with it responses that are at lower developmental levels of thinking, and contain malevolent content. It is primarily in the inaccurately perceived responses, when idiosyncratic interpretations of reality are given, that psychotic patients can portray a world that is more differentiated, well-articulated, integrated, and benevolent.

These findings suggest that there are at least two major dimensions in the psychotic experience. First, when contact with conventional reality is maintained, the psychotic individual functions at a developmentally lower level and perceives and experiences the world as distorted, undifferentiated, fragmented, malevolent, and destructive. The second dimension indicates that, though psychotic patients have a great proclivity for experiencing the world unrealistically, within these unrealistic experiences they can function at developmentally higher levels and represent the world as benevolent and kind. Psychotic patients appear more disorganized when they are struggling to deal with and integrate a painful reality and less disorganized when absorbed in unrealistic experiences. The findings that some seriously disturbed patients have a significantly greater number of human responses which are inaccurate but at higher developmental levels than normals, raises a number of complex and important issues about the nature of the psychotic experience.

First, the data are consistent with our previous findings[12-15] that schizophrenic patients have primitive and impaired representations. Many of the responses of the patients contain indications of boundary disturbances, and they generally portray human figures as malevolent and at lower levels of differentiation, articulation, and integration. Highly inconsistent, rejecting, and destructive relationships with primary caretaking figures very early in life have created impairments in the development of representations so that the schizophrenic patient is profoundly vulnerable to later experiences of rebuff, rejection, and abandonment. The impairments in the development of representations in schizophrenia are severe and involve the most fundamental dimensions of mental representation—the basic differentiation and definition of objects. These impairments in object representation in schizophrenia evolve from a transaction between the child's basic biological capacities and predispositions and the degree of organization and structure provided by the environment. Although genetic and biological factors are predispositional in a nonspecific way, it is the failure of the environment to provide consistent care and affection and the degree of organization and structure required by the particular developing child, that is the primary cause of the impairments in representation that we observe in schizophrenia.

The instability of the schizophrenic patient's capacity for the representation of boundaries creates a profound vulnerability to experiencing stress as a disintegration of reality and as a destruction of the self, especially in bodily terms. There are intense experiences of disorganization[16-18] and fears of fragmentation and annihilation. Frightening, persecutory hallucinations and delusions are expressions of the schizophrenic patients' chaotic, destructive experiences in reality, as well as expressions of their being overwhelmed by their own rage and anger. Schizophrenic patients have an omnipresent fear of disorganization, dissolution, disintegration, and annihilation. Tenuous boundaries of self and object make it difficult for the patient to maintain a sense of himself and of others which is stable and enduring. Psychotic symptomatology can be understood as either a serious disorganization and fragmentation or a desperate struggle to maintain contact with objects and reality in order to preserve a sense of self as a psychological entity.[16] Schizophrenic patients are apprehensive about internal disintegration as well as about being overwhelmed, engulfed, and devoured. They desperately seek contact with objects in an attempt to maintain a sense of being, but they also dread contact because they fear that they will be annihilated by the object.[19] These apprehensions and fears of disintegration and annihilation are expressions of profound early traumatic experiences with significant love objects that seriously interrupted psychological growth early in the developmental process.

The schizophrenic patient's profound vulnerability to experiences of an unstable world in which things can collapse, disintegrate, and disappear, requires the therapist to be aware of the patient's desperate need to experience a very stable, consistent, highly dependable relationship. The impaired concept of the object and of the self of the schizophrenic patient requires the therapist and the therapeutic community to provide organization and structure early in the therapeutic process.[20-22] The schizophrenic patient needs a highly stable and predictable environment. The organization that the environment and the therapist provide is internalized by the patient as a sense of cohesion, and this is essential for the establishment of more mature psychic structures.[23] Early in therapy there is a need to focus on reality relatedness; the "real relationship" between patient and therapist becomes a vehicle for aiding the patient to establish a stable sense of the therapist and object constancy more generally.[24-27] The patient initially needs to establish rudimentary identifications with the therapist and to rely on aspects of the therapist's behavior and responses as guides for his own behavior because the patient's fundamental psychological structures have been fragmented or partially lost in the psychosis.[28] Schizophrenic patients initially need to establish real relationships with reliable and predictable objects before they can enter into an exploration of more subtle psychological dimensions. Concrete assistance with reality adaptation, assistance with the control of instinctual outbursts, appropriate psychological and physical distance within a reliable, regular, and dependable relationship, and communication and understanding facilitate the development of object relationships and the establishment of object representation. It is only with the development of object constancy that the patient can experience and explore in depth realistic and unrealistic aspects of his interpersonal relationships.[28]

Our data also suggest that there is a second major dimension in psychosis in which the psychotic patient deals with his experiences of a disorganized, chaotic and destructive reality and his fears of annihilation and disintegration by retreating into an unrealistic fantasy world. What is surprising and important to stress, however, is that our findings indicate that this unrealistic fantasy world is not as primitive and autistic as is often assumed. These fantasies are often well structured and at a high developmental level. They are well defined, articulated, and integrated idyllic representations. It seems paradoxical that seriously disturbed patients with such profound proclivity for amorphous and diffuse thinking can also establish and maintain representations that are well-differentiated, highly articulated, integrated, and stable. We must ask how a seriously disturbed patient can establish some representations at a high developmental level, and we need to explore the role of these unrealistic but developmentally advanced representations in the patient's pathology and understand how they are expressed and can be utilized in the therapeutic process. These idyllic fantasies may also provide us with further understanding of the psychological experiences of schizophrenic patients—their libidinal orientation, defensive structures, level of cognitive organization, and the nature of the interactions that are available for reality-relatedness and interpersonal relationships.

Our data suggest that schizophrenic patients experience the external world as chaotic, confused, fragmented, and destructive and that they seek comfort and solace in thoughts of blissful satisfaction in a highly stable fantasy world in which there is order, predictability, and organization. In actual interactions, schizophrenic patients feel bombarded by stimulation and flooded by sensations and ideas. They have difficulty maintaining a separation between various experiences and events and easily become confused.[13] Schizophrenic patients seem to have failed to internalize adequate cognitive schemata which allow them to integrate a diversity of perceptions and experiences and to maintain a sense of order, predictability, consistency, and continuity. In normal development, the cognitive schemata necessary for understanding and organizing experiences are established in the internalization of consistent, stable, predictable action sequences around gratification of fundamental and basic needs. What is impaired in schizophrenia is not only the image of the good mother,[17] but also the internalization of the action sequences of a predictable caring agent. The lack of reasonably well-organized and predictable action sequences in the basic caring relationship creates impairments of the congnitive schemata, which places limits on the capacity to appreciate and understand interpersonal relationships and to deal effectively with reality. These difficulties become most apparent during intense interpersonal relationships when the schizophrenic patient feels bombarded and flooded by excessive stimulation, and becomes confused and disorganized.

Difficulties in establishing order, cohesion, and continuity force the schizophrenic patient to find organization in rigidly held, preformed images, which are split off and removed from the unpredictable multiplicity of experiences in external reality. Preformed social stereotypes provide the basis for rigid, fixed, unreal images of a desired, nurturant, blissful relationship with a constant, consistent, and stable caring agent. The idyllic narcissistic fantasies not only offer comfort and solace for painful and destructive experiences, but they provide order and cohesion. Intense investment in a common, well-defined, preformed image or myth which is separated from the real world diminishes the need to deal with the confusion experienced in variable, and at times unpredictable, interpersonal interactions.

In many ways our findings offer support and further understanding of the classic observation[29-34] that schizophrenic patients resort to grandiose, narcissistic fantasies as replacement for relationships in external reality. Our data indicate that a second major aspect of psychosis is the restitution attempts which occur subsequent to experiences of psychic disaster and inner catastrophe. In this restitution process, fantasies of relationships, based on preformed social stereotypes, are established as replacements for real and current relationships. Often there is an urgent orality and hypersexuality in these fantasies. These urgent restitutive efforts often involve overvaluation of the self and the object in bodily terms, and in themes of world salvation, creativity, power, and beauty. The investment is in remote symbols of safe, neutral, and idyllic objects, far removed from reality, so that they cannot be disrupted by reality events. Restitutional fantasies are a partial solution to the problem of painful experiences in reality and a loss of object representations. Because of impaired object constancy, these restitutional fantasies are fixed, rigidly maintained, and held with great tenacity.[35,22] Schizophrenic patients seek refuge in restitution fantasies in which powerful forces bring bliss and a sense of peace and order. The world is no longer chaotic, unpredictable, destructive, or empty, but instead full of new and grand meaning. Everything has a purpose and a place, and there is meaning everywhere. The content of these fantasies is often passive-receptive and narcissistic, and contains themes of oral reunion. The fantasies are an attempt to create a new reality as a replacement for the malevolent, destructive, unpredictable, chaotic external world.[36] It is important to emphasize, however, that our data indicate that these grandiose restitution fantasies should not be considered simply as primary process thinking or as autistic. Although the content of these images is frequently narcissistic, passive-receptive, and contains themes of oral reunion, it is important to note that in formal or structural terms these fantasies are at a high developmental level. They have an internal consistency and logic and seem to offer organization and order as well as feelings of safety, comfort, peace, and solace in a chaotic and destructive reality. They seem to express a wished-for idyllic state which is split off from the more reality-based representations of malevolent, destructive, and chaotic experiences.

One frankly psychotic adolescent patient, for example, somewhat late in therapy began to discuss a very precise, elaborate, and highly stable fantasy that his biological mother, who placed him for adoption immediately after his birth, was "blond and plump," and that he would be reunited with her in a specific place and at a specific time—in "the Spring in the Garden of Eden." The themes of Paradise Lost, and the hope for reestablishing a happier, earlier time before he was expelled from the "Garden of Eden," emerged in the therapy only after a major consolidation of the therapeutic relationship had taken place. Initially in treatment he was much more comfortable discussing his general fantasies that women were destructive, seductive vampires, who would suck his blood, semen, and mind, envelop and consume him, and leave him a "blob on a rock." The more positive fantasy of a blond and plump mother who was beautiful, loving, and kind, and with whom he would be reunited during the springtime in the Garden of Eden, was highly specific, well-defined, and stable. It seemed to have provided him with hope and promise for the future and to have sustained him through considerable turmoil and stress. While his Garden of Eden fantasy could also possibly contain unconscious thoughts that it was his sexuality which disrupted an earlier idyllic state and destroyed his mother, many of these more negative thoughts and feelings were expressed more directly in his relationship with his adopted mother. He believed, possibly somewhat realistically, that she had often tried to seduce him. She was often drunk at night, and he reported that she would sit on his bed wearing a revealing nightgown. At times he would find her attractive and pinch "her bottom." He was angry and agitated about these experiences and freely discussed them in therapy. In contrast, the positive image of a reunion with is biological mother was a very precious fantasy that he was reluctant to reveal and discuss. It clearly seemed to have an organizing function, and to provide him with hope and promise. It was impressive how he was able to sustain this well-articulated, stable, though highly unrealistic fantasy of a reunion with his biological mother, despite periods of florid psychosis in which he was unable to maintain any level of sustained attention because of the continual intrusion of inappropriate ideation and affect, particularly when he was involved in interpersonal contact.

Certainly, everyone has idyllic fantasies, myths, and images which provide comfort and solace at times of stress and anxiety. As Willie Hoffer commented (oral communication from G. Pollack), we all have our secret little garden which we cultivate and go to in moments of stress and pain. But what is unique and pathological about idyllic fantasies in schizophrenic patients is their fixed, rigid, monolithic, stereotyped, repetitive nature, and the intensity with which they are maintained. They are split off from reality and from any input from the real world. The intensity with which these idyllic fantasies are maintained indicates their importance to schizophrenic patients' equilibrium, not only as a replacement for traumatic experiences in a world filled with confusion and chaos, but also as a defense against the recognition of the fury and rage felt about the deprivations they have experienced in the basic caring relationship.[37]

There seem to be relatively few comments in the literature on the constructive and positive aspects of unrealistic, idyllic fantasies. Most comments and discussion focus on the autistic, restitutive, or defensive dimensions.[32,36,38] Smith[38] recently has discussed a specific hidden golden fantasy which can be seen in all patients, but is seen most starkly in infantile, narcissistic, and schizophrenic patients. The content of this fantasy is always passive and "tied to the conviction that somewhere (there is) a person capable of fully meeting one's needs." The patient feels that the fantasy touches on the deepest issues of his life and that his very survival may depend on its preservation. Smith discussed these fantasies primarily as the basis for significant resistance in treatment and as evoking particular counter-transference problems. But our data suggest that these idyllic fantasies also provide comfort, a sense of meaning, self-definition, and hope; that they can be a positive dimension in psychosis and can have a central and constructive role in therapy. Burnham, Gladstone, and Gibson[19] have discussed the schizophrenic patient's inability to maintain relatively constant object representations and how the schizophrenic patient attempts to achieve a "temporary pseudo-constancy" through "object redefinition" in which idealization leads to a construction of a reliable, good object—a magic helper and constant companion, filled with goodness, trustworthiness, and helpfulness. This idealization is sustained by primitive defenses, such as denial and splitting. The idealization can be maintained if the fantasy has little or no contact with reality: "Such an autistic, totally unilateral relationship may persist for years and serve as a source of great comfort and pseudo-stability

. . ." (p. 38). When the idealization disintegrates, the adoration is replaced by hatred. Burnham et al. discuss the therapeutic process as aiding the patient to place more reliance upon real, meaningful, and currently available objects and less reliance on distant and autistic objects.

Jacobson[39] has also discussed the course of psychotic episodes as involving the fragmentation of object and self representations and their restitutional reorganization in new, composite, pathological images. She discussed, for example, a schizophrenic social worker who planned to set up an international social agency which would prevent war and save the world from destruction. The patient also maintained the delusion of having a secret adversary in the government who tried to ruin all his plans. The omnipotent destructive image was split off and projected onto an imaginary outside evil adversary and maintained as separate from the image of an omnipotent, loving, "rescuer of mankind." Jacobson saw the omnipotent destructive images as arising from a painful destructive reality and from a perception of disintegration and the dissolution of both object and self representations. The positive delusional ideas she considered as restitutional processes which attempted to reintegrate fragmented images and attach them to external objects in a positive and constructive form.[39]

The idyllic fantasies of schizophrenic patients can play a central role in the therapeutic process. The fantasies seem to express a wished-for symbiotic reunion with the mother (or her substitute) in narcissistic bliss—a deeply held hope to find a safe, blissful, caring relationship in which a loving, concerned mother provides nurturance, support, and affection. These fantasies seem to represent the last vestiges of hope for the schizophrenic patients in what they experience as a hostile, destructive reality. They seem to provide the patients with organization and a sense of meaning and hope which has sustained them, at least in a limited way, in a chaotic and destructive reality. They also indicate the patient's potential for organization and for interpersonal relatedness. In the early stages of therapy, these often unspoken idyllic fantasies silently provide a basis for the establishment of a therapeutic alliance. Often they can be expressed in a partially unconscious idealized transference through which the patient attempts to defend against the apprehensions that therapy will be another destructive interpersonal experience.

Because of their profoundly painful and traumatic experiences in reality, schizophrenic patients must protect their idyllic fantasies and are often reluctant to reveal and discuss them for fear the therapist will destroy the dream and shatter the illusion. Though the patient is often most reluctant to reveal and discuss these idyllic fantasies, it is precisely these fantasies that provide the basis for the therapeutic alliance and the patient's eventual ventures to seek realistic, appropriate, satisfying relationships in the external world. In the midst of a chaotic and destructive world, the idealized fantasy serves as a refuge in the storm, but eventually the patient must relinquish it and begin to use it as a basis for seeking more appropriate and realistic modes of gratification. As these fantasies are considered in the therapy, the idyllic fantasy and the idealized transference can become a bridge[37] between the patient's primitive, chaotic, destructive experiences and his potential to become constructively involved in a realistic world.

In therapy, the closed system of the idyllic fantasy slowly begins to open to include the therapist as a substitute for the maternal figure. Initially, the patient apprehensively anticipates that the therapist will be another unrealible, destructive, potentially devouring figure. The therapeutic relationship, like any other interpersonal encounter, is fraught with danger similar to those originally experienced in the painful, destructive, traumatic experiences in an unpredictable and chaotic reality. The patient tests the therapist in numerous ways and tries to reduce his apprehensions about a possible repetition of the trauma and chaos experienced in painful, sado-mashochistic early life experiences. As the schizophrenic patient experiences consistency, continuity, and safety, the closed idyllic fantasy system slowly extends to include the therapist.

At first the therapist is included in the idyllic fantasy as a representation fused with the maternal figure. The patient experiences a blissful sense of well-being with the therapist—a sense of union and at-oneness which obliterates boundaries. Within the therapeutic relationship, the experiences of blissful reunion need not threaten the patient with annihilation. The therapist can allow the patient, when necessary, to establish distance and differentiation in increasingly constructive forms without the apprehension and fear of being rejected, abandoned, or even destroyed in the process. Slowly, the therapist begins to provide a realistic relationship which can offer some hope for realizing some aspects of the idyllic fantasy. The therapist, through the idyllic fantasies, enables the schizophrenic patient to replace his perception and experience of a traumatic, chaotic, destructive reality, with a realistic hope for closeness and affection.

Eventually the idyllic fantasy and the idealizing transference become a major issue in therapy.[38] The patient must confront the unreality of the fantasy and the ultimate disillusionment and disappointment[37] that no relationship can provide the love, support, succor, protection, and warmth of the idyllic fantasy. In the rage experienced over the disillusionment that is inevitable in the therapeutic relationship the patient reexperiences the rage over earlier failures to establish a satisfying, caring relationship. Within the therapeutic relationship, the patient can examine and understand current disappointments as well as the intensity of the rage originally experienced over the earlier failure to establish and maintain a blissful, satisfying caretaking relationship. It is essential in the treatment of schizophrenic and borderline patients that the idyllic fantasies emerge in the therapeutic rela-

tionship and the patient express the rage over the inevitable disillusionment within the therapeutic relationship. This disillusionment is experienced
not by interpretation, but by the therapist's natural failure to always be
available, understanding, and comforting. The therapist's failure to meet the
demands of the idealized symbiotic fantasy allows the patient to work
through the rage over profound narcissistic injuries that have been so carefully warded off and so intensely defended against. If the therapist can aid
the patient to tolerate and manage the disappointment and rage experienced
in the therapeutic relationship, the patient may be in a position to
experience and consider the rage over the disappointments in the original
caretaking relationships. As the patient is able to experience, tolerate, and
manage disappointment and rage within the therapeutic relationship, he
may be able to begin to risk establishing more realistic and mature modes
of relating, first within the therapeutic relationship and, eventually, more
generally. He can begin to risk investment in appropriate relationships to
find gratification for some aspects of his symbiotic needs while being able to
relinquish other aspects of these needs. The idyllic fantasies and
transference can provide the bridge for the transition back to reality rather
than serving as the defense against reality. It is only with therapeutic
progress that the patient can come to place reliance upon a more accurate
appraisal of himself and upon real, meaningful, and currently available
objects, and relinquish his ties to unrealistic, idyllic fantasies. But it may
require several years of therapy for the patient to articulate the symbiotic,
idyllic fantasies, to open the closed fantasy system to include the therapist,
to reexperience and work through the storms of ambivalent rage within the
therapeutic relationship, and to begin to make the transition back to reality,
at first tentatively, and hopefully eventually, in a consolidated and sustained
fashion. The idyllic fantasies provide the basis for the therapeutic alliance,
and they can become the vehicle for the eventual working through of basic
issues and conflicts, for establishing realistic interpersonal relationships, and
for developing appropriate plans and goals.

In summary, it should be stressed that these considerations about the
nature of the therapeutic process with schizophrenic and borderline patients
are based on a series of unexpected, yet highly consistent and replicated
findings about two primary modes of representation in psychosis. We
found that when seriously disturbed patients are able to maintain contact
with conventional reality, their concepts of the object are at developmental
levels lower than normal. Their representations are fragmented, poorly
articulated, lack cohesion and integration, and contain malevolent content.
These images seem to be representations of a hostile destructive reality in
which the patient has been exposed to overwhelming, traumatic, and even
catastrophic experiences in an unstable, unpredictable, destructive reality.
The second mode of representation in these patients occurs when they relin-

quish contact with conventional reality. Surprisingly, these idiosyncratic responses are at higher than normal developmental levels—the representations are well-differentiated, articulated, and integrated and usually have benevolent content. These representations appear to be rigidly held, preformed images based on social stereotypes which are split off from a painful, destructive, chaotic reality. These idyllic fantasies of schizophrenic patients can play a central role in the therapeutic process. The schizophrenic patient's wish for a well-ordered, coherent, consistent, caring relationship forms the basis for the therapeutic alliance. The idyllic fantasy provides the bridge through which the patient moves from an investment in his inner world to an involvement in the outer world. It provides the basis for the patient's tentatively venturing out into the real world, first within the therapeutic relationship and then more generally.

These findings about the nature of psychoses, and their implications for therapeutic process, offer further support for the importance of carefully considering both the content and the structure of the concepts of the self and of the object world.[7] It is these dimensions of the representational world that express man's unique symbolic capacity and aspects of his complex, interpersonal experiences. These dimensions provide insight into aspects of the organizing principles that determine and shape manifest behavior. Further understanding of these underlying structures and principles of organization not only can provide insight into aspects of schizophrenia, borderline states, and other types of psychopathology, but it may also enable us to understand many aspects of the more general and complex process of personality development.[40]

ACKNOWLEDGMENT

Earlier versions of this paper were presented at the Austen Riggs Center, Stockbridge, MA (10/76) and the Institute for Psychoanalytic Training and Research, New York, NY (5/78). We are endebted to Drs. Robert Rosenheck and Daniel P. Schwartz for their comments on this paper.

REFERENCES

1. Piaget J: *The Construction of Reality in the Child* New York, Basic Books, 1954. (Original French ed., 1937).
2. Werner H: *Comparative Psychology of Mental Development.* New York, International Universities Press, 1948.
3. *Werner H, Kaplan B: Symbol Formation: An Organismic-Developmental Approach to Language and the Expression of Thought.* New York, John Wiley & Sons Inc., 1963.

4. Decarie TG: *Intelligence and Affectivity in Early Childhood.* New York, International Universities Press, 1965.

5. Freud A: *Normality and Pathology in Childhood: Assessments of Development* New York, International Universities Press, 1965.

6. Wolff P: The developmental psychologies of Jean Piaget and psychoanalysis. *Psychological Issues*, Monograph 5. New York, International Universities Press, 1960.

7. Jacobson E: *The Self and the Object World.* New York, International Universities Press, 1964.

8. Mahler MS: Symbiosis and individuation: The psychological birth of the human infant. *Psychoanal Study Child* **29**:30–106, 1974.

9. Fraiberg S: Libidinal object constancy and mental representation. *Psychoanal Study Child* **24**:9–47, 1969.

10. Blatt SJ, Brenneis CB, Schimek J, et al: Normal development and psychopathological impairment of the concept of the object on the Rorschach. *J Abnorm Psychol* **85**:364–373, 1976.

11. Ritzler BA, Wyatt D, Harder D, et al: Psychotic patterns of the concept of the object on the Rorschach. *J Abnorm Psychol*, **89**:46–55, 1980.

12. Blatt SJ, Ritzler BA: Thought disorder and boundary disturbances in psychosis. *J. Consult Clin Psychol* **42**:370–381, 1974.

13. Blatt SJ, Wild CM: *Schizophrenia: A Developmental Analysis.* New York, Academic Press, 1976.

14. Blatt SJ, Wild CM, Ritzler BA: Disturbances of object representations in schizophrenia. *Psychoanalysis and Contemporary Science* **4**:235–288, 1975.

15. Brenneis CB: Features of the manifest dream in schizophrenia. *J Nerv Ment Dis* **153**:81–91, 1971.

16. Frosch J: Psychoanalytic considerations of the psychotic character. *J Am Psychoanal Assoc* **18**:24–50, 1970.

17. Klein M: Notes on some schizoid mechanisms. *Int J Psycho-Anal* **27**:99–110, 1946.

18. Schwartz DP: Aspects of schizophrenic regression: Defects, defense and disorganization. In the proceedings of Sixth International Symposium of Psychotherapy of Schizophrenia. Netherlands, *Excerpta Medica*, 1979.

19. Burnham D. Gladstone A., Gibson R: *Schizophrenia and the Need-Fear Dilemma.* New York, International Universities Press, 1969.

20. Boyer LB: Psychoanalytic technique in the treatment of certain characterlogical and schizophrenic disorders. *Int J Psycho-Anal* **52**:67–85, 1971.

21. Giovacchini PL: The influence of interpretation upon schizophrenic patients. *Int J Psycho-Anal* **50**:179–186, 1969.

22. Wexler M: Schizophrenia: Conflict and deficiency. *Psychoanal Quart* **40**:38–99, 1971.

23. Hartmann H: *Contributions to the Metapsychology of Schizophrenia. Psychoanal Study Child,* **8**:177–198, 1953.

24. Wexler M: The structural problem in schizophrenia: Therapeutic implications. *Int J Psycho-Anal* **32**:157–166, 1951.

25. Wexler M: The structural problem in schizophrenia: The role of the internal object, in Brody E, Redlich F (eds): *Psychotherapy with Schizophrenia.* New York, International Universities Press, 1952.

26. Wexler M: Hypothesis Concerning ego deficiency in schizophrenia, in Scher S & Davis H (eds): *The Outpatient Treatment of Schizophrenia.* New York, Grune and Stratton, 1960.

27. Bak RC: Object-relationships in schizophrenia and perversion. *Int J Psycho-Anal* **52**—235–242, 1971.

28. Greenson RR, Wexler, M: The non-transference relationship in the psycho-analytic situation. *Int J Psycho-Anal* **50**:27–39, 1969.

29. Freud S: *Neuropsychoses of defense* (*1894*). The Standard Edition of the Complete Works of Sigmund Freud, 3. London, Hogarth Press, 1962, pp 25–68.

30. Freud S: *Psycho-analytic notes on an autobiographical account of a case of paranoia* (*Dementia Paranoides*) (1911). The Standard Edition of the Complete Works of Sigmund Freud, 12, 3–82. London, Hogarth Press, 1958, pp 3–82.

31. Freud S: On narcissism: An introduction (1914). The Standard Edition of the Complete Work of Sigmund Freud, 14, 73–102. London, Hogarth Press, 1962, pp 73–102.

32. Freud S: *The unconscious* (1915). The Standard Edition of the Complete Works of Sigmund Freud, 14. London, Hogarth Press, 1962, pp 166–215.

33. Freud S: *Neurosis and psychosis* (1924a). The Standard Edition of the Complete Works of Sigmund Freud, 19. London, Hogarth Press, 1961, pp 149–153.

34. Freud S: The loss of reality in neurosis and psychosis (1924b). The Standard Edition of the Complete Works of Sigmund Freud, 19. London, Hogarth Press, 1961, pp 183–186.

35. Wexler M: Working through in the therapy of schizophrenia. *Int J Psycho-Anal* **46**:279–286, 1965.

36. Fenichel O: *Psychoanalytic Theory of Neurosis*. New York, WW Norton & Co, 1945.

37. Searles H. *Collected Papers on Schizophrenia and Related Subjects*. New York, International Universities Press, 1965.

38. Smith S: The golden fantasy: A regressive reaction to separation anxiety. *Int J Psycho-Anal* **58**:311–324, 1977.

39. Jacobson E: Contribution to the metapsychology of psychotic identifications. *J Am Psychoanal Assoc* **2**:239–262, 1954.

40. Blatt SJ: Levels of object representation in anaclitic and introjective depression. *Psychoanal Study Child* **29**:107–157, 1974.

Chapter 10

Problems Inherent in the Study of Psychotherapy of Psychoses

Conclusions from a Community Psychiatric Action Research Study

YRJÖ O. ALANEN, VILJO RÄKKÖLÄINEN, JUHANI LAAKSO, and RIITTA RASIMUS

The methodological problems inherent in the study of psychodynamics and psychotherapy of the psychoses deserve a critical examination because of the influence they have on the results achieved. Our research culture, based, as it is, on the methodologies of natural science, easily devaluates observations which rest on a case-specific approach difficult to confirm by experimental methods. Still, much of the most creative and clinically useful work in this field has been based on penetrating observations of individual cases relatively few in number; an excellent example of this being the classic study of seventeen families of schizophrenic patients carried out at the Yale University Department of Psychiatry by Lidz, Fleck, and Cornelison.[1] Such a study, inseparably linked with an extended clinical situation, would not have been possible to execute by making use of simultaneous and matched control material. Employing a natural scientific method, the observational angle would have been more narrow and superficial, of necessity. While saying this, we do not deny the significance of experimental research design (e.g. in verifying the observations based on a case-specific approach).

YRJÖ O. ALANEN, VILJO RÄKKÖLÄINEN, JUHANI LAAKSO and RIITTA RASIMUS • Department of Psychiatry, University of Turku, Turku, Finland.

Similar constellations occur in studying the results of psychotherapy. Here the restricting influence of an experimental research design is also obvious, not only by making the observational level superficial, but sometimes also distorting it as we are going to indicate later. On the other hand, the dangers of subjectivity's leading to faulty appraisal are actual, particularly when the therapists are themselves also investigating the effects of treatment.

In the following, we attempt to elucidate certain salient problems concerning explicit research objectives and attitudes relative to the psychotherapeutic treatment of psychotic patients, considering them in the framework of the problems we have encountered in our own work and have attempted to solve.

THE TURKU COMMUNITY PSYCHIATRIC SCHIZOPHRENIA PROJECT

Background and Objectives

Our research is carried out in Turku, Finland, by a four-person team of two psychiatrists, a psychologist, and a nurse with special training in psychiatric work. The background of our work is based on the experience gained, during a period now exceeding ten years, from the development of a broadly based psychotherapeutic treatment approach in the care of schizophrenic patients at the Turku University Department of Psychiatry, and from the research activities connected with it. This approach combines the psychotherapeutic and social psychiatric views reflected in the individual studies published earlier.[2-8]

Our present project started in the spring of 1976. It centers on two objectives.

1. We want to find out what activities and resources should be required in a model of schizophrenia treatment which could be realized in an ordinary community psychiatric setting and which would also be optimal according to our family-centered and psychotherapeutically oriented views of schizophenia and its treatment.

2. We are also interested in the effects of our treatment model on the prognosis of the patients.

It is important to emphasize that we are not studying the results of psychotherapy compared with other kinds of treatment, but the possible effects achieved by a global psychotherapeutic treatment orientation of schizophrenic patients. Our concept of schizophrenia is multifaceted, emphasizing, however, the interactional origin, and the psychologically comprehensible nature of this disorder.[6,9,10]

The emphasis laid on community psychiatry in our project is concordant with the public health policy of our country. It also reflects our views that opportunities for psychotherapy should not be restricted to a few socially and economically privileged patients. There is reason to point out, in this connection, that many recent studies concerning the prognosis of schizophrenic patients in community psychiatry clearly indicate the limitations of current treatment approaches in improving the prognosis of schizophrenia from its present level. This also indicates an increasing demand for finding new treatment approaches. For example, follow-up studies of schizophrenic first admissions in Helsinki, Finland, carried out on samples from 1950, 1960, 1965, and 1970, with a follow-up interval of five years,[11-13] showed that the favorable development found in the outcome of treatment in the transition from the 1960s was no longer observable in the transition from the 1960s to the 1970s. Although hospital stays had become shorter, the clinical and psychosocial status of the patients was found to be somewhat poorer than before (Cf. also chapter 3 of this volume.)

The Community Psychiatric Circumstances

The city of Turku, which has 165,000 inhabitants and an additional population of some 15,000 students, forms its own mental health district. It proves a particularly good setting for research concerning community psychiatry, since its system of communal services also includes the teaching hospital of the Department of Psychiatry of the University of Turku (called the Psychiatric Clinic) which receives its patients from the catchment area of this district and works in close cooperation with the other treatment units of the district. These units are illustrated more clearly in the following Table.

TABLE I. Community Psychiatric Treatment Units of the Mental Health District of the City of Turku

Hospitals	
Psychiatric clinic (University Hospital)	111 beds
Psychiatric clinic (University Hospital)	18 day patients
Kupittaa Hospital	364 beds
Other hospitals (chronic patients)	139 beds
Altogether 3.7 beds per 1000 inhabitants	

Open Care
Two Mental Health Offices
After-care activity of the Psychiatric Clinic
Psychiatric Outpatient Clinic of the University Central Hospital (General Hospital)
The Outpatient Clinic for Alcoholics and the private sector included, there were altogether 408 psychiatric outpatient visits per 1000 inhabitants 15 years of age and over in 1977.

The resources of the communal outpatient treatment system are inadequate. This is compensated for by the facts that there are in Turku, as elsewhere in Finland, also psychiatrists engaged in private practice. There is also a foundation-based psychotherapeutic outpatient clinic, as well as a mental health service for students. Cooperation between the field of community psychiatry and the private sector functions well, and we have been able to rely also on the latter in developing our action-research-oriented project. According to recent studies, Turku can be regarded as an area of relatively abundant outpatient services, in terms of Finnish conditions.[14]

The General Design of the Present Project

Our present research project includes all those patients, a total of 100, aged 16 to 45 and living in Turku, who entered treatment for a schizophrenia-type disorder for the first time at an outpatient or inpatient treatment unit operating in the sector of community psychiatry in the Turku Mental Health District during a period extending from April 1, 1976 to October 31, 1977.

Three of our team members work at the Psychiatric Clinic, and one in a Mental Health Office of the district. We carried out a psychiatric and psychological investigation of these patients, and also interviewed the patients' closest relatives (the parents, the spouse, and in certain cases siblings or other persons close to the patient). The central data obtained from the psychiatric investigation, which was thus extended to the family as a whole, were entered on a research questionnaire. This questionnaire is a modification of one constructed at the psychiatric Department and designed as an aid to both research and everyday clinical work.[6,8] It includes 163 multiple-choice items, covering, in addition to the usual information on the patient's clinical status and social background, assessments based on psychodynamic and family research on schizophrenia. The last part of the questionnaire includes a place for a recommendation of an optimal treatment plan consistent with available psychiatric services.

According to the "action research" nature of our study, the caretaking personnel in both hospital and outpatient services have been stimulated to provide psychotherapeutic treatment as part of the treatment plans. The team has held consultative meetings and provided supervision and guidance for their work. Only part of the patients and/or their families have been under direct care of the team members.

The first follow-up survey of the patients was scheduled to take place two years after entrance into treatment and is currently being carried out. This part of the study includes again both psychiatric investigation and psychological tests.

The family members are also reinterviewed. A multidimensional assessment of prognosis, as well as an evaluation of the effects of the treatment on the outcome, are carried out for each patient. The second follow-up survey will be carried out seven and a half years after the beginning of the treatment.

In investigating the outcome of treatment, the following five dimensions are considered:

1. The descriptive-psychiatric dimension (clinical symptoms)

2. The psychodynamic dimension (the development of interpersonal relationships with the family and other social environment, the intrapsychic status of the patient)

3. The psychosocial dimension (social adjustment, working history, survey of incidence, frequency and length of hospital stays)

4. The socioeconomic dimension (sick-leave compensations, disability pensions, social assistance, etc.)

5. The phenomenological dimension (the way in which the patient and his family experienced the disorder and its treatment)

THE APPROACH: METHOD ORIENTATION VERSUS PROBLEM ORIENTATION

Distorting Effects of the Method-Oriented Approach

In planning the therapeutic and research procedures to be used in the project, we have deliberately given up certain methodological designs which in our opinion are in conflict with our present knowledge of the psychotherapy of psychotic patients.

One such question concerns the "method-oriented" versus "problem-oriented" approach in research. Many studies of the effectiveness of various forms of treatment in psychosis which have been based on a model derived from the natural sciences are, by their very point of departure, method-oriented in such a way that they cannot give an adequate picture of the possibilities of psychotherapeutic treatment modes. Typical of these studies (e.g. May,[15] May et al[16]) is that different forms of treatment have been applied to different patient groups, set up randomly, and thus rendered mutually comparable. Findings concerning the effectiveness of the various treatment modes are then obtained in the form of undifferentiated, statistically significant facts, easy to condense, to read, and to interpret.

We shall not discuss the criteria postulated for psychotherapy in these studies, or the problems inherent in their methods of measuring the patient's improvement or "cure." Instead, our intention is to show, by means of observations and solutions of our study, how that type of method-oriented approach may, from the very outset, introduce factors which influence and distort the results obtained, thus already rendering their value dubious, at least as far as the possibilities of psychotherapeutic activities are concerned.

TABLE II.   Distribution of Patients by Age and Diagnostic Group

Age	Schizo-phrenia	Paranoid psychosis (near) schizo-phrenia)	Acute schizo-phreni-form psychosis	Schizo-affective psychosis	Border-line psychosis	Total
16–25	20	1	2	3	8	34
26–35	17	1	9	9	10	46
36–45	7	2	7	1	3	20
Total	44	4	18	13	21	100

We know, for example, that an unselected group of schizophrenic patients is, in terms of both their clinical pictures and their psychological problems, a highly herterogeneous group of individuals whose life situations also vary largely from patient to patient. As an illustration of this, the distribution of our present sample by age and diagnostic groups is shown in Table II.

The diagnostic and psychodynamic heterogeneity has very direct relevance and practical implications for the psychotherapeutic management of schizophrenic patients. The therapeutic challenge created by, say, an isolated nineteen-year-old hebephrenic boy living with his parents is very different from that created by a forty-year-old married woman fallen ill with an acute schizo-affective psychosis, or from the challenge created by a paranoid schizophrenic man living alone. *The psychotherapeutic treatment approach should be individually planned in each case*, taking into consideration the nature of the disorder and of the patient, as well as the constellations formed by his most significant interpersonal relationships and their dynamic effects on the disorder. This kind of critical examination of therapeutic strategies is usually omitted in the frames of formalistic method-oriented research plans.

The Problem-Oriented Approach: Determining the Indications for Different Modes of Psychotherapy

On the basis of the therapeutic diagnosis referred to above, we have in our study assigned the patients to various treatment categories following a problem-oriented approach. The following table shows the pattern of indications for different forms of psychotherapy, determined on the basis of our initial examination (cf. Alanen et al.).[17] Besides the clinical and psychodynamic constellation, an assessment of the possibilities of motivating the patient and/or his family for treatment were taken into account.

Individual therapy with psychotic patients, which takes place in a dyad consisting of the patient and his therapist, has a long tradition beginning with Sullivan,[18] Federn,[19] and Sechehaye,[20] and, as the table shows, it plays an important role in our treatment orientation as well. The same tradition, however, has revealed also the limitations of the dyadic treatment setting. Positive results cannot be obtained with all patients, as was shown by the catamnestic studies of Müller[21] and Schulz.[22] In our project, the most important indication for "intensive individual psychotherapy"—meaning, in our case, a minimum frequency of one session per week—was the investigator's view of whether the patient would be able to benefit from a therapeutic process working toward conscious developmental goals in a two-person relationship, and whether there would be adequate motivation for realizing this in the particular case. Although it was decided that psychotherapy was indicated in one fourth of our patient sample, a possibility for a less differentiated individual contact with a caretaking person was considered as needed in almost all cases.

Due to the findings of Lidz's group[1,23] and other family investigators (e.g., Alanen,[24] Wynne et al.,[25,26] Stierlin[27]) the very important role played by the family environment in the etiology of psychotic disorders and their treatment has been recognized over the last few decades in all its significance. Although problems related to the family are also relevant in other psychiatric disorders, the disorders of the family environment in schizophrenia are particularly severe and the concomitant pathology of the intrafamilial relational network more aberrant than, for example, in neuroses (Alanen et al.).[28] Therefore, in the case of many schizophrenic patients, individual therapy for the patient is impossible unless treatment is provided for the family too.*

TABLE III. Number of New Schizophrenic Patients Indicated for Different Forms of Psychotherapy (Alanen et al., 1979)

	$N \, (= \%)$
1. *Individual psychotherapies*	
Intensive individual therapy	25
Other individual contact	71
2. *Family therapies*	
Conjoint family therapy	16
Marital or couple therapy	26
Other contacts with the patient's family	55
3. *Group Therapy* (Open Care)	10
4. *Psychotherapeutic community in the hospital ward*	63

* Alanen[10] has recently, in another connection, given a survey of his studies of the interactional pathogenesis of schizophrenia, examining especially the parents' relations to their children, and the transactional defense mechanisms characteristic of these relationships.

A conjoint family therapy is often necessary with the families of the youngest patients, in whom the developmental disturbance and the onset of the patient's psychosis is usually most intimately connected with intrafamilial interpersonal relations in the form of unsolved mutual separation problems. Our experience indicates that there is an urgent need for a *conjoint couple therapy* in the case of most of those patients who became schizophrenic after marriage (cf. also Alanen & Kinnunen).[29] The preventive psychiatric implications concerning the following generation are also usually considerable, and must be taken into account.

According to our assessments, a more global family-centered treatment, based on contacts with our patient's family members, was indicated also in nearly all of the other cases. The great importance of the problems involving the family revealed by our approach would lead us to contend that those studies of the psychotherapy of schizophrenic patients in which the treatment has been provided without any contact with the patient's family and his other environment outside the hospital (e.g., the study of Grinspoon et al.)[30] must be regarded as highly inadequate.

Table III also shows the importance we have placed on *the psychotherapeutic community** in the case of these patients who are in treatment for the first time. Regressed psychotic patients as a rule are particularly in need of hospital treatment in a wider therapeutic milieu, where the patient can be taken care of and approached in an empathic way outside the scheduled and planned therapy hours as well as in them. In many cases, this kind of broadly based therapeutic encounter is a prerequisite for the successful initiation of subsequent psychotherapy, helping the consolidation of the motivation of both the patient and the family. We consider this shared empathic attitude toward the patients and their families one of the basic hallmarks of the psychotherapeutic community formed by our hospital ward for psychotic patients. Another hallmark is the development of individual therapeutic relationships between the staff members and the patients, often based on the spontaneously arising contact.[9]

On the basis of the above, it is probably easy to understand what serious difficulties we would have encountered in actual treatment practice and what problems would have resulted in trying to "measure" the treatment results in order to assess the effectiveness of different modes of psychotherapy if we had, for instance, divided our sample rigidly into four groups and tried to treat each group by means of either individual therapy, family therapy, group therapy, or drug treatment without other form of therapy. It may be noted that the research team as well as the caretaking staff shared the view that such a procedure would not only lead to poorer

---

* We use this term to emphasize the caretaking, parental attitude of the personnel (cf. Alanen).[9]

treatment results, but would also exert a destructive effect on the basic hallmarks of our psychotherapeutic community, and on its whole therapeutic atmosphere.

PROBLEMS INHERENT IN THE ASSESSMENT OF TREATMENT RESULTS

Solution of the Problem of Control Materials in the Turku Project

Our problem-oriented approach to research and therapy does not solve the problems posed by the assessment and comparison of treatment results which are great indeed. For the reasons just referred to, we are not using control materials consisting of patients treated without psychotherapy. There are some possibilities, however, for comparing our results with contemporaneous follow-up data based on studies carried out elsewhere in our country and outside of its borders. Especially relevant are the follow-up studies of first-admission schizophrenics treated in Helsinki, another urban Finnish mental district.[11-13] In Helsinki, the psychotherapeutic treatment orientation plays a lesser role than in Turku, in terms of the number of patients involved.

In the Turku schizophrenia project, we have chosen a solution which is integrated into the overall design of our project, and made possible by the local circumstances. It is illustrated in Table IV.

The psychotherapeutic orientation in the treatment of psychotic patients was first introduced in Turku in the years 1967–1968; in the former year, the Psychiatric Clinic was established to operate as an independent hospital unit. The psychotherapeutic orientation has thereafter developed gradually, centering first on hospital treatment, and then extending also to the sector of outpatient treatment. We have gathered data on three samples

TABLE IV. The Overall Design of The Turku Community Psychiatric Schizophrenia Project

First admission of the sample	Number of patients	Phase of psychotherapeutic treatment orientation	Follow-up investigations
1965–1967	100	not organized	1973–1974
1969	68	scattered, hospital-centered	1971
			1976–1977
1976–1977	100	more broad and explicit, open care included	1978–1979
			(1983–1985)

of new cases of schizophrenia drawn from the same basic population. These groups correspond closely in terms of age distribution, social structure, and diagnosis. Their therapy has been provided in the setting of the same community health-care system, but they represent different stages in the evolution of this system toward an increasing and explict emphasis on a psychotherapeutic orientation as the basic framework for treatment, both in theory and in practice.

At the end of all the follow-up periods, we shall have three mutually comparable samples. For each succeeding sample, the proportion of psychotherapy they received as part of the treatment has increased in comparison with the sample that preceded it. The extent of psychotherapy used in each case is relatively easy to measure in terms of the time required by the various forms of psychotherapeutic activities, frequency of visits, and hours in supervisions and guidance of the work. If the treatment results of the different samples also differ from each other, we shall be able to draw certain conclusions as to the usefulness of psychotherapy in schizophrenia in general, as well as in the particular case when the aim is the adequate utilization of various treatment modes in existing conditions of community psychiatry, providing a viable basis for such work.

Advantages and Problems

This research setting brings with it both advantages and problems. From the viewpoint of comparative research, a special advantage may be mentioned, arising from the conditions of our country: the fact that in Finland patients are generally easily reached for research purposes. Thus, 88 out of a total of 100 patients were reached in the follow-up study carried out on our first sample after seven and half years; as nine patients had died, only three subjects were lost to the follow-up for other reasons.[8] Information was obtained on these subjects, as on those who had died, from family members and treatment units, as well as from different kinds of social institutes.

One of the problems connected with our research setting is that the samples from 1965–1967 and 1969 consist of new hospital patients, whereas in the case of the 1976–1977 sample, the patients came to either an outpatient or a hospital treatment unit operating in the section of community psychiatry. Methodological problems that arise from this circumstance may, however, be relatively easy to solve in connection with the processing of the data.

Another problem connected with the evaluation of treatment results is the part played by *drugs* in our treatment approach. An assessment of the indications for drug treatment, too, was made in our newest patient sample, and we are measuring the amount of drug treatment actually used in all of the samples. There is a typical if not very strict difference between the samples of new schizophrenic patients drawn from 1965–1967 and 1976–1977 in this respect. The patients from the former sample had received neuroleptic drugs in somewhat larger doses than those in the latter. In the former sample, drugs formed the basis for treatment, and all the patients received them. However, nearly all of the patients in the latter sample likewise received neuroleptics at least in mild doses, during some phase of their treatment,' often provided as a support to psychotherapy. Another difference between the nature of the treatment of these two samples was that the first hospitalization was on the average somewhat shorter in the former than in the latter sample, in keeping with goals of the psychotherapeutic community. Both of these differences may be regarded as typical contrasts between a more directive therapy of schizophrenic patients which rests heavily on drugs, on one hand, and treatment centering primarily on psychotherapy, on the other. As pointed out previously, we are comparing the results of different treatment orientations rather than those of different treatment modes. Our psychotherapeutic approach does not exclude a moderate use of neuroleptic drugs.

During the ten-year period that separates our samples from each other, certain changes have taken place in social conditions and attitudes toward mental illness in Finland. It is not easy to estimate their exact influence on the treatment results, but, in our opinion, it may be regarded as relatively slight. The most important of these changes is probably the change in the criteria for disability pensions, which became more relaxed in the early 1970s.

A central part of the work of our new project is the investigation of the *suitability of different forms of psychotherapy and family-centered approach for various kinds of patient groups*, taking into consideration such variables as the patient's sex, age, social class, marital status, family-dynamic constellation, and diagnostic group (whether nuclear schizophrenia or other). Our results concerning indications of different treatment modes in relation to background variables of this kind have been published in another report.[18] The assessment of the results of psychotherapeutic treatment modes will be largely based on the empirical, clinical observation of individual cases; the values of this method in psychiatric research should not, in our view, be underestimated.

The Caring Team versus an "Independent" Investigator in the Follow-Up Survey

A classic problem in the psychotherapeutic research—which we have referred to already in the beginning of this paper—is that of the "objectivity" of the psychotherapeutically oriented investigator who has entered into close contact and relationships with the patients in assessing possible correlations between treatment and outcome. At present, nearly three years have elapsed from the beginning of the study, and the first follow-up survey is under way. A total of 24 patients included in our present project have been under the direct care of the four team members who have provided either their individual or family therapy. In addition, we have participated in the treatment of many of our patients through the supervision and guidance of clinical work, support provided for family members, meetings to outline treatment plans for patients, and the solving of many administrative problems.

This is the situation we have deliberately aimed at from the very beginning, since we have wanted to influence actively the treatment received by our patients in accordance with the principles of action research. Though we think it is somewhat paradoxical that the persons who actually know the patients best may be considered disqualified for making certain important follow-up assessments, we are ready to admit that this is partly the case. We would like to emphasize, however, that the position of noninvolved investigator is not without its problems either. His findings may easily remain superficial if he is not able to establish empathic contact—the principal instrument of observation in psychotherapeutic research—with the patient he is dealing with. And this is again impossible for him unless he gives up his external, measuring approach, at least temporarily. In order to be able to understand sufficiently what he is studying, he should have an implicitly therapeutic attitude toward the human being involved. This is particularly true in the case of psychotic patients whose inner world cannot normally be approached without a specific empathy. The question of how the procedures pertaining to treatment and those pertaining to research can be implemented without adverse effects on the meaningfulness of the study on one hand, and reliability of the results on the other, represents, in fact, a central problem in research concerning the psychotherapy of psychotic patients.

We have solved this problem in the following way: the psychiatric follow-up examination is carried out both by the original research team, and by a psychiatrist (Dr. Ritva Järvi), independent of the team, who has not otherwise participated in the study and has not met the patients earlier. The team members who met the patients and their families in the early phase of the study possess, just because of this acquaintance, important knowledge which contributes to the value of their assessments. On the other hand, the more outside position of the independent psychiatrist gives to her estimates an uninfluenced background.

Both the independent psychiatrist and the original investigating team have, accordingly, their own significant contribution to make to the follow-up study. Each of them has his own follow-up questionnaires which partly overlap, making possible two independent follow-up investigations. This methodological approach also makes it possible to examine the problem of objectivity in a research design in which a basic research instrument is precisely that of "subjectivity," or, in other words, empathic observation on the part of the investigators who have influenced by their knowledge of the subjects and by their treatment relationships with them.

COMMENT

In the present paper, certain typical problems inherent in the study of psychotherapy with schizophrenic patients are dealt with in the light of the work of our own research project.

Given a conception of schizophrenia as a psychologically comprehensible disorder of personality growth and adjustment, interactional in origin, the psychotherapy must be planned individually for each patient, taking into consideration both the nature of the disorder itself, and the patient's life situation. Of central importance are the effects of the interactional psychodynamics of the family unit, as well as the other significant interpersonal relationships of the patient. Only when these factors are taken into account in planning the research approach is it possible to obtain a relevant picture of the possibilities of psychotherapeutic activities in the treatment of schizophrenic patients. In spite of their apparent "objectivity," rigidly method-centered research projects may introduce factors which influence and distort the results achieved. It is also essential that the investigators have an adequate knowledge of the specific nature of psychological problems of schizophrenic patients, elucidated by psychoanalytic and family dynamic investigations.

The results of our own study are not reported in the paper, since the first follow-up survey is not yet complete. We have already come to the conclusion, however, in agreement with the Norwegian, Ugelstad,[31] that the implementation of individually planned psychotherapeutic forms of treatment (individual therapy, family therapy, group therapy, treatment in a psychotherapeutic community) is possible in the setting of community psychiatry without an inordinate increase in resources. What this does require is an integrated, psychotherapeutically and also family-oriented, broadly based approach to treatment, shared by the members of the caretaking staff and reinforced by supervision and guidance.

REFERENCES

1. Lidz T, Fleck S, Cornelison AR: *Schizophrenia and the Family.* New York, International Universities Press, 1965.
2. Alanen YO, Laine A, Räkköläinen V, et al: Evolving the psychotherapeutic community: Research combined with hospital treatment of schizophrenia, Paper presented at the Conference on Schizophrenia: The Implications of Research Findings on Treatment and Teaching. Washington, D.C., NIMH, 1970.

3. Alanen YO, Laine A: Development of hospital centered community psychotherapy service for schizophrenic patients: Evaluation of the first phase, in Wing JK, Häfner H (eds): *Roots of Evaluation: The Epidemiological Basis for Planning Psychiatric Services.* London, Oxford University Press, 1973, pp 309–327.

4. Salonen S: On the technique of the psychotherapy of schizophrenia, in Jorstad J, Ugelstad E (eds): *Schizophrenia 75.* Oslo, Universitetsforlaget, 1976, pp 115–133.

5. Räkköläinen V: Psychodynamic and interpersonal aspects of the onset of psychosis, in Jorstad J, Ugelstad E (eds): *Schizophrenia 75.* Oslo, Universitetsforlaget, 1976, pp 1–70.

6. Räkköläinen V: Onset of Psychosis: A clinical study of 68 cases. *Ann Univ Turku Ser D,* **7:**1–70, 1977.

7. Salokangas RKR: Skitsofreniaan sairastuneiden psykososiaalinen kehitys (The Psychosocial Development of Schizophrenic Patients). *Kansanelakeläitoksen julkaisuja* Sarja AL 7, Turku 1977, English summary pp 329–377.

8. Salokangas RKR: Psychosocial prognosis in schizophrenia. *Ann Univ Turku, Ser D,* **9:**1–174, 1978.

9. Alanen YO: The psychotherapeutic care of schizophrenic patients in a community psychiatric setting, in Lader MH (ed): *Studies of Schizophrenia. Br J Psychiat* Spec Pub 1 No 10, 1975, pp 86–93.

10. Alanen YO: In search of the interactional origin of schizophrenia. The Stanley R Dean Award Lecture, in Hofling CK, Lewis JM, (eds): *The Family: Evaluation and Treatment.* New York, Bruner/Mazel, 1980, pp 285–313.

11. Achté KA: On Prognosis and Rehabilitation in Schizophrenic and Paranoid Psychoses. *Acta psychiatr Scand* **43** (suppl 196): 1–217, 1967.

12. Niskanen P, Achté KA: *The Course and Prognosis of Schizophrenic Psychoses in Helsinki: A Comparative Study of First Admissions in 1950, 1960, and 1965.* Monographs from the Psychiatric Clinic of the Helsinki University Central Hospital, No 4, 1972.

13. Achté KA, Niskanen P, Lönnqvist J: The prognosis of schizophrenic psychoses in Helsinki, first admission in 1950, 1960, 1965 and 1970 with five-year follow-up, in *Psychiatria Fennica, 1980* (Yearbook), in press.

14. Lehtinen V, Salokangas RKR, Holm H, et al: Need and realization of the open care of mental health disorders. *Sosiaalilääketieteellinen Aikakauslehti* (Journal of Social Medicine in Finland) **16:**280–291, 1979 (with English summary).

15. May PRA: *Treatment of Schizophrenia.* New York, Science House, 1968.

16. May PRA, Tuma AH, Yale C, et al: Schizophrenia: A follow-up study of results of treatment. *Arch Gen Psychiatry* **33:**474–486, 1976.

17. Alanen YO, Räkköläinen V, Rasimus R, et al: Indications for different forms of psychotherapy with new schizophrenic patients in community psychiatry, in Müller C (ed): *Psychotherapy of Schizophrenia. Excerpta Med Int Cong Ser* No 464, pp 185–202, Amsterdam-Oxford, 1979, p. 185.

18. Sullivan HA: The modified psychoanalytic treatment of schizophrenia. *Am J Psychiatry* **88:**519–540, 1931.

19. Federn P: Psychoanalysis of psychoses. *Psychiatr Q* **17:**3–19, 246–257, 470–487, 1943.

20. Sechehaye MA: *A New Psychotherapy of Schizophrenia.* New York, Grune & Stratton 1956 (French original in 1947).

21. Müller C: Die Psychotherapie Schizophrener an der Zürcher Klinik. Versuch einer Vorläufigen katamnestischen Übersicht. *Nervenarzt* **32:**354–368, 1961.

22. Schulz CC: A follow-up report on admissions to Chestnut Lodge: 1948–1958. *Psychiatr Q* **37:**220–233, 1963.

23. Lidz T, Cornelison AR, Fleck S, et al: The intrafamilial environment of schizophrenic patients: II. Marital schism and marital skew. *Am J Psychiatr* **114:**241–248, 1957.

24. Alanen YO: The mothers of schizophrenic patients. *Acta Psychiatr Neurol Scand* 33 (Suppl 124): 1–361, 1958.

25. Wynne LC, Ryckoff IM, Day JR, et al: Pseudomutuality in the family relations of schizophrenics. *Psychiatry* **21**:205–220, 1958.
26. Wynne LC, Singer MT, Toohey ML: Communication of the adoptive parents of schizophrenics, in Jorstad J. Ugelstad E (eds): *Schizophrenia 75*. Oslo, Universitetsforlaget, 1976, pp 413–451.
27. Stierlin H: Family dynamics and separation patterns of potential schizophrenics, in Rubinstein D, Alanen YO (eds): *Psychotherapy of Schizophrenia*. Amsterdam, *Excerpta Medica* 1972, pp 169–180.
28. Alanen YO, Rekola JK, Stewen A, et al: The family in the pathogenesis of schizophrenic and neurotic disorders. *Acta psychiatr Scand* 42 (suppl 189): 1–654, 1966.
29. Alanen YO, Kinnunen P: Marriage and the development of schizophrenia, *Psychiatry* **38**:436–465, 1975.
30. Grinspoon L, Ewalt JR, Shader R: *Schizophrenia: Pharmacotherapy and Psychotherapy*. Baltimore, Williams & Wilkins Co, 1972.
31. Ugelstad E: Possibilities of organizing psychotherapeutically oriented treatment programs for schizophrenia within sectorized psychiatric service, in Müller C (ed): *Psychotherapy of Schizophrenia. Excerpta Medica Int Cong Ser* No 464, pp 253–258, Amsterdam-Oxford, 1979.

Chapter 11

Insight and Self-Observation

Their Role in the Analysis of the Etiology of Illness

ALFRED H. STANTON

ON READING MINDS

The subtitle, "On Reading Minds," is not without risk in a symposium of experts on schizophrenia, particularly if it suggests a cookbook set of directions. However, the way one reads minds is clear; it is similar to the way one reads books. One listens to what someone else has to say, and hears what that person has in mind; not everything in his mind, and not necessarily accurately what is in his mind, but something of what he has in mind. This is a wonderful and improbable set of phenomena: that thoughts are quickly transferred back and forth between two organisms in a universe which, at first glance, would not seem to be a likely place for such an occurrence.

The psychiatrist or any other student interested in schizophrenia knows of the manifestations of schizophrenia, its associated suffering, the course of the disturbance, indeed, even of its very existence, only, in the final analysis, by being told of the experience by the person suffering it. From this "raw data" the student develops his theoretical concepts regarding the disorder

ALFRED H. STANTON • Department of Psychiatry, Harvard Medical School and Senior Consulting Psychiatrist, McLean Hospital, Belmont, Massachusetts 02178.

and its treatment, using more or less systematic methods as carefully as he can. In this procedure, he is doing the same type of analysis which occurs in those disciplines generally lumped together as the humanities—history, the social sciences, psychology, linguistics—which are united by the fact that their data is in large part, or exclusively, drawn from human communications, in contrast to the "natural sciences," where the contrary is the case—where data are drawn in large part or exclusively from other sources than human communications.

A great deal of attention has been given to the analysis and creation of methods for developing the data of the natural sciences—Nobel prizes have been given for highly specialized measuring instruments alone. Considerable study has also been given to the methods of the humanitites, although much less, and most of it less well developed. There has, of course, been some borrowing of methods, mostly from the natural sciences by the humanities, but there are limitations to the amount which can be borrowed with profit.

How the student of schizophrenia elaborates the long and often confused interview material is critically important. Psychoanalysis has made exclusive use of patient or subject reports as its source material, and has developed an elaborate and sophisticated technique for dealing with this material—largely for clinical purposes—with much less attention given to how to use the data to develop new knowledge. Those scholars interested in the psychodynamic or sociodynamic analysis of schizophrenic patients for scientific purposes have been forced, whether they would or not, into a familiarity with psychoanalytic methods and have used these methods for scientific purposes. A more explicit consideration of the methods used should therefore be useful.

Ricoeur[1] has recently given a penetrating analysis of the nature of proof in Freud's writing. The humanities represent systematic disciplines aimed at the fullest possible understanding of what people say, write, or paint; in contrast, the methods of the natural sciences are heavily based upon explanation—developing and testing hypotheses and theories which provide causal and predictive information.

Ricoeur emphasizes that we must use both methods of analysis together, even though various scholars have tried to assert that they are discontinuous, a nonintersecting language game; indeed, the usual American solution is to divide what an interviewer does into two parts—a scientific one and the clinical one, the clinical taking usually a second-class status. While the psychoanalyst may insist that his psychoanalysis is indeed research, he often does so with an inner reservation, and he is not likely to be widely accepted in this role. The systematic elaboration of the semantic precision, organization, stability, and coherence of generalizations—which would move the individual experience of understanding someone toward a more stable and generalizable knowledge—has indeed proceeded within psychoanalysis, but the process is discouragingly complex.

Ricoeur points out that even Freud found himself using increasingly unsatisfactory metaphors when he arrived at an intersection between the elaboration of his analysis of *understanding* and the provision of *explanation* with its cause and effect formulations; his metapsychology never did illuminate his technical papers. But, however unsatisfactory, the metaphors were unavoidable for Ricoeur, uniting the processes of understanding and of explanation in an ongoing complex process of "interpretation."

There are two reasons why it is appropriate to discuss this topic here. First, the contributions of Ted and Ruth Lidz are excellent examples of clinical and investigative application of the methods of the humanities in a medical discipline. In a singularly clear way, the work of Lidz, Fleck, and Cornelison changed the conception of schizophrenia. There had been smoke before, of course—discussions of the mothers of schizophrenics, the relation of the disorder to social disorder in general, and social class relations were being established, but with the Lidz work it was clear that the family, not one particular member, was the proper subject—that the family structure and the structure of the patient's disorder were systematically related to each other in ways which could not be seen unless one looked at it the way they did. Experimental methods were not only impossible—had they been possible, they would have been wrong. Their work was a significant underpinning of a whole new method of treatment which has grown in importance, and their work is known to everyone, even to those who are so resistant to the humanities that they cannot bring themselves to examine exactly what the Lidz study reported.

A second reason for introducing the issue here is its pertinence to our topic of research in psychotherapy, a field where many think of research method versus clinical method. There has recently been a spate of discussion about why the practice of psychotherapy has benefitted so little from research in psychotherapy. I am not certain that the premise is as clearly warranted as the question states, but many have seemed sure of it. It is true that most psychotherapists believe that what they have learned about patients comes primarily from clinical rather than from organized research efforts. If one pushes hard for more objective procedures in psychotherapy, he will be certainly thought of by many of his colleagues as abandoning psychotherapy, at least to some extent. And psychotherapists do tend to stick to their work, and their convictions. At the same time, those students most emphatically skeptical of the effects of psychotherapy on "research" grounds seek to find indirect ways to recommend it clinically.

This is not a sign of chaos, gullibility, or cupidity. The coherence and intelligibility of the events of psychotherapy and of the emotional disorders studied in psychotherapy act as continuing reinforcers for psychotherapists. After it was first shown that schizophrenic patients were understandable, and something of how to understand them, such patients have never been left alone in the same matter-of-fact way they were before. This is, in principle, the same kind of coherence which Lidz showed in the families he studied, which Roman Jakobson brought to the distinctive features of phonemes, Champollion to the grasp of the nature of hieroglyphic writing, or Turner to the understanding of the influence of the frontier on American life—it is the observation of a coherent structure, in every case derived from the human understanding of the scholar.

INSIGHT

Insight, the goal of psychoanalysis and of much of dynamic psychotherapy, condenses into itself both the values of therapy and those of research. The identification and analysis of relationships, of structures previously unrecognized, represent insight, for instance, into family structure and psychotic limitation. I should like, however, to restrict the term insight, here, sharply, to any grasp *by the patient* of his own inner life; reserving other terms for anything learned by the therapist or others. Insight, in this sense, is particularly pertinent to our topic of schizophrenia. But the concept has a long history in psychology, especially among the Gestalt psychologists (Wertheimer), and in psychoanalysis. For some time, the attaining of insight was not often mentioned directly in psychoanalytic writing, but was indicated, for instance, in the term to "analyze" a symptom—leaving unspecified whether "analyzing" meant the analyst's putting a problem together, telling the patient, having the patient hear and accept it, having the patient put together some observations about himself, or some uncertain mixture of these.

Refinements in understanding insight have grown since the thirties, a growth which has been reviewed by Richfield[2] and by Hatcher.[3] The old problem of intellectual insight (where the patient decides something *must* be so on logical grounds) and the complementary confusing concept of emotional insight have been replaced on the basis of Bertrand Russell's[4,5] distinction between knowledge by acquaintance (where one knows something by direct cognitive grasp of it), and knowledge by description (where something is defined or described for one). Insight, of the acquaintance sort, is never "admitted," "confessed," or "proclaimed"; it is recognized, seen, taken as something one has always known, or should have always known; although it may be lost by the next hour, it is likely to return. It is noncontroversial. In contrast, apparent insight (based on knowledge by description) may result from a patient's more or less thoughtful conclusion that some-thing must be so. Insight may occur dramatically, but much more often it is progressive and gradual. A few examples will illustrate:

> A sophisticated male patient in analysis had been stopped by a policeman for speeding on the way to his hour. Even later than he would have been, he was furious, a not unusual state for him regarding the police. As he was expressing himself violently, he started the sentence, "God, how I hate them" but it came out, fluently, "God, how I love them." A several-minute pause, while he seemed to be thinking furiously, led to his recog-nizing his longstanding, ambivalent, not purely hostile, wishes, not only regarding the police, but proctors at school, and other authorities of importance. The analyst was substantially silent. This type of event is a somewhat unusual moment of insight.

> After months of talking often about his sister as a demanding and overbearing woman spreading gloom about her, a sophisticated male patient remarked to himself one hour: "You know, I guess I really don't like her," said with a mild tone of wonder and surprise. After recognizing his dislike, he proved much more able to deal with her, changing his auto-matic avoidance tactics, and recognizing, again with some surprise, that she was chronically depressed. (His choice of the phrase "I really don't like her," rather than speaking of his "hostility" or his "angry feelings," helps to show that this type of insight was by acquaintance, not an intellectualized conclusion about himself.)

> A year after an acute schizophrenic panic in which a patient drove up and down the streets of Boston in terror of either her or her family's being shot by foreign agencies, the patient had completely cleared except for recurrent periods of short-lived suspicions, each of which she quickly brought to the hour. She had broken down in the service of the state, and her fees were being paid by the state. She first connected the fears with times when the continuity of the treatment was interfered with, a dis-covery she made away from the hour and then brought in to review it, as it were, and see if it passed inspection. The fears were related to the ever-present anxiety that something would interfere with the treatment and she would lose her therapist and have an unmanageable recurrence. Two months later, she brought the same problem back, saying she had found that the fears were also related to money—not only did she need money for her treatment, but she had in fact been very poor as a child, and had had many situations where she could have quite reasonably feared the loss of her father; her mother had died when the patient was at an earlier age.

These examples illustrate the variation of incidents of insight; they also suggest that certain ideal-type images of insight are never so, and are often misleadingly expressed. Insight is never complete; it encompasses only one area in a patient's experience, although a sense of wholeness may accom-pany a formulation. Insights vary in importance and in depth—Bibring's "clarification" may lead to a superficial (not necessarily unimportant) insight if it refers to oneself. I recently reported[6] a hierarchy of depths of insight into illness, which report is being used as the basis for a scale to measure it in typescripts of interviews with psychotic patients.*

One especially important aspect of the development of insight is the way the patient manages the discovery. We have oversimplified the patient's mental activity in a way which is all too usual. A patient's most effective use of insight, indeed its actual occurrence, depends upon his being able to observe his own mind effectively. This entails some distance from himself conceptually, some reasonably discriminating critical facility, some awareness of things missing and of potential relationships in his mind, some interest, and a modicum of self-confidence. It is in this area that some of the most critical issues in the psychotherapy with schizophrenic patients occur, and differently than among psychoneurotic patients.

> A "post-psychotic" patient came into the office in a frenzy of despair and agitation—he noted that months before he had "wanted to kill Julie," his girlfriend. What was he to do, when he was terribly dependent upon her, loved her, and still was this sort of man? Questioning showed that he had been reflecting upon his earlier delusional fears of his family's being killed, including the girlfriend, and had assumed that this meant he had wanted her dead. Questioning and reflection on his fears of the rest of his family's deaths led to the observation that this was another manifestation of an anxiety over the control of his own mind.

> The silence of the analyst with the patient angry at the policemen was possible only because the general condition of the patient and the therapist's knowledge of it made it almost certain that he was managing his insight by altering his self-conception. But he could have been pictured as wondering who put that thought into his head, or into his mouth, or that he was homosexual and hopeless (with suicidal thoughts developing), or a host of other possibilities.

When a patient achieves an insight, either with the therapist's interpretation or without it, it is instructive to note quite carefully how the patients deals with the information. He may agree with a therapist's interpretation, nod politely, and go on. He may admire the therapist's presentation, and go on. He may agree, with some reservations, and go on. He may occasionally say "Oh, yeh," pause, and then go on. He may blush, stammer, and "confess." He may receive the interpretation with some appreciation as his due. He may openly or quietly resent the implications of the comments, he may withdraw into a suspicious regard of the therapist, and all but ask what he is doing here, etc. Each of these behaviors might be explored—they only hint at his management of the insight. It is unusual for a therapist to

* A group of us in Boston are studying intensive psychotherapy with schizophrenic patients. The group includes Peter Knapp, M.D., John Gunderson, M.D., Robert Schnitzer, Ph.D., Howard Katz, M.D., William Boutelle, M.D., Beverly Gomes-Schwartz, Ph.D., Marsha Vannicelli, Ph.D., and Norbett Mintz, Ph.D. It is supported by N.I.M.H. grant #MH25246-05.

catalogue the patient's reception of an idea as carefully as he does what led up to his own remarks. If he does, he uses the remarkably general and vague criterion: Does it lead to new material? How soon? How is new material different from changing the subject? Few therapists settle as a matter of course into an unreserved study with the patient of his reception of the interpretation, of what the interpretation signified to him, what it brought to mind, does he think it is so, and, if so, what difference does this make to his thinking about himself and the treatment. And, by the way, exactly what did the patient understand the therapist to say? If the patient grasped only half of what was said, and got that partly wrong, it would be understandable, since, if the patient is psychotic, he suffers a combination of difficulty in cognitive function, often great social anxiety, and a moderate to profound disinterest in what is said, be this for defensive or other reasons. Understanding how the patient manages new information is usually overlooked in the literature, but is often a most rewarding topic to explore.

> One patient, some months out of a paranoid break, had profitably noted her tendency to defend particular beliefs as if they were challenged when she was in therapy. She began to use this to gain perspective, and many times aborted what she feared might otherwise be an overwhelming return of psychosis. She had attended to this process aspect of her reception of alternative suggestions with persistent up-hill hard work, which gained her mastery over this particular defense, and incidentally over the formation of delusions.

Pressman[7] has emphasized the implications of the earlier heavy reliance upon free association in psychoanalysis, as if insight were simply given, came from someplace in a finished and final form, and was then used. This picture of a spontaneous and more or less effortless noncognitive process, he believes, is inadequate; in fact, it has never been the way patients understood themselves. He describes a "cognitive attitude," indicated by the style of the patient, in which the patient is scanning his mental content while reporting it to the analyst and at the same time integrating his newly discovered material, combining his experiencing ego and integrating ego, primary process and secondary process. He emphasizes that the patient may need to be taught, not only free association, but also how to understand himself and his associations, how to increase his attention and his grasp, not only of what he has said, but of what its implications and contexts are. Pressman's emphasis is upon the indispensability of education and cognitive working into the insight for maximum effect.

Pressman's recommendations are timely and accurate for psychoanalysis—they are, however, particularly appropriate for our consideration of psychotherapy with schizophrenic patients, where ego processes counted upon by the therapist with psychoneurotic patients cannot be taken for granted. The ways psychotic patients observe themselves are often different from those of non-pychotic patients in many unpredictable ways. They include particular difficulties in taking emotional distance from oneself, unexpected rigidities in interpretation, obscure difficulties in recognizing contexts which lead to failures in appreciating figurative remarks—all have their effects upon patients' interpretations of themselves, as well as of others. They can only be suggested here, but their frequency and importance underscores the value of noting the way patients incorporate new insights.

SELF REPRESENTATION

The special difficulties in interpretation mean, necessarily, resulting difficulties in self representation.

Here I must pause for semantic clarification, needed because crucial terms are used differently by experts, and may lead to different conclusions because of these different usages. These usages also have significant effects clinically, and in the understanding of clinical phenomena as sources of scientific information.

Much difficulty stems from the early psychoanalytic use of "ego" interchangeably with "self" and with "self-representation." As the concepts are now used most helpfully, the two concepts are from entirely different levels of discourse. The ego is a pattern of processes controlling perception, action, defense, thought—a structure in the mind—while the "self-representation" is the (reflexive) image each person has of his own person. The "self" *is* one's own person, everything of one's own person. This usage follows that of Hartmann,[8] Jacobson,[9] and Sandler and Rosenblatt,[10] and contrasts sharply with usage by Kohut[11] (who seems to have proposed a new department of the mind to be called the "self"), with usage by Sullivan[12] (who uses the term "self" and "self system" in an entirely different way), and with many others. Hartmann's usage has the advantage of clarity and consistency, and unravels a number of tangles in the theory of narcissism.

Self-observation, then, means only the perception, study, observation of some aspect of the self, of one's own person. Although usefully heightened in some circumstances—psychotherapy, for instance—it may be assumed to be going on a great deal of the time in a less focused way, contributing to the development of a self representation—the (reflexive) representation of one's self to one's self—an interpretive construct, more or less clear, more or less consistent, more or less a unit, more or less satisfying. Some aspects of the representation of the self are subjectively felt to be more real, solid, fixed, more essentially part of oneself, whereas others are felt as less part of one's core self. One's confidence in one's self-representation is usually high, but psychotic experience often jars this confidence.

The self-representation is not only a part of one's perceptions; also it has a motor function. It is part of the mechanism of control of behavior and of shaping it, so that we speak and act according to what we believe ourselves to be; personal integrity may refer precisely to the degree to which we perceive our behavior to be in accord with our background assumption of what we are. In psychotherapy, we take it for granted that the patient expresses himself in how he says something, as well as in what he says, but the place of the self-representation in this is rarely made explicit. A recent study by Fontana and Klein[13] showed the way a prolonged reaction time, classically the deficit of schizophrenic patients, could be eliminated in a setting appropriate to a different type of self-presentation. I believe we would profit greatly by much more attention to the self-representation of the patient, as such, and certainly not by confusing it with the patient's self.

Schizophrenic patients tend to oversimplify their self-representation. Observation and full acceptance of contrasting or contradictory themes of experience in oneself is a luxury usually of complex and generally sophisticated minds, where contrast can be counterpoint, not inconsistency or insanity, where discontinuities can be sources of interest and potential growth, not threats of tearing the fabric of the mind apart. This state of mind was not available to the patient who knew he wanted to kill his girlfriend, nor to many other schizophrenics who can hardly pause to notice the actual complex content of their mind when threats arise.

But therapists often—usually?—reenforce patients in this type of misleading interpretation. We so usually use the shorthand "ego" or "self" for self-representation, even to ourselves, that we often compound anxiety with confusion for our patients.

> A patient slowed in his therapy, with progressively less to say. Finally the therapist said, "Are you afraid of my going away on vacation?" The patient reluctantly said he was—and lapsed into silence. After reassuring him that he, the therapist, would be back, the matter ended.

The therapist actually misled this patient, I believe, by oversimplifying his experience. He overlooked the degree to which the patient wanted not to be afraid of the vacation, what his fear meant to him, and ended by simply underlining to the patient that he was dependent.

The occurrence of a conflicting wish in partial awareness is often interpreted by "What you really want to do is to get even with me," or whatever—the statement being made that the patient "really wants" only one of the two or more wishes at conflict in his mind. On a broader scale, the continuing activity during psychosis of the residual intact ego of psychotic patients took many years to identify, and the degree to which patients work with their therapists even while "out of contact" is only still partly known and accepted.

> The patient mentioned earlier who had recurrent controllable fears, usually mild and transient but reminiscent of, and fitting in with, her earlier paranoid delusions, learned to note her own motivation in defending the suspicions and their reasonableness. Although at first discouraged over what she could do about recurring fears of this sort, which required, she thought, the physician or her boyfriend to banish them—she came to note her own argumentativeness, and used it as a cue to examine the origin of the fear. While she has succeeded only once or twice, the maneuver itself now often suffices to banish the fears.

This represents a great increase in the awareness of, tolerance of, and use of, the complexity of her mind, a complexity quite inconceivable to her while sicker. The change shows insight at work.

One special relationship should be mentioned:—insight, inasmuch as it is new, is likely to occasion some surprise, and, as a corollary to this, to mean a change of some significance in the self-representation. A new feature of the self can be brought out by the patient in relationship to it. These are all aspects of the patient's readiness for insight and for interpretations. Ego activity is more handicapped, and in different areas, with psychotic patients than is often obvious or expected. Testing by finding out what the patient's response to one's interventions is an obvious and practical way of watching the growth in the patient's competence in self-observation, in cognitive processing of insight, in maturity and sophistication of self-criticism, in freedom of exploring alternative consequences, imagery, and possibilities—and, together, they indicate his level of competence in managing insight.

The absence of information in the case of patients treated with early deep interpretations about the patient's attitudes toward the interpretations shows one aspect of the therapist's oversimplification. His attention to only one side—the primitive fantasy or image—and not to its meaning to the patient, implies, I believe, that much of this "insight" (in the patient) is either a panic-driven incorporation of the therapist's apparent ideas, or actually a special form of schizophrenic intrusion or delusion, which may replace delusional self-interpretations.

THE VALUE OF INSIGHT IN EXPANDING KNOWLEDGE

I should return here to the nature of the self-representation. We must assume that, however, "genuine," "honest," or "accurate" a patient's picture of himself may be, it cannot be more than a very partial and specially oriented image. Not only is there no possible "complete" self representation, it is *systematically* incomplete—no matter how deep the insight, it will never reveal that the patient has a cerebellum, although the cerebellum plays a part in the overall activity which comprises his person. A highly informative account of the image of the mind was offered some years ago at the Ernest Jones Lecture in London by Richard Wollheim.[14] He concludes with some considerations concerning the spatial image of the mind, its having an inner and an outer aspect, borders, and other geographical characteristics, which are relevant to such imagery as that of Federn (and others) regarding "ego boundaries." Certainly patients do have various disorders in their representation of the boundaries of their self, and the elements which give rise to or maintain these alterations in self-imagery are, potentially, open to patients to study. But are these "boundaries" themselves real, aside from the patient's representation of them? When splitting occurs, what is split? The patient's representation of himself, or his mind, or him, his "ego"—or simply his image of himself?

This type of question cannot be answered categorically and immediately. To accept as fact an honestly achieved insightful reorganization of the patient's self-representation is to ignore that it still represents, as it were, only the opinion of the patient, however honest, and probably only one of several possible opinions at that. To discard it as "mere opinion" is to ignore its observable effect on the patient's behavior as real, its consistent immediacy as "real" to the patient, and, almost certainly, ignore selectively those aspects of the patient's report which do not fit our own preconceptions, retaining those which do. What is required is that the place of the insight in the patient's experience, or in his disorder if you will, be as accurately outlined as possible, using both humanistic and natural-science types of analysis. To ignore the first is to risk missing the problem, or analyzing a miscast problem; to ignore the second is to risk being lost in a nightmare which just possibly might turn out to be psychotic.

EXPLANATION, UNDERSTANDING, INTERPRETATION

Ricoeur[15] examines this dilemma in some detail. The search for understanding (the "Verstehen" of Dilthey) characteristic of the humanities—and of the psychological side of psychiatry—rests upon our ability to found understanding on our ability to transfer ourselves into another's psychic life on the basis of signs the other gives us; but it must be elaborated beyond this to become part of a science, in an organized body of knowledge, with some stability and coherence.

Specifically, in the study of the action of persons, the problem of the nature of causation and of motives for action becomes significant. Analysis of causation has rested heavily upon Hume's type of "cause," where the cause must be logically separable from the rest of the effect—as a match is from the cigarette. The interpretation of violence in Freudian terms fits with this definition fairly well—what incited the behavior, what drives "caused it"; in contrast, many actions—of which a move in chess is offered as a clear example—have to be analyzed in terms of their "reasons"—which are not separable from the action itself. Most human behavior falls between these two extremes—the tacit concept of cause is more Aristotelian than Humian, since the cause is formally a part of the action—a motive, a sense of desirableness, or a similar concept.

For our purposes, what this entails is the necessity of retaining analytic abilities of both sorts—explanatory and understanding—and to note that, where they meet, they need both to be submitted to an interpretation which is not the prisoner of one or the other form of thought.

A hypothetical example will permit clarification of the nature of the interpretation required. One type of emotional disorder is featured by a child's compulsively repeating, in "play," some terrible experience that he has had; the experience, usually a single one but of hideous intensity, is reenacted by the child, in the usual interpretation, in order to experience the event as under his own control, and often, therefore, to make it come out differently and better, at least in fantasy. The recall and reporting of the experience may often be followed by a rapid disappearance of the behavior; there is usually a convincing similarity between the original experience and the reexperienced fantasy.

It would be quixotic to discard this insight into the child's disorder and its cause, until one could subject some twenty children to the experience, and a matched group of twenty to a similar but not unpleasant experience, and examine the outcome. It would even be misleading to ask whether, if the event had not occurred, the child still might have had an emotional disorder; he would not have had one of the particular form he did. "Understanding" is the principal tool of the investigator in this case, and any "explanatory" description of repression, the nature of a traumatic experience and its effects, will have to *include* the fruits of our "understanding" in its material. The relation between the two types of analysis of the cause cannot be reduced, even in thinking about it, to such empirical formulae as how much of the variance is accounted for by one or the other; their relations are not of this alternative type.

It would be dangerous also, if not quixotic, to ignore the manifold possibilities of suggestion, hypnotic states, anxiety to please the therapist, selective attention of the therapist, folklore and myth, parental guidance, possible law suits, and similar phenomena, as contributors to the disorder. The methods of the humanities require methodical and skeptical therapists whose, sensitivity and ingenuity are encouraged, but also controlled and directed. The development of quantification and rigorous methods of testing statistical inference is a major successful development in empirical scientific method; it is not adequately in place as a method for the humanities, nor is an equally satisfactory substitute. Many efforts to make the humanities scientific have involved the deliberate sacrifice of the understanding characteristic of our work—the superficial operationism, the emphasis upon repeatability (reliability before validity), have meant that the motivation and intentions of our patients have often been relegated to either nonexistence, redefinition into something else, or into a never-never land some centuries away when we hope to be ready for it.

One of the better methods of controlling the study of "understanding" is the development of intensive psychotherapy, with its greatly extended interview, the special training of the therapist, the detailed study of the ways of deception and self-deception among human beings; and how to help recognize and avoid them. Erikson[16] has described this method and its advantages, limitations, and techniques with some care not to abandon the analysis of understanding in the process of trying to describe it.

Erikson emphasizes appropriately the receptivity of the therapist, the "disciplined subjectivity," as he participates in a free-floating attention which

> turns inward to the observer's ruminations while remaining turned outward to the field of observation and which, far from focusing on any one item too intentionally, rather waits to be impressed by recurring themes. These will first faintly but ever more insistently signal the nature of the patient's distress and its location. To find the zone, the position, and the danger, I must avoid for the moment all temptations to go off on *one* tangent in order to prove it alone as relevant. It is rather the establishment of strategic intersections on a number of tangents that eventually makes it possible to locate in the observed phenomena that central core which comprises the "evidence." (p 80)

He returns several times to "disciplined awareness," to the full use of the therapist's personal responses to the patient's presentations, and includes the importance of the patient's efforts as a collaborator with the therapist in assessing the interpretations of the observations. The paper is an excellent introduction to the nature of a therapist's experience as it contributes to the development of science. It is not possible here to follow these methodological problems beyond calling attention to the need for their further analysis.

The subjective experience of psychotic patients presents a specially interesting and promising area for such clinical analysis, and for understanding the nature of illness and recovery.

> A nonpsychotic physician patient returned to an hour with a complaint I have almost come to regard as characteristic of physician patients—he had had a bad migraine at the beginning of the last hour, and when he left, it had completely disappeared. He was annoyed and felt slightly cheated because he did not know why it had left—and made some

penetrating remarks about my profession—ending with, "It's like the old cultist folklore—you think you have that headache, but you're wrong; it isn't really you."

There are reasons to suspect that he had begun to answer his own question with his fable; but, if so, how different was his experience from that of a psychotic patient facing the same problem.

REFERENCES

1. Ricoeur P: Explanation and understanding, in Regan CE, Stewart D (eds): *The Philosophy of Paul Ricoeur: An Anthology of His Work*. Boston, Beacon Press, 1978, p 181.
2. Richfield J: An analysis of the concept of insight. *Psychoanal Q* **23**:390–407, 1954.
3. Hatcher RL: Insight and self observation. *J Am Psychoanal Assoc* **21**:377–398, 1973.
4. Russell B: *Human Knowledge, Its Scope and Limits*. New York, Simon & Schuster Inc, 1948.
5. Russell B: *Mysticism and Logic*. New York: WW Norton & Co, 1929, p 209.
6. Stanton AH: The significance of ego interpretive states in insight directed psychotherapy. *Psychiatry*, **41**:129–140, 1978.
7. Pressman MD: The cognitive functions of the ego in psychoanalysis: I. The search for insight. *Int J Psycho-Anal* **50**:187–196, 1969.
8. Hartmann H: Comments on the psychoanalytic theory of the ego. *Psychoanal Study Child* **5**:74–96, 1950.
9. Jacobson E: *The Self and the Object World*. New York, International Universities Press, 1964, pp 6, 19–23.
10. Sandler J, Rosenblatt B: The concept of the representational world. *Psychoanal Study Child* **17**:128–145, 1962.
11. Kohut H: *The Restoration of the Self*. New York, International Universities Press, 1977.
12. Sullivan, HS: Beginnings of the self system, in Perry HS, Gawel ML (eds): *The Interpersonal Theory of Psychiatry*, WW Norton & Co, 1953, pp 158–171.
13. Fontana AA, Klein EG: Self-presentation and the schizophrenic "deficit." *J Consult Clin Psychol* **32**:250–256, 1968.
14. Wollheim R: The mind and the mind's image of itself. *Int J Psycho-Anal* **50**:209–220, 1969.
15. Ricoeur P: Explanation and understanding: On some remarkable connections among the theory of the text, theory of action, and theory of history, in Reagan CE, Steward D (eds): *The Philosophy of Paul Ricoeur: An Anthology of His Work*. Boston, Beacon Press, 1978, pp 149–166.
16. Erikson EH: The nature of clinical evidence, in Lerner D (ed): *Evidence and Inference*. Free Press of Glencoe, Ill, 1959, pp 73–95.

Chapter 12

Discussion

A. HUSSAIN TUMA

Three general themes emerge from these papers. The first is the very distinct emphasis on the importance of more information regarding the nature of schizophrenic psychopathology, and the use of this information in designing appropriate therapeutic interventions. We are currently witnessing the beginnings of a greater use of data on the nature of psychopathology in schizophrenia in the context of treatment.

Second, as a consequence of greater awareness of the potential usefulness of multifaceted comprehensive approaches to treatment, we note the clear signs of integration and rapprochement between biological, psychological, and social environmental interventions in the effort toward treatment, rehabilitation, and prevention of relapse.

The third main theme is a greater recognition of the role of psychosocial stress in the etiology and course of schizophrenic disorders, in addition to the already established genetic contribution to this type of psychopathology. Consequently, we note a greater weight being placed in research on the role of family and social support systems, both in an effort

A. HUSSAIN TUMA • Clinical Research Branch, Division of Extramural Research Programs, National Institute of Mental Health, Rockville, Maryland 20857.

toward treatment and rehabilitation, and also in the search for determinants of schizophrenic illness.

If we truly recognize the significance of environmental stress in precipitating schizophrenic breakdowns, then Dr. Goldstein reminds us of the necessity to pay attention to, and capitalize in treatment on, social support factors, including the family. The major implications of Drs. Goldstein and May's presentations, for me, are that our approach to treatment of schizophrenic patients and their reintegration into community life should utilize a range of treatments, each treatment being used to its optimal level of specific and nonspecific effects. Hence, the data suggest a general research strategy that can ultimately show us how to use pharmacological, psychological, social, and other therapeutic approaches effectively and prudently to achieve very specific and targeted goals of intervention in an additive way.

Dr. May challenges the clinician, the theoretician, and the technologist in us to make psychotherapy work. He very carefully identified some of the roadblocks, and also prescribed several specific strategies for the future. He and all of us aim to achieve the same goal, the development of an adequate knowledge base for treating schizophrenic patients in effective and helpful ways.

Dr. May very aptly pointed out that the social dynamics of the treatment system tend to encourage and perpetuate a fragmented approach. I agree with this observation. If I can be a bit more direct, I must point out that the preoccupation and overinvolvement with one or another theory of schizophrenia or one or another approach to its treatment has unfortunately too often helped perpetuate this fragmented approach, frustrating the emergence of a comprehensive psychobiological and social approach to the understanding and treatment of mental disorders.

Dr. Blatt focused on the compelling need to examine the basic cognitive processes that characterize schizophrenic patients, and through this to identify the issues related to methods of treatment, as well as issues related to the content of the psychotherapeutic process.

I am comfortable with Dr. Blatt's emphasis on the patient's desperate need to experience a very stable, consistent, highly dependable relationship, and a highly stable and predictable universe. Much of our clinical experience, regardless of theoretical framework, clearly supports this position. Moreover, I found no difficulty in viewing the establishment of such a reliable, predictable, and safe relationship as a prerequisite to the patient's readiness to explore more subtle psychological dimensions.

I noted that, in reporting past work on perceptual processes in relation to developmental factors, he very aptly stayed with the data as much as possible. I personally experienced some problems in following him when he these new scales in their new empirical controlled studies and treatment of schizophrenia. They can show whether or not these concepts work.

Dr. Alanen and his colleagues describe studies that have been going on in Finland for a number of years. Their work is extremely interesting and potentially productive from a research vantage point. In my opinion, their investigations do not represent an experiment in the strict sense of the word, but rather a naturalistic study taking advantage of significant historical developments in the psychiatric treatment of schizophrenic patients. They aim to provide information on the use and value of various types of psychiatric treatments. Given their design and style, they can indeed provide careful observations on complex processes on a case-by-case basis, and, hopefully, on sizable subgroups from their different cohorts.

I agree wholeheartedly with Dr. Alanen and his colleagues on the importance of therapist attitude toward the patient. This includes open and free communication among the caring personnel, development of individual therapeutic relationships between staff and patients, and the use of family-oriented therapeutic work that is aimed at the patient's closest relatives. However, I would like ever so gently to question the need for the polarities that he presented about psychotherapy versus drugs, method versus problem-oriented approach, and caring versus independent investigators. I wonder whether, in this day and age, it is productive or even necessary to pose these matters as representing opposite values. Can we view these matters as elements that are central to both a comprehensive approach to treatment and an open, flexible framework for research?

I would like now to move to an entirely different issue, that is critical to the problem of research in psychotherapy. I hope that we, as individuals and members of organizations and institutions, can do something about this problem. The problem I am referring to is that of clinical research manpower, and the lack of a critical mass of researchers in this area.

Schizophrenia is estimated to be one of the most prevalent and severe major disorders. The rapid expansion of mental health services, the increase in the ranks of psychotherapists of all persuasions and backgrounds, and the enormous growth in the number and types of psychotherapies offered, do not correspond at all with the rather modest magnitude of research efforts in this area. Empirical research and the comparative efficacy of the various psychotherapeutic interventions have not developed or expanded at the same rate as the vast number of constructs, theories, and speculations about how these various treatments can and should be working.

Our most gifted clinicians and experienced practitioners do not, for the most part, engage in clinical research careers that are directly relevant to the understanding, diagnosis, and treatment of schizophrenia. Only a few do. The vast majority of young professionals, psychiatric residents, doctoral candidates in clincial psychology, postdoctoral fellows, students of psy-

got into the area of relating these empirical observations to the treatme
process. He presented to us a large number of concepts and theoreti
constructs. I would like to ask a few questions about these constructs.

First, from the viewpoint of parsimony, are all these constructs equa
needed for designing and carrying out psychotherapy research in this ar
Which ones are more essential, and which ones are secondary?

Second, could the concepts be translated into operational terms, int
language so that other researchers could find themselves able to use th
concepts? For example, how can we identify or develop replicable resea
evidence for the assumption that "these fantasies provide the basis
therapeutic alliance, and for the patient's eventual venture to seek realis
appropriate, and satisfying relationships in the external world?" How
we validate the existence of such states as "the initial fusion of the thera
with the maternal figure, and the resultant experiences of the patien
blissful reunion?"

These and other formulations, I assert, have and will continue to pro
a framework for the daily therapeutic transactions of many dyna
psychotherapists with their patients. To the extent that these formulat
provide a belief system, a source of confidence, and a sense of mastei
the therapeutic relationship, they can, I am certain, help the therapi
dealing with the schizophrenic patients in a helpful manner. My conce
simply with the relative necessity of some of these constructs and
potential usefulness for empirical research on the process and outcon
treatment.

Dr. Stanton changed the title of his paper twice. If I may chan
once more, I would like to label it "Insight: A Large Step Forward."
ceptually, I found Dr. Stanton's paper particularly interesting and si
cant. To me, it represented a profound approach to concepts that al
exist in the psychoanalytic vocabulary. He questions some of these con
and attempts to redefine them for purposes of his own research, con
like insight, self, and self-representations. To paraphrase Dr. May, St
is attempting to make these concepts work; that is, he first defined
concepts, or rather, redefined them. For example, in the case of insig
called it a gradual, progressive, and new grasp by the patient, a perce
that is, of his own inner life. He then proceeded to develop a hierarc
depth of insight about the illness, and illustrates this by concrete cl
examples.

Finally, he and his colleagues at McLean and Boston Universi
moving forward to develop a measure, a scale, that can be used by clin
and researchers to assess patient change and improvement on this part
criterion. The McLean and Boston University investigators who ar
rently engaged in a major psychotherapeutic research can indeed

chiatric social work, attempt to stay away from research careers. Those few who choose research as a career prefer basic laboratory work.

As you all know, the problem of severe shortage in clinical research manpower is not a simple one. Its complexity stems from several factors such as inherent conceptual and methodological difficulties in the research area itself, and the multidisciplinary prerequisites for diagnostic, therapeutic, and clinical methodological expertise for such research. There is a very limited number of research centers that can provide this type of expertise to individual investigators. There is often a considerable length of time required before treatment results are at hand and published, rather modest social and economic rewards offered to career scientists in general and to those in the field of psychiatry in particular, limited access to adequate patient populations, and the availability of a vast number of more attractive career opportunities. I could go on.

It seems to me that we face a very difficult situation. We are unable to attract young investigators to this field and to keep them active in it for any significant period of time.

We also face difficulties in motivating and persuading senior and established researchers in basic science areas to become interested in problems of treatment in schizophrenia. To illustrate, I would like to provide you with two indices from the NIMH funding for extramural research. One index relates to research support on the treatment of schizophrenia. Currently this includes only 25 projects at a total cost of approximately 3 million dollars. This is a country that spends billions on other areas of research. The 3 million dollars covers all treatment research relevant to schizophrenia, including psychopharmacology, psychotherapy, family therapy, milieu therapy, behavior therapy, hemodialysis, rehabilitation, and evaluation of several community-based treatment programs. This amount represents less than 3% of the total extramural research support dollars that are spent at the NIMH on over a thousand projects.

My second index is that the NIMH currently supports 124 individual investigators within the framework of the research scientist development program. None of these scientists—none—designates treatment of schizophrenia as his or her main theme for research. Only one career scientist awardee focuses on psychotherapy, but not in schizophrenia. One specializes on precursors of psychopathology in vulnerable children, and one on characterizing the schizophrenic patient and his relationship to his family.

What is distressing is both the relatively small proportion of research efforts on the treatment of schizophrenia and the fact that there has been a slight but steady decrease in the level of research support for this area over the past several years.

I would like to end by reminding all of us that our collective ability to deal with specific research questions is very highly dependent on the number and quality of research projects that can be undertaken on them at any given time. And the very existence of these projects is entirely dependent on the number and quality of investigators who are interested in, and also receive support and encouragement to work on, the problems discussed in this conference.

Chapter 13

General Discussion

OPEN DISCUSSION

DR. BLATT: Dr. Tuma raised an interesting question, to which I would like to respond. I am not sure what Dr. Tuma was referring to in his comments about a large number of concepts and whether they could be operationalized, but he did cite one particular concept, and let me respond to indicate its importance, and how one might operationalize it. He questioned the concept of the schizophrenic's wish for reunion and fusion; was this a necessary construct, could it be operational, was it of any utility in the study of schizophrenia. He asked if there was any evidence to support the importance of this concept.

I think these questions really tap into a central issue that has pervaded much of this conference, the issue of clinical versus research approaches. I think that this is an artificial and false dichotomy. What has been referred to as research is often the studies with large Ns, where there is a single, isolated empirical variable which can be quantified. And what has been referred to as the clinical enterprise is a nonresearch modality. I would argue that the clinical enterprise can be, and must be, a research endeavor. It may have limitations in the sense that it has limited control and possibly limited generality, but, on the other hand, with multiple observations over a long period of time, you can identify configurations which may have much greater meaning. The question is not one of a research versus a clinical approach, but an integration of the two.

There is considerable evidence in the clinical and theoretical literature about the importance of fears of, and wishes for, fusion in the schizophrenic patient—the wish for reunion with the symbiotic object. A few central references would include the work of Searles, Lidz, Burnham, Gladstone and Gibson, and Freeman, Cameron, and McGhee. All these contributions have been made within the last ten to 15 years, all attempting to evaluate systematically the observations made in the clinical context of the kinds of experiences reported by schizophrenic patients. I would argue that this is research, meaningful research that must be supported, research that has to be encouraged, and research that must be integrated with more limited, focused, empirical research designs.

How to achieve this integration is a difficult issue. In terms of the fear of and wish for fusion, the question is a provocative one. Let me respond briefly. The issue is, how do you operationalize a preverbal phenomenon, a phenomenon that patients often can't really put into words, one which they often can only enact? One way we have tried to approach this issue in our research was based on the theoretical assumption that cognitive structures evolve from interpersonal interactions, and that cognitive structures and modes of cognitive organization reflect the level of interpersonal relatedness. What we tried to do was take the boundary phenomena, not try to get patients to verbalize what is a very difficult phenomenon for them to express, but rather ask what are its derivatives, expressions, and manifestations. Based on the research of Ainsworth and others on cognitive processes and interpersonal relationships, we expected that, if schizophrenic patients struggled with issues of fusion and merging, this would be expressed in their cognitive structures. Wild and I, in our book (1976), reviewed a number of perceptual cognitive-interpersonal studies which demonstrated that one of the major underlying structures that could account for a host of seemingly diverse, isolated, and at times disparate findings was that many perceptual cognitive disturbances could be understood as disturbances in boundary formation. The wish for and fear of fusion was expressed by an instability of being able to maintain a representation of oneself and others, and even of inanimate objects as separate and distinct. It seemed to us that these could well be an expression of the interpersonal issue of a fear, and a wish for symbiotic fusion which clinicians have reported so consistently.

The issue, when operationalizing a concept, is often a matter of trying to utilize observations made in the intense, long-term clinical process to obtain data which may have limited generality but important meaning, and to use these observations to establish more systematic and circumscribed laboratory investigations.

DR. MAY: I was given a question which I had a chance to duck owing to the courtesy of our moderator, but I really shouldn't duck it. Somebody says that they're disturbed by what I said, and they ask if I ever really worked with a schizophrenic patient, and was I aware that there was some terribly good work being done at the Menninger's and the Austin Riggs and Chestnut Lodge, demonstrating rather remarkable results with the use of long-term psychotherapy.

Now, I would like to reply to that. I am very well aware that there are a lot of people at those institutions who have worked very hard in a very dedicated manner with schizophrenic patients and have very clearly done outstanding work in the field. No doubt about that at all. And there are a large number of case reports and descriptions of individual cases and anecdotal material.

What there is *not* in the literature at all is any controlled study to show that these particular people got better results than a comparison group. Now, I want to tell you an anecdote. To answer the question as to whether I ever saw a schizophrenic patient, at one time I had an experimental ward of my own, in which I dealt only with schizophrenic patients, paranoid schizophrenics mostly. At that time, I was deeply convinced that the kind of treatment which would work best with schizophrenic patients was not drug treatment, but milieu treatment. So I wrote a paper that I presented at UCLA—and I remember it very well—in which I said what marvelous results you got with milieu therapy when I did it. And thank goodness I never published that paper because I had the wit to realize that I didn't have a control group. If I had had a control group, which I did in our later study, I would have found the results that I thought were so good could have been gotten with a control group. We have to be terribly cautious not to be misled by individual cases, and that is why I am a complete believer in scientific evidence. We ourselves can be so caught up in what we believe—and we have to believe to do the work we do—but I think we have to watch our claims and ourselves.

MODERATOR: Are there any other comments on that point?

DR. ALANEN: Sometimes it is possible to cure a schizophrenic during a very long therapy, so that even without any controls you can see how this person is growing. With some other patients, this may not be possible. I think that his kind of evidence also has its value.

DR. MAY: Of course I don't agree with you. The difficulty is that when you deal with one case, you never know what would have happened if you had done something else.

DR. BLATT: The question is, what do you want to control for? If you propose a control group, what is it that you are proposing needs to be controlled for? Let me clarify why I ask the question. It seems to me that, for example, you could control for judges' distortions by having independent assessments of the same patient over time. This could be a reasonable research design which would answer a series of questions about treatment efficacy without necessarily having a control group which received no treatment at all. The issue is a question of type of research design, rather than a simple cliché demand for "a control group."

Some of the problems in conducting research on long-term therapy are the amount of time required in the treatment process and the difficulties of being able to gather adequate numbers of cases and establish procedures for processing the data for systematic study. There is a desperate need for developing research designs which utilize the data in the clinical files that have been compiled in good clinical facilities throughout this country, and finding ways of evaluating these data in a systematic fashion. These data contain valuable observations that could be systematically assessed and provide considerable new insight and understanding into the nature of schizophrenia and its treatment.

DR. GOLDSTEIN: I just have one comment. I don't know if you want to persevere on this issue. I think the dead horse is sitting right out on the table becoming dismembered. But in the volume on the psychotherapy of schizophrenia that Gunderson and Mosher compiled from a previous conference, they asked psychotherapists who had a lot of experience with schizophrenic patients to list the attributes of those patients with whom they thought they could be most successful. And indeed, they compiled a list that had a moderate degree of consensus, and that reduced to what many people who have done research on schizophrenia would call patients with good premorbid histories with many psychosocial assets and resources. I think that perhaps the issue is, not "does long-term psychotherapy work," but rather "is it perhaps more appropriate for people with certain developmental resources"?

An important issue that has to do not only with long-term therapy is, "what is really the critical component of therapy"? I think one thing we have heard today from people who have done long-term psychotherapy is the importance of a long-term emotional commitment to these individuals, that it's open-ended, that it involves, of course, specific skills, but it also involves this very basic commitment over the long haul to ride out problems and stick with the individual. I don't think we know whether it is in fact this deep and abiding and long-term emotional commitment that is the important therapeutic agent, or whether it has to do with other specifics. It's that level of question that I think we might profitably explore in psychotherapy research.

DR. STANTON: Phil (May), the implication of what you said is that if there is no control group, then it's not worth publishing, that there are no data at all. I think that is to throw out all of the issues about the humanities. For instance, is it worthwhile doing any study of history, if it's not possible to control it? You only have a single case. On the contrary, there is much to be gained by describing and analyzing. I think one has to have the intellectual discipline to know that the question of cause and effect is not answered. But I think it is damaging to have the assumption that, unless you can do a relatively fully controlled experiment, you really shouldn't do anything at all, the way it often turns out.

Critics often say there are no data on such-and-such a problem. But there often are data, and sometimes they are very valuable. They may be inconclusive data. There has been a lot of therapy, not just in psychiatry, which rests on other observations than controlled experiments.

DR. MAY: When you're proceeding on the basis of what you think is evidence, you have to know how firm and how hard the evidence is. I am well aware that clinicians are often faced with situations where they have to do something when there is no scientific evidence whatsoever. The critical issue is that when you do whatever you do, you should be able to distinguish between when you're acting on the basis of hard scientific evidence, when you're acting on the basis of case example, and when you're acting on the basis of sheer hope and faith.

QUESTION FOR DRS. GOLDSTEIN AND MAY: Since dyskinesia is on the increase, and may already involve over 30% of patients on long-term use of antipsychotic drugs, we may not be able to use them as maintenance treatment over a prolonged time. Yet there are far too few clinicians to conduct psychotherapy with schizophrenic persons. What do you see as a future method of dealing with this dilemma, both in terms of medication and of psychosocial issues?

DR. GOLDSTEIN: Tardive dyskinesia appears to relate to the duration of phenothiazine treatment. It may very well be that short-term use like the six-week critical period that we had in our study is where the risks may be reduced and at the same time the benefits may be considerable. I think that there are very serious problems with long-term maintenance on phenothiazines and many people are really questioning the viability of that approach.

How to find alternatives to this, it seems to me, is going to require more creativity than simply saying that we need more individual psychotherapists because there is no question that the costs of chlorpromazine versus an individual psychotherapist are not exactly equal. I do think that the idea of imaginative psychosocial treatment models which can be delivered to the large number of schizophrenics that need them is a critical issue at the present time.

DR. MAY: Tardive dyskinesia with long-term phenothiazine treatment is a serious problem, as indeed is long-term treatment with any form of medication for any illness whatsoever. To some extent, the answer lies in the development of drugs that don't cause such toxic effects. To some extent, the solution lies in finding out the mechanism that leads to these side effects, and seeing if we can find some way around them. To some extent it involves developing entirely new forms of treatment. It isn't necessarily saying that one treatment can substitute for another. The effects of drug treatment do not substitute for psychotherapy, any more than the effects of psychotherapy substitute for drug treatment. I think we just have to do the best we can, and at the moment the best we can is to try to give patients the smallest possible dose for the shortest possible length of time we can, trading off the potential risks against the potential benefits.

Part III

The Practice of Psychotherapy with Schizophrenics

Comments on the 'Elements' of Schizophrenia, Psychotherapy, and the Schizophrenic Person

OTTO ALLEN WILL, JR.

INTRODUCTION

We are concerned in this conference with the process of psychotherapy as it is related to certain patterns of behavior referred to as evidence of a grave psychosis, schizophrenia. These phenomena are common in our society, and appear in one form or another in a variety of cultures. They are generally bothersome to all concerned, and most people who pay any attention to them would like to get rid of them or, at least, get them out of sight. They tend to be embarrassing because they appear as strange imitations, distortions, caricatures, and extravaganzas of humanity, related in some vague, haunting, and painful way to those forms of living which we may wish to cherish as normal, or as "normally idiosyncratic." In addition, they are costly in terms of the money required to do anything about them—useful or not. We—the citizens—would prefer to invest in something other than the madness which has been with us so long and persists despite our ignorance and knowledge, defying both our loving and our hateful efforts to change or eliminate all of its manifestations. If, by chance, misfortune, or intention,

---

OTTO ALLEN WILL, JR. • 307 Western Drive, Richmond, California 94801.

we notice these events, we are likely to feel uncomfortable and put upon without good reason, and yet strangely guilty.

During the past sixty years there has been an increasing amount of observation and systematic research concerning the schizophrenias. The results of all of these activities are varied, but the name persists, and with it the myths and prejudicies of the past. Adolf Meyer insisted that dementia praecox (schizophrenia, parergasia) should not be equated with a "living death." But the dread of the malady continues. In the years in which I have had something to do with these matters, there has been an aura of mystery and threat about psychotherapy and schizophrenia. There is also an ill-defined suspiciousness related to them, as if there were something dirty, unclean, and immoral in their very existence and operation. The disorder and the treatment are not easy to define, and it is difficult to hold them within the limits of hard science. But the basis of the distaste does not simply lie there.

Here I shall attend to only some of the possible reasons for the persistence of this attitude which combines feelings of fascination and dread.

• Schizophrenia and psychotherapy are not defined easily and are thus subject to many definitions. Their identities are unclear, even within a professional group. The person who seeks to deal with the complexities of schizophrenic behavior through personal exploration of its psychological-social manifestations will discover to his discomfort that in this process his own identity is threatened and becomes muddled.

• Personal contact with a schizophrenic person over along period of time will lead to the exposure of loneliness in both patient and therapist. To my knowledge, true loneliness even more than anxiety is an experience that we seek to avoid, ignore, and forget.

That which cannot be identified clearly lies close to the realm of the unknown, inviting the elaboration of fantasy and the attempt finally to explain the phenomena, or to consign them to discard as inexplicable or governed by magic. Schizophrenic behavior cannot be pushed aside as a form of peculiarity or craziness derived only from the seeming imper-sonality of chemical–tissue activities. Could they be looked upon in this grossly oversimplified fashion, they would not be so feared or dealt with in such strange ways.

In terms of my own experience as a psychotherapist, I shall mention briefly the following matters which are currently of particular interest to me in my work:

1. The problem of identity as related to the concept of schizophrenia.
2. The problem of identity as related to the patient.
3. The problem of identity as related to the therapist.

4. The experience of loneliness.
5. Dread and schizophrenia.
6. A grossly oversimplified comment about disorder and treatment.
7. Cost and the choice of options.

THE IDENTITY OF SCHIZOPHRENIA

The history of the treatment of schizophrenia is informative in terms of the identity of this disorder. I shall refer here only to my personal contacts with the problem, which have been both peripheral and direct for about fifty years, and more specifically professional for the past forty. During that time I have learned something, but not enough to make me feel comfortably expert (or expert in any sense), and perhaps of greatest importance to me has been the necessity to escape from certain of my prejudices, and to unlearn some of the ideas which I once held to be obvious truths, yet which interfered with my gaining any useful grasp of what went on in my efforts to be a therapist.

The treatments to which I refer were directed toward the alleviation or elimination of a disease within the afflicted person. Evidences of the disease were exhibited by someone in the form of crazy behavior which most of us did not recognize—or like to admit—as being part of our own living; reference is to delusions or "false" beliefs, hallucinations of various kinds, suspiciousness that appeared to be excessive and beyond one's own, muteness, extreme withdrawal, self-mutilation, and other activities that commonly invited attention, and often led their perpetrator to become a public nuisance, and, in some social groups, a patient. The nature of the disease, its pathological changes in tissue, and its origins were not understood, but its outlook was considered to be grim. Therapy tended to mimic what was being done for sicknesses that were more easily fitted into the structure of classical medical practice. Treatment included the following:

1. Surgical removal of foci of infection in an effort to remove sources of toxic material.
2. Injection of horse serum intrathecally to produce a sterile meningismus.
3. Intravenous injection of gold salts, as in the then treatment of arthritis.
4. Hyperthermia—artificially induced fever—a form of treatment for syphilis of the nervous system.
5. Insulin coma and subcoma, with or without convulsions.
6. Metrazol-produced seizures.
7. Nitrogen with associated oxygen reduction.
8. Electroconvulsive treatment.

9. Surgical interference with selected neural pathways in the brain.

10. Implantation of electrodes—or bits of metal—in the brain as receptors of externally produced electrical stimuli in the service of controlling or modifying behavior.

11. The administration of massive doses of vitamins—megavitamin therapy.

12. Dialysis of the blood, as in the treatment of renal failure.

13. Multiple drugs that affect the functioning of the brain, and other drugs to inhibit certain side effects of medication.

The list is not complete, and I am confident that other treatment forms will be developed in the future. What is reported here is well-known, but is repeated because of its relevance to the problem of identity.

Schizophrenia has been—and is—viewed from several positions:

1. It is a form of disease in the more traditional medical sense, its precise etiology and pathology as yet undetermined, its cause and outcome varied, its physiology and biochemistry perhaps beginning to be illuminated, and its treatment inadequate in the sense of not being curative. Means for its prevention are, at best, speculative.

2. It is a reflection, in part, of an undetermined genetic trait associated, perhaps, with increased susceptibility to stress.

3. It is to a large extent a reflection of experience—developmental, family, social, cultural.

4. It is a term applied to a variety of behaviors not necessarily related to each other or to common causes.

5. It is a combination of these factors.

6. It is a "way of living"—a form of existence which is both a product of learning and of personal choice.

7. And—perhaps there is no such "thing" as schizophrenia, in which case the term should be abandoned, as some say.

Struggles can—and do—develop about the problem of conceptualization, reflecting differences in beliefs, methodological approaches, experiences in living, professional training, and opportunities for working with patients, personal bias, etc. The investigator may discover in the pheomenon of schizophrenia some support for his own preferences, whatever they may be. The presence and influence of the observer—at least I speak for the psychotherapist—cannot be eliminated from the field of treatment and study.

During the past forty years, the understanding of human behavior in general—and of schizophrenic behavior in particular—has been furthered through the following approaches:

1. Studies of the "milieu"—the hospital and other social systems.

2. Investigations of the structure and functions of the human family.

3. The refinement of concepts of the social field, communication networks, and general systems theory.

4.   Interdisciplinary studies with emphasis on cultural patterns in the moulding of behavior.

5.   The extension of personality theory.

6.   Recognition of the idea that the human being, no matter how grossly disordered he may become, shares to varying degrees in the griefs and pleasures of each of us; in his "sickness," or his "wickedness," or "depravity," he retains his human status.

It is difficult, for me at least, to pull together into a meaningful operational unity these various ideas about the ways in which some human beings, schizophrenics, are fated—or formed by circumstance—or choose by odd design, to live. In my discomfort at uncertainty and the lack of clear and persistent identity of the cluster of behaviors in which I attempt to involve myself, I may seek an evanescent security in embracing wholeheartedly, and perhaps blindly, one point of view, and ignoring or discounting others. I often wish that I could say, and believe with assurance, something like: "We do not know the answer now, but as knowledge is increased and techniques refined, we shall find it. Then another of mankind's maladies will be understood and eliminated." I have no such hope, nor, in truth, do I have such a wish. I think that the lack of definition and precise identity may be preferable to some "solutions" that might turn out to be the constraints of conformity and control rather than the freedom that we both desire and fear. I hold no brief for the schizophrenic misery: I have observed in it no great delights. But if it is one of the complicated and obscure ways of escape and rebellion, its closure through ignorance must lead to the seeking, finding, and invention of other routes of release. We know more—and are learning more—about the control of human behavior than we do about its cure in a benign sense. The therapist—the one who applies the knowledge available to him—cannot avoid the problem of ethics. That which he does has consequences; there is for him no truly neutral act.

THE PATIENT

The schizophrenic person's sense of identity if fragile, unstable, and unclear, as are his relationships with other human beings. It is in adolescence that formation of identity is accelerated, and, to a large extent, consolidated. At this time there is experienced the powerful need for intimacy, requiring trust and confidence in another person. This bringing together of two personalities is too great a task for the preschizophrenic adolescent; the challenge to his identity is threatening to its integrity. The problem may be met by anxiety, withdrawal, and various acts which will become known as schizophrenic. The person is then in transition to a new and strange identity—that of patient.

If the young person acknowledges that he is a patient, he may well ask: "What kind of patient am I?" In the light of earlier remarks in this account, the answer is not necessarily apparent. There are choices to be made—borderline, narcissistic personality, pseudonarcissism, latent schizophrenia, and so on. Let us suppose that in this unreal conversation the response is: "We call you schizophrenic." The reply to the question might well be: "What's that? And what do you plan to do about it?"

A patient may not ask such questions at first, usually being too preoccupied with matters of survival to pay much attention to the niceties of naming and the magics of professional intervention in his troubles. Relatives and others interested in the patient's welfare do, however, ask the questions, and they should receive understandable replies. As a therapist, I often review with the questioner the history of the disorder and treatment, and the problems associated with these. I shall recommend a course of action, and I want those concerned to know the reasons for my doing so.

Not long ago I heard a colleague state his advice to a schizophrenic patient. To the patient he said, "You have a disease which interferes with your thinking and feeling. We don't know its cause, but we can help you, although we can't cure you. You must learn to live with it, and to keep its symptoms under control, you must take medicine for the rest of your life. When you get very sick, come into the hospital for a time, and we'll see that you get better."

That's a fair enough statement, but it isn't mine. I tend to be a little less certain about this matter. I do not hesitate to explain what is known about the situation as best I can. Such an open expression of views—a sharing—is, in my opinion, a small step toward the development of trust and personal identity.

The uncertain identity of the patient is then confronted with the continuing uncertainty of identity of his troublesome behavior and the methods available for dealing with it. I see no way of escaping from this situation; I prefer to acknowledge it, and then to get on with the business of making what sense we can of the disorder, and doing what we can about it.

THE THERAPIST

I remember well that in my adolescence I suffered greatly because I could not get clear about who I was. I admired and envied those people who seemed to be more clearly defined than I was—the athlete, the musician well on his way to a career, the boy who built model airplanes and was going to be a "flyer"—anyone who apparently knew what he was about, and could extend that knowledge into a view of his future. I did what I could to conceal my own doubts and formlessness with a facade of confidence that in my private hours was likely to dissolve away. After many wanderings, I entered upon the study of medicine, and my anxieties subsided as I acquired the identity of physician. I held to it as best I could, but I carelessly stumbled into the field of psychiatry. Then I discovered that I was no longer, in the eyes of many people, a "real doctor." I was a "crazy doctor." I sought identity in psychoanalytic training, but became involved somehow with patients who were schizophrenic. The old doubts as to self were revived. I do know that I am a form of psychiatrist and psychoanalyst, but I don't fit precisely or easily into a well-defined and accepted professional category.

Not infrequently in my work as a therapist, I feel the need to identify, at least to myself, who I am. I reach for some feeling of recognizable certainty. If I am for the moment not recognizable as physician, psychiatrist, or psychoanalyst in the traditional sense, then who am I? Perhaps, I think privately for a brief moment, I am simply a good, compassionate, and understanding person whose very presence can, in some inexplicable fashion, be healing to the sick. I don't waste much time on that idea; all the evidence is to the contrary. The answer to this false problem is not impossibly complicated, and I find it acceptable. I am a therapist attempting to make some sense of the behavior of people whose identity is unclear, and who suffer from a disorder, the identity of which is also unclear. In such dealings, it is not remarkable that my own identity is challenged, explored, revealed as unclear in some ways, and required to be subject to change.

LONELINESS

I shall comment briefly on the experience of loneliness, as it is a major aspect of my work with schizophrenic patients. I mean that this sentiment is felt by both patients and therapists, although it is unpleasant, frequently denied, hidden by anger and other emotions, and difficult to discuss, except in retrospect or in greatly attenuated form. The following comments by Fromm-Reichmann[1] are relevant to our purposes at this juncture.

> Real loneliness . . . leads ultimately to the development of psychotic states. It renders people who suffer it emotionally paralyzed and helpless. . . . People who are in the grips of severe degrees of loneliness cannot talk about it, and those who *were* there seldom do so either. Because of the extremely frightening and gruesome character of the experience, they try to dissociate the memories of the sense of loneliness, including their fear of it. This frightened secretiveness and lack of communication about their loneliness seem to increase the threat entailed in it for the lonely ones,

even in retrospect; it produces the sad conviction that nobody else has
experienced or ever will sense what they have experienced or what they
have submerged.

The experience of loneliness in the sense that the word is used here
appears in adolescence along with the development of a sense of intimacy;
that is, only as another human being becomes important and recognizably
meaningful in those years, can loneliness exist—an awareness of the need
for friendship and love, and the possibility that they cannot be gained or
held. The psychotherapeutic process is designed to expose this need, and to
encourage the formation of trust in another person. The feeling of loneliness will thereby be awakened. This is a major reason why the exploration
of human relationships is painful; but his form of pain cannot be avoided.

DREAD

The concept of schizophrenia is marked by a quality of dread. Reasons
for the arousal of this uncanny emotion include the following ideas.

1.   The history of the disorder, with associated myths of deterioration
and unresponsiveness to treatment.

2.   The identity problems of patient, disorder, and forms of treatment.

3.   The strangeness of some of its outward manifestations.

4.   The fear of motivations that exist beyond awareness.

5.   The vague and unpleasant apprehension that someone is to blame
for the trouble, or that it represents punishment for personal evil and
wickedness, hitherto concealed but now to be revealed in the display of
madness.

6.   The fear of contamination through association with the afflicted
person.

7.   The revelation of a loneliness of human existence.

A PERSONAL AND SIMPLIFIED CONCEPT OF THE
PATIENT

As a psychiatrist, it is necessary for me to have some idea about the
patient's identity, and some formulation of his troubles. Simply stated, I
think of the patient and his disorder as follows:

1.   Whatever there may be of obscure and unidentified defects of
genetics and physiology, he (or she) can learn through experience and
undergo change.

2.   To a large extent his behavior, pathological or otherwise, is
learned and reflective of the social systems within which he has so far
developed.

3. Behavior has purpose and is goal-directed, although both purpose and goal in many instances may remain unclear.

4. There is present both a great need for, and fear of, intimacy.

5. The patient has not been able to deal adequately with the tasks of adolescence.

6. He is isolated in a terrible loneliness,

7. He is not a case just like other cases; he is to me a stranger, and my conceptions about him must be subject to observation and modification.

8. There is nothing "inhuman" about this person.

9. The trouble is to be taken seriously; it is no object for false pessimism or optimism; it is a subject for learning.

10. Schizophrenia can be defined—to an extent—and I use the term. It is important to me, however, *that the patient define it for me* in terms of his own life, and that I do not attempt to define his life in terms of the concept, or in terms of my own ideas of how one "ought to live."

A SIMPLIFIED CONCEPT OF PSYCHOTHERAPY

A great deal has been said about psychotherapy, and there is a great deal more to be said—and learned. For me, these are the "bare essentials"—necessary "openers," if you will.

1. The therapist shall be there, physically and otherwise. The process cannot be carried on well in absentia, unless one is willing to substitute malleable fantasies for the data—accurate or not—of observation.

2. Consistency—that is, there should be no great or obscure discrepancies between the therapist's words, gestures, appearance, emotions, and ideas. It is not his job to puzzle the patient unnecessarily.

3. Patience and the ability to tolerate difference and paradox.

4. No great fear of uncertainty and the extravangances of psychosis, and no particular reverence of them or fascination with them.

5. The ability to listen and observe, even at the expense of keeping one's views to oneself—at least for a time.

6. The therapist works to enable the patient to become effective as his (the therapist's) teacher. In teaching the therapist what all the fuss is about, the patient is likely to learn something about himself, to his profit.

7. It is a good idea to keep with one a leavening of hope; not blind hope, but a confidence in the power of the human relationship to produce changes, for better or for worse.

8. A recognition that psychotherapy—a form of human relatedness—is not a bland concoction that can be applied without knowledge, skill or experience, and that if it does not produce good results, is at least neutral. Not so. It can produce both benefit and hurt; it is no inconsequential force.

IN CONCLUSION

What is the future for this psychotherapy with schizophrenic patients? I do not know. I do know—as do you—something of the costs in time, money, and effort that are included in this enterprise—and the many social needs that demand to be met. Psychotherapy is, for me, a process of growth and learning, and is not subject to significant shortcuts with which I am familiar. That it is of great help to some patients I have no doubt. I also have no doubt that its principles can be applied to other forms of less intensive interpersonal treatment.

Of course, we may come to a world in which these patients— schizophrenic people, largely expressions and products of our culture—are considered to be too expensive to maintain, study, or treat. Such an attitude would presage disaster; it would open the gate to a hell for the destruction of all of us in our efforts to destroy schizophrenia—that contorted, yet accurate image of ourselves.

This last from Sullivan:[2]

> I [plead] . . . the urgent necessity for much broader investigation as to adolescence and as to schizophrenia than has been anywhere so far recorded. . . . I say this because I am convinced that in the schizophrenic processes and in the preliminaries of schizophrenic illness—so common among adolescents who are having trouble in the social adjustments—can be seen, in almost laboratory simplicity, glimpses which will combine as a mosaic that explains many more than half of the adult personalities that one encounters.

These remarks were written fifty years ago. A great deal of careful and useful work in the field has been done since then, as evidenced by presentations in this conference. There is more to be done.

REFERENCES

1. Fromm-Reichmann F: *On Loneliness, in Psychoanalysis and Psychotherapy.* Chicago, University of Chicago Press, 1959, pp 326–328.
2. Sullivan HS: Research in schiophrenia, in Perry HS (ed): *Schizophrenia as a Human Process.* New York, WW Norton & Co Inc, 1962, pp 201–202.

Chapter 15

Comprehensive Psychosocial Treatment

Beyond Traditional Psychotherapy

GORDON L. PAUL

A psychosocial orientation to assessment and treatment of people called schizophrenics is shared by nearly all participants of this conference—more for some than for others. For me, the "psycho" component of "psychosocial orientation" reflects assumptions that the particular excesses or deficits in cognitive and ideational, emotional, or motoric behavior of focus are those that are traditionally referred to as psychological, rather than physical or biological. Similarly, the "social" component reflects the importance of the social environment as the context in which: (a) most of the relevant activity occurs, (b) the appropriateness or inappropriateness of functioning is defined, and (c) changes in conditions may be expected to produce changes in behavior. From a psychosocial orientation, nearly any clinical intervention outside of surgery, shock, and chemotherapy could be considered "psychotherapeutic."

However, I would like to focus upon a patient population whose severity in terms of office-based interchanges between a professional therapist and one or more patients for one to five hours per week is inade-

GORDON L. PAUL • Psychology Department, University of Houston, Houston, Texas 77004.

quate to the task—even though a broader concept of psychosocial treatment is not. Namely, the severely disabled institutionalized mental patient. Intramural treatment of these patients in public mental hospitals, mental health centers, and community residential facilities remains the most expensive mode of treatment generally available.[1] Until recently, no intramural treatment had been documented to show differential long-term benefits for patient functioning, release, or eventual stay in the extramural community.[2]

Given the notorious lack of reliability and validity of traditional diagnostic practices, I have explicitly adopted the strategy of experimental-behavioral science as the guiding framework for both assessment and treatment of any client.[3] In general, this strategy requires specification of particular motoric, emotional, and ideational behaviors that pose problems because of excesses or deficiencies in their frequency, intensity, or timing of occurrence in the physical and social environment in which the client is ultimately to live. The functional relationships between specific problems and events in the physical-social environment and other aspects of the client's behavior are then sought, followed by change efforts within a hypothesis-testing model. Even if a specific subset of diagnostic criteria produces a reliable categorization of "schizophrenia," none of the current or proposed approaches[4] will be useful for treatment-disposition decisions from an applied experimental-behavioral approach, since they lack the specificity of assessment needed for functional analyses. Thus, while the treated patients to be described below were all diagnosed as schizophrenic, I do not consider the approach to be treatment of schizophrenia, but, at most, treatment of problems in schizophrenic clients.[5]

MINIMAL GOALS FOR RESIDENTIAL TREATMENT

In the absence of useful information from current diagnostic practices, I undertook a review of followup studies of released mental patients about 12 years ago to see if there were any consistencies in individual behavior, environments, or the interaction between the two in determining conditions for rehospitalization.[6] That analysis of empirical associations with the act of hospitalization or rehospitalization led to the identification of four areas of focus required as minimal goals for intramural treatment to return institutionalized mental patients to the outside community:

1. *Resocialization*—including development of self-maintenance, interpersonal interaction, and communication skills.

2. *Instrumental role performance*—including provision of salable vocational skills and housekeeping skills—at a minimum of "on task" and "on time" components of performance necessary to interact freely with the local community, and participate in future training programs.

3. *Reduction or elimination of extreme bizarre behavior*—including appropriate changes in frequency, intensity, or timing of individual acts or mannerisms consensually identified as distressing.

4. *Provision of at least one supportive "roommate" in the community*—including either a spouse, relative, parent, or friend.

It is reassuring to see that the reviews and prospective studies of Strauss and Carpenter and their colleagues[7]—from a different conceptual approach—result in conclusions that are quite compatible with the first three identified goals. Similarly, recent research has emphasized the importance of the social network which underlies the fourth goal identified in the earlier review.[8] In addition to these areas of focus, intramurally, both treatment and assessment operations should ultimately focus upon the transition from institution to community, and the particular community of release, to assure that situationally determined requirements are met.[2,9]

THE SEVERITY OF DISABILITY IN RESIDENTIAL POPULATIONS

As noted earlier, the severely disabled institutionalized mental patient's problems are such that traditional psychotherapy cannot logically provide the needed impact for achieving minimal goals. This is becoming even more true as "deinstitutionalization" of the less severely disabled takes place.[10] Before presenting specific information on the severity of those problems, some familiarity with the assessment systems employed is needed. One system that has proven to be an exceptionally reliable and useful system for assessment and ongoing monitoring of patient functioning in any residential setting is the Time-Sample Behavioral Checklist (TSBC).[11]

The TSBC is a direct observational system in which data are obtained by trained observers with computer summarization. In practice, professional observers record the presence or absence of 69 specific behavioral codes, or one of three control codes, following a standardized instance of patient observation each waking hour. Each observation also specifies the time, location, and nature of activity during which the observation occurred. A computer summary program then combines the discrete hourly codes to provide scores for each patient and treatment unit over time periods desired. These scores include the relative frequency of actual occurrence for each of the 72 codes for individual clinical evaluation, programming, and treatment monitoring, including: physical location (e.g., bedroom, living area), physical position (e.g., walking, lying down), whether eyes are open or closed, facial expression (e.g., smiling with apparent stimulus, neutral with no apparent stimulus), social orientation (e.g., alone, with staff), engagement in normal elective appropriate activities (e.g., talking normally to others, personal grooming), and performance of bizarre behaviors. The computer-summary program also combines the discrete behaviors into higher-level scores reflecting overall adaptive and maladaptive functioning, as well as component scores characteristic of those obtained form more expensive psychiatric interviews.

Since the TSBC provides the only known means for continuous assessment of most clinically relevant bizarre behavior, better understanding of the instrument may be gained by examining the codes entering the higher-order maladaptive behavior scores presented in Table I. The grouping of data into higher-order scores was based upon factors found from earlier studies of rating data.[12] However, it should be clear that the TSBC data base does *not* consist of ratings, but simply "presence–absence" judgments of low inference codes.[13] In fact, due to the low level of inference, the reliabilities of higher-order scores regularly range from 0.90 to 1.00, with a median $r = 0.97$.[2] Thus, in addition to the relative frequency of each class of behavior provided by the computer summary, a Schizophrenic Disorganization Index provides the sum of the relative frequencies of nine bizarre

TABLE I. Time-Sample Behavioral Checklist Components of Higher-Order Maladaptive Behavior Scores

Schizophrenic Disorganization Index (Bizarre motoric behavior)	
Rocking	Blank staring
Repetitive & stereotypic movements	Lying down
Posturing	Eyes closed
Shaking, tremoring	Neutral facial with stimulus
Pacing	

Cognitive Distortion Index (Bizarre verbal and facial behavior)	
Chattering, talking to self	Crying
Verbalized delusions, hallucinations	Smiling, laughing with NO stimulus
Incoherent speech	Grimacing, frowning with NO stimulus

Hostile-Belligerence Index (High-intensity aggressive behavior)	
Screaming	Injuring self
Swearing, cursing	Physical intrusion
Destroying property	Verbal intrusion

Total Inappropriate Behavior Index
All behaviors of above indices, plus:
Seclusion location
Unauthorized absence
"Other" crazy concurrent behaviors

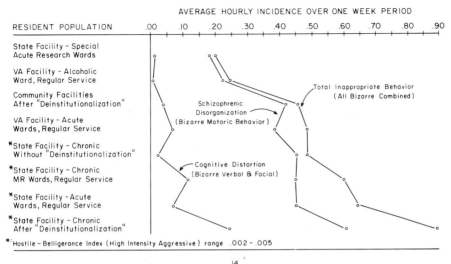

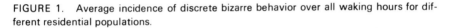

Note: Data from Time-Sample Behavioral Checklist (see Paul)[14]

FIGURE 1.   Average incidence of discrete bizarre behavior over all waking hours for different residential populations.

behaviors that are primarily motoric, while the Cognitive Distortion Index provides the sum of the actual occurrence of bizarre verbal and facial behaviors indicative of thought disorder. The Hostile-Belligerence Index totals observed incidence of high-intensity aggressive behaviors. Unlike the other higher-order scores, this index is less adequate for individual clinical monitoring, since *any* occurrence of these behaviors is critical, and requires continuous event recording for individual clinical use. The Total Inappropriate Behavior Index sums all bizarre behaviors, including a category for "other" crazy behaviors which do not fit the previous codes.

As part of a multiinstitutional generalizability-normative study of the TSBC, full week observations are available on about 1,200 patients over 36 different sites covering the full range of adult residential settings and populations.[14] A sampling of that data, presented in Figure 1, should assist in clarifying the nature of the problem. The resident populations in Figure 1 are ordered from the least to the most bizarre in terms of actual incidence over a full week period. The "VA–Alcoholic" ward was included to provide a normative base of an institutionalized population that was expected to be essentially psychiatrically normal. In fact, the average resident of a VA–Alcoholic ward performed only one bizarre behavior of any sort less than 25% of the time during all waking hours over a full week, and nearly all were inappropriate motoric behaviors. To our surprise, even less bizarre behavior occurred on special acute wards in a research facility, although the average patient did show slightly more incidents of cognitive distortion. The screening of patients for acceptance into these restricted wards obviously resulted in a very select group for investigation. Contrast the latter group of patients—about 90% of whom were diagnosed as schizophrenics—with those on regular service wards for acute patients, in which the average patient was performing at least one bizarre behavior about 65% of the time, or for those chronic patients remaining after the less severely disabled were "deinstitutionalized"—all of whom were diagnosed as schizophrenic—where the average patient performed at least one bizarre behavior about 90% of all waking hours. These are clearly different groups in terms of traditional concepts of symptomatology. In fact, those residents of community extended-care facilities, after "deinstitutionalization," were performing more bizarre behaviors of every sort, except high-intensity aggressive behaviors, than the two least disabled populations—even though the residents of those community facilities were demonstrably performing at levels tolerated by the outside community.

Nearly parallel findings emerge on examination of the actual incidence of competent performances, presented in Figure 2. Acute psychiatric patients in regular state service wards showed more bizarre behavior than any of the groups other than the chronic patients remaining after deinstitutionalization. However, Figure 2 shows that these patients still perform more

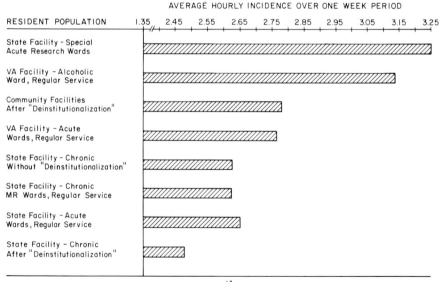

Note : Data from Time-Sample Behavioral Checklist (see Paul)[14]

FIGURE 2.   Average incidence of discrete appropriate ("normal") behaviors over all waking hours for different residential populations.

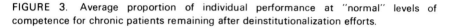

PROPORTION OF COMPETENT FUNCTIONING

CLASS OF PERFORMANCE   .00   .10   .20   .30   .40   .50   .60   .70   .80   .90   1.00

Total Appropriate Behavior   ▨▨▨▨ (range .00 - .56)

Interpersonal Skills   ▨ (range .00 - .30)

Self Care   ▨▨ (range .00 - .42)

Instrumental Roles   ▨▨▨▨▨▨ (range .00 - .92)

Note: Data from Clinical Frequencies Recording System for Social - Learning Group at Program Entry (see Paul & Lentz)[2]

FIGURE 3. Average proportion of individual performance at "normal" levels of competence for chronic patients remaining after deinstitutionalization efforts.

competently than either adult retardates or chronic patients without "deinstitutionalization." Nevertheless, I suggest that the deficits in competent performance of the bottom four population groups shown in Figure 2, combined with the extent of bizarre behavior for those four groups—which ran from nearly 50% of all waking hours to about 90% on the average (Fig. 1)—are such that nothing less than a 24 hour per day, seven day per week, comprehensive treatment program is likely to make a significant impact. I can report this with assurance for the most severely disabled population, whose average appropriate behaviors were nearly two and a half standard deviations below the most competent, since this is a group on which we have done extensive controlled research and treatment.[2]

For this population, in addition to performing at least one bizarre behavior about 90% of the time, data from the Clinical Frequencies Recording System (CFRS) provide a clear picture of the extreme deficits in competent functioning which the earlier review of the literature had suggested as a necessary focus for minimal goals of residential treatment. These data are presented in Figure 3. Unlike the TSBC, the CFRS is a program-specific means of assessment, in which time-place-situation-specific performances of each patient are recorded by clinical staff.[9,14] Such recordings require that the opportunity for patients to demonstrate each critical class of performance and for staff to assess that functioning reliably and practically must be scheduled on a regular basis. Reliability coefficients of 0.95 and above have regularly been obtained for recordings of each discrete performance.

The data presented in Figure 3 show the average terminal-level performance (i.e., competency indistinguishable from "normal") on computer-summarized higher-order scores for one group of patients the week before introduction of a comprehensive psychosocial treatment program. Over all areas of social and instrumental functioning these patients failed to perform competently on over 80% of opportunities. The interpersonal interaction and communication skills reflected in the Interpersonal Skills Index (e.g., normal conversations at meetings, informal interaction) shows severe deficits, with the average patient failing at competent performance on 96% of opportunities over a full week. Similarly, the Self-Care Index shows only 13% normal maintenance of appearance, meal behavior, bathing, or any other self-maintenance activities. The only area of competent functioning that occurred at a greater than 20% rate was instrumental roles, primarily reflecting the fact that some patients did attend scheduled meetings and activities. Overall, the severity of deficits for this group of patients, who had spent nearly two-thirds of their adult lives in mental institutions, was such that institutional control was, in fact, necessary for their survival. Additionally, the extensiveness and amount of bizarre behavior was so extreme that they simply frightened "outsiders." This is the population that will become more and more representative of the residents of our public mental institutions as "deinstitutionalization" continues.[2]

COMPREHENSIVE PSYCHOSOCIAL TREATMENT

At the time of the earlier review of the literature from which the minimal goals were determined, I also reviewed the treatment literature to see if any approach offered promise for effecting change in those areas of functioning.[6] At that time, only two approaches appeared to offer promise at all. They were both unit-wide psychosocial treatment approaches, rather than the traditional approaches of psychotherapy or chemotherapy, and neither had yet been systematically evaluated for specific effectiveness in improving functioning to the point allowing community tenure for the chronically institutionalized. My colleagues and I, therefore, proceded to construct two explicit, comprehensive unit-wide psychosocial programs for comparative evaluation, based upon the empirical promise suggested by the earlier literature. The programs, design, and outcomes of that comparative study, including a traditional hospital control group, are detailed by Paul and Lentz.[2]

Basically, both programs were constructed to focus specifically upon the areas identified as necessary minimal goals for residential treatment, with continuous assessment of both staff and patient functioning following the applied experimental-behavioral strategy. Staffing was established at the level initially existing in state hospitals. Including administrative personnel, the total staff/patient ratio averaged less than 0.57, with about 80% being nonprofessional technician-level staff. Equal focus was established for both programs with the same staff conducting each on a counterbalanced schedule; however, the specific psychosocial principles and interactional technology differed: the Milieu Therapy Program based structure, verbal content, and staff–resident interactions on communication theory and therapeutic community principles; and the Social Learning Program based structure, verbal content, and staff–resident interactions on social learning theory and principles of instrumental and associative learning.

Over 85% of every patient's waking hours was specifically scheduled for formal psychosocial focus on skills acquisition to overcome identified behavioral deficits, while maladaptive and bizarre behaviors were systematically dealt with on the basis of specified principles at all times. About 3% of waking time was scheduled for drug administration (as compared to over 6% in the traditional hospital wards), but much less actually occurred as patients in the most effective program were withdrawn to the point that fewer than 11% were on any drugs at all. Meals and morning and evening routines provided a time for explicit training in self-care skills, with ongoing assessment systems providing detailed, step-by-step focus for each individual at his/her particular level of current competence. Three to four periods each day and evening consisted of assessment and training in interpersonal and communication skills in the context of informal interaction around recreational activities. At lowest levels of functioning, two activity periods each weekday used physical exercise, arts and crafts, and practical self-care training as a means to activate patients, and to train them to focus on external stimuli. Three periods of formal classes each weekday focused upon functional arithmetic, reading, writing, speaking, homemaking, and grooming, or the minimal attentional skills necessary to participate in those content areas. Large and small group meetings during days and evenings were scheduled for practice in problem identification and solution, as well as further social skills training. Individual behaviors were monitored for each patient, with a step system increasing responsibilities, such that higher levels of performance resulted in more time devoted to prevocational and vocational training. Increasingly greater exposure to the outside world was systematically introduced as competence was demonstrated in each lower-level component.

OUTCOME AND CONCLUSIONS

Space limitations preclude detailed presentation of process and outcome analyses and findings. Since these are available elsewhere,[2,9,14] I will present only highlights of outcome, and note a few process findings that are particularly relevant to the more traditonal mode of in-office psychotherapy. A major result is that, even with such comprehensive programs with identical staff, focus, and goals, the interactional treatment techniques differ markedly, and these turn out to be critical variables for effective treatment. The Social Learning Program emerged as remarkably effective on an absolute level, and significantly more effective for every identified minimal goal of residential treatment.

The overall reduction in the average absolute incidence of maladaptive behavior in both psychosocial programs is presented in Figure 4. Although the Milieu Therapy Program did produce significant reductions in every class of maladaptive behavior, the Social Learning Program was significantly more effective for all except Cognitive Distortion. The absolute reduction in bizarre behavior for patients treated by the Social Learning Program was to levels below those of all but the two least disabled populations presented earlier (Figure 1) for every class of bizarre behavior except Cognitive Distortion. The absolute level of Cognitive Distortion was reduced to approximately that of the acute populations. However, that level was low enough that independent raters in the community failed to discriminate level of functioning on this basis, whereas all other classes of maladaptive behavior during the week prior to release predicted rated functioning in the community to at least 18 months after discharge.

More dramatic differences were obtained in overcoming severe deficits, as seen in Figure 5. Here the psychosocial procedures of the Milieu Program were only minimally effective, while those of the Social Learning Program were remarkable, indeed. Major and significant improvements were obtained for every patient in every class of behavior identified as a minimal goal for institutional populations. On an absolute level, about a quarter of the people treated by the Social Learning Program—previously among the most severely disabled schizophrenic patients ever subjected to systematic study—were functionally indistinguishable form the "normal"

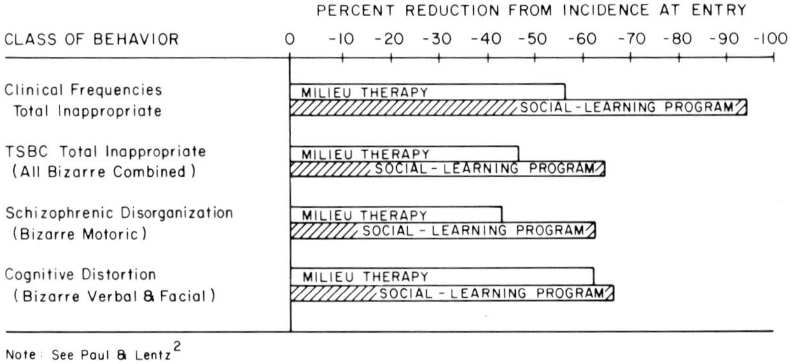

FIGURE 4. Percent reduction in average objectively assessed maladaptive behavior from program entry to release or program termination for original equated groups in two psychosocial programs. (*N* = 28 each)

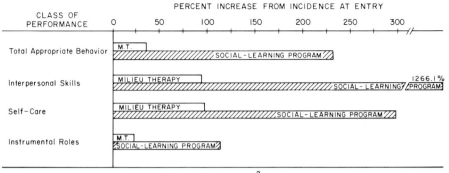

Note: Data from Clinical Frequencies Recording System (see Paul & Lentz)[2]

FIGURE 5. Percent increase in average objectively assessed incidence of competent performance from program entry to release or program termination for original equated groups in two psychosocial programs. (*N* = 28 each)

population of the same social class. Although the group as a whole was still functioning at a marginal level, the average incidence of appropriate behaviors had improved to approximately that of the VA–Alcoholic population presented earlier (Figure 2).

Practically speaking, every patient who was physically capable of participating in the Social Learning Program not only improved in all areas of focus in the relative absence of psychotropic drugs, but achieved release with continuing community stay for the minimum follow-up period of 18 months. Nearly 11% of the original group treated by the Social Learning Program improved to the point that allowed independent release with self-support and continuing community stay without rehospitalization—as compared to about 7% for the Milieu Therapy Program and, none for traditional hospital treatment. Any such release for this population was remarkable, but some ex-residents from the Social Learning Program had been successfully functioning in the community for over five years at project termination. All remaining patients who achieved community placement went to board-and-room facilities. Of course, community stay is dependent upon follow-up procedures. However, declining-contact aftercare consultation based on social learning principles was provided for releases from all programs. This aftercare consultation prevented recidivism in over 97% of cases.

Since the Social Learning Program treated more patients and was more effective (over 92% released with continuing community stay) than the Milieu Therapy Program (71%) or traditional hospital programs (about 48%), it was nearly four times as cost effective as traditional practices, even considering only direct costs. Employing those social learning procedures now known to be most effective, the most severely disabled mental patient who is physically capable of participation could reasonably achieve minimal goals, allowing community placement in 26 to 30 weeks, while improvement to a level of relatively independent self-support would likely require two to three years.

Based upon the expense of institutional treatment and its restrictions for clientele, Bob Lentz and I have recommended that public mental institutions not only focus upon the identified minimal goals required for release, but limit intramural work to the achievement of levels of functioning that will allow safe survival in less restrictive community environments, without serious burden to self or others.[2] "Optimal goals" are defined as further enhancement of social functioning and instrumental role skills, and further reductions in distressing maladaptive behaviors, to allow greater freedom of choice, autonomy, and satisfactions in the social and economic areas. Focus on optimal goals appears appropriate for work starting or continuing on an extramural basis.

Our findings show little promise for in-office modes of psychosocial treatment with the more severely disabled. Even focusing on specific tasks within the Social Learning Program produced no demonstrable effects from group therapy to "real life" functioning until patients had improved in attentional components of being "on time" and "on task" through continuous and consistent focus in the psychosocial environment.[2,15] The severe deficits in self-care, interpersonal interaction, and communication adequacy, as well as deficits in prevocational, vocational, and housekeeping skills, all required continuous, consistent, concentrated focus in the ongoing environment to bring patients to a level meeting minimal goals. Similarly, all classes of bizarre behavior except Cognitive Distortion and a few other bizarre behaviors based upon excessive stress reactions were found to require ongoing, continuous, and consistent contingencies directly within the psychosocial environment for their reliable reduction or elimination.

However, the different situational specificity of cognitive versus social behaviors, and of some stress reactions, does provide guidance for more precise use of in-office procedures. Specifically, cognitive dysfunction shows little situational specificity, and does respond to continuous, consistent, concrete information transmission,[2,16,17] whereas excessive conditioned stress reactions have been found to respond to specific in-office techniques.[2,18] Thus, only after severely debilitated patients have been brought to a level of minimal functioning are in-office procedures effective or efficient modes of intervention within comprehensive psychosocial treatment, and then with a specific focus. Such a mode of treatment appears more feasible for work on optimal goals with the higher functioning patient who no longer requires residential treatment, or who never did. In any case, the outlook for schizophrenic patients no longer need be viewed as one of continuous deterioration, requiring life-long care. We have no "breakthrough," but we do have data-based hope, and where there is hope—

REFERENCES

1. Ozarin LD, Redick RW, Taube CA: A quarter century of psychiatric care, 1950–1974: A statistical review. *Hosp Commun Psychiatry* **27**:515–519, 1976.
2. Paul GL, Lentz RJ: *Psychosocial Treatment of Chronic Mental Patients: Milieu versus Social-learning Programs.* Cambridge, Harvard University Press, 1977.
3. Paul GL: Experimental-behavioral approaches to schizophrenia, in Cancro R, Fox N, Shapiro L (eds): *Strategic Intervention in Schizophrenia: Current Developments in Treatment.* New York, Behavioral Publications, 1974, pp 187–200.
4. Spitzer RL, Andreasen NC, Endicott J: Schizophrenia and other psychotic disorders in DSM–III. *Schizophr Bull* **4**:489–511, 1978.
5. Hagen RL: Behavioral therapies and the treatment of schizophrenia. *Schizophr Bull* **13**:70–96, 1975.
6. Paul GL: Chronic mental patient: Current status—future directions. *Psychol Bull* **71**:81–94, 1969.
7. Strauss JS, Carpenter WT: The prognosis of schizophrenia: Rationale for a multidimensional concept. *Schizophr Bull* **4**:56–67, 1978.
8. Beels CC: Social networks, the family, and the psychiatric patient: Introduction to the issue. *Schizophr Bull* **4**:512–521, 1978.
9. Paul GL: Social competence and the institutionalized mental patient, in Smye M, Wine J (eds): *Identification and Enhancement of Social Competence.* New York, Guilford Press, in press.
10. Paul GL: The implementation of effective treatment programs for chronic mental patients: Obstacles and recommendations, in Talbott JA (ed): *The Chronic Mental Patient.* Washington, DC, American Psychiatric Association, 1978, pp 99–127.
11. Paul GL, Power CT, Engel KL, et al: The Time-Sample Behavioral Check-list Observer Manual, in Paul GL (ed): *Observational Assessment Instrumentation for Institutional Research and Treatment.* Cambridge, Harvard University Press, in press.
12. Lorr M, Klett CJ, Cave R: Higher level psychotic syndromes. *J Abnorm Psychol* **72**:74–77, 1967.
13. Fiske DW: *Strategies for Personality Research.* San Francisco, Jossey-Bass, 1978.
14. Paul GL (ed): *Observational Assessment Instrumentation for Institutional Research and Treatment.* Cambridge, Harvard University Press, in preparation.
15. Paden RC, Himelstein HC, Paul GL: Video-tape vs. verbal feedback in the modification of meal behavior of chronic mental patients. *J Consult Clin Psychol* **42**:623, 1974.
16. Mariotto MJ: The interaction of person and situation effects for chronic mental patients: A two year follow-up. *J Abnorm Psychol*, in press.
17. Mariotto MJ, Paul GL: Persons versus situations in the real-life functioning of chronically institutionalized mental patients. *J Abnorm Psychol* **84**:483–493, 1975.
18. Paul GL, Bernstein DA: *Anxiety and Clinical Problems: Treatment by Systematic Desensitization and Related Techniques.* New York, General Learning Press, 1973.

Chapter 16

All-or-None Phenomena in the Psychotherapy of Severe Disorders

CLARENCE G. SCHULZ

The phenomenon of splitting, referring to "good" and "bad" attitudes toward others or toward oneself, is a prominent feature in borderline personality disorders, as well as in the schizophrenias. My thesis is that splitting is only one aspect of the broader concept of the all-or-none phenomenon. Our diagnostic abilities and therapeutic efforts will improve if we recognize the many clinical manifestations of all-or-none phenomena. Among these I will present examples of cognitive aspects, affective features, narcissistic manifestations, and aspects of superego- and ego-ideal functions. In addition, I will cite a few references about all-or-none phenomena appearing in the psychiatric literature, and will consider developmental relationships to splitting. Finally, I will focus on some implications for psychotherapeutic techniques with these patients.

Since they occur in neurotics and normals, all-or-none phenomena are not pathognomonic of severe disorders, but become significant for diagnosis when combined with the other features of borderline personality so well detailed by Kernberg.[1]

CLARENCE G. SCHULZ • The Sheppard and Enoch Pratt Hospital, Towson, Maryland 21204.

CLINICAL EXAMPLES

I shall illustrate a variety of all-or-none features as these occur in different patients.

My first example comes from a psychological report on a 15-year-old adolescent patient. The initial diagnosis of phobic neurosis was later changed to borderline personality disorder. She did very well on the Wechsler Adult Intelligence Scale (WAIS) with a verbal IQ of 133. She was described as not liking to make decisions, and passivity was prominent. The responses to the projective tests had a bizarre flavor. The following all-or-none features were evident. "Patient quickly recognizes that complete understanding and control will not be possible for her. When she senses this lack, her current tendency is to avoid dealing with the problems altogether." In describing the Thematic Apperception Test (TAT) story, two examples that are relevant for this presentation were: (a) the first sign of failure on the part of the person in her story leads to a termination of that activity; and (b) when the patient needs to explain why a person is sick, she makes the person dead. This same patient informed her therapist that if she tells everything about herself she will have nothing left and therefore may as well be dead.

A patient may present the all-or-none concept as an extreme situation that is a "case of life and death," or "I either must control or I will be controlled." Fears revolve around giving in completely, with the only alternative being to resist everything. Sometimes when these patients are facing transfer to the state hospital, they view the future as "hopeless," with the notion that no one gets out—which, of course, is not true. Patients with all-or-none attitudes will become extremely stubborn and dogmatic, maintaining a very fixed position, declaring "that's the way it is going to be," with an inability to crawl in off the limb to seek compromise, negotiation, or resolution. Another phrase enhancing resistance to treatment might be, "That is the way I am; don't try to change me." One patient, in a quite resistive way, said "I don't want to connect anything. You want to connect things together." Another aspect of all-or-none manifesting itself as a resistance in treatment occurs when the patient defiantly says "I will work it out myself."

All-or-none may become related to *narcissistic* aspects. From this perspective, any flaw or criticism of a part immediately tends to include the whole. Any difficulty, instead of being partial, becomes experienced as total and devastating fluctuations in self-esteem. If one is not perfect, one is nothing at all. The patient in an all-or-none attitude might, instead of idealizing a few traits, become totally infatuated with the other person, as evident in a severe "crush." Ambitions and ambitious striving can have an all-or-none grandiose dimension. As an example, only a Ph.D. thesis can be considered important, rather than any lesser contribution. Another patient thought he should know what was in the textbook at the beginning of the course. A person decides to drop a course when he doesn't like the teacher, when he cannot master the subject perfectly, or get a perfect mark in the course. These unreasonable total expectations will become important later on when I take up treatment approaches.

In the *time* dimension, incidents from the past loom up with a vividness that seems to flood the present. In this way, present perspective is disrupted by feelings and events from the past. Patients, unable to tolerate any delay, insist on leaving the hospital, with the attitude "it is now or never." Even voluntary patients who have submitted a notice are often unable to wait the legally prescribed three days, and may impulsively run away. If the person is late for an appointment and cannot make up the time, the situation becomes worse, so he reaches the point of cancelling altogether.

Sometimes these patients are really quite threatened by physical illness. Even a minor ailment arouses fear of death and dying. This is especially true if the illness or ailment occurs without having been self-inflicted.

Ambivalence or indecision itself is viewed by the patient in an extreme way as intolerable. He anticipates that, if he has mixed feelings about a thing, he will be unable to decide anything, and will end up in a helpless paralysis. A patient had difficulty making choices in selecting a program for a music recital, since some pieces were favored by some friends, whereas others would be favored by other friends. In this way, the patient was unable to please everyone, and the need to make choices then became impossible. This same patient hated to come to treatment, because it was degrading, and, at the same time, since not everyone was receiving therapy, "I shouldn't receive it."

Sometimes the patient wishes for and provokes a stronger external force to deal with ambivalence. For example, with the demand, "Why don't you commit me?", the ambivalence is dealt with by attempting to externalize one-half of the conflict, and perpetuate the split.

An all-or-none attitude related to object constancy is the concern of the patient who has unescorted responsibilities. If not accompanied by staff, he fears he will be forgotten by staff—out of sight is truly out of mind in this instance.

In *affective* aspects of splitting, the fear of anger equals the fear of an explosion. All-or-none is experienced like a trigger of a gun, with an inability to modulate the experience and express a partial affect.

Hallucinations are sometimes a reflection of splitting in the psychotic patient. For example, a patient was trying to decide whether or not she felt ready to leave the hospital. She felt better, but then she felt she would like to stay longer. This was then followed by hallucinating her former therapist's voice saying that, by remaining, she was "taking the easy way

TABLE I.   Two Constrasting Patient Approaches

All or none	Integrated
Splitting into either "good" or "bad"	Ambivalence
Rigid overcontrol vs. loss of control	Modulated expression of affects
Attack entire problem vs. avoidance of problem	Approach by breaking down into manageable parts
Now or never	Ability to tolerate delay
Murderous rage or total denial of anger	Partial expression of anger
Infatuation (crush) or denial of dependency	Mature object dependency
Either my way or your way	Shared responsibility, cooperation
Either this way or not at all	Able to consider variety of options
Perfect health vs. death	Tolerate illness or defect
Complete optimism vs. hopelessness	Realistic appraisal of limitations
Impulsivity vs. failure to act	Appropriate decision making
Extreme attachment vs. rejection of object	Stable interpersonal relationships
Harsh disapproval, self-injury vs. absent moral constraint	Fairly consistent moral regulations
Narcissistic ideal expectations vs. despair of accomplishing anything	Reasonably stable goals
Overeating vs. starvation	Moderation in caloric intake
Severe alcohol intoxication vs. abstinence	Self-control in drinking
Instant recovery vs. no progress	Improvement by small increments, working through
Special patient or feels overlooked	One individual among many

out." Here her own uncertainty was expressed in the form of splitting as a former therapist's voice, rather than an ambivalent attitude. It was as though she could not integrate and hold into awareness opposite attitudes, but instead had to take one position, and have someone else (via a hallucinated voice) take the opposite viewpoint. Instead of the psychotic's hallucination, the borderline patient experiences the contrary attitude as a strong thought, such as a prominent obsession. Yet the borderline still accepts the thought as his own.

I attended a conference where the interviewer, in summarizing, pointed out to the patient the various ways in which he was using an all-or-none approach in his attitude. The patient listened, paused, and replied, "I agree with you 100%." The following table, in summary form, presents the contrasting all-or-none attitude with the more mature, integrated approach.

REFERENCES TO THE PSYCHIATRIC AND PSYCHOANALYTIC LITERATURE

For a phenomenon which is rather widespread in psychological experience, there are relatively few references in the psychiatric literature.

By contrast, much has been written in recent years about the concept of splitting. I will cite some of those references which seem pertinent to our topic.

Sullivan[2] described various syndromes in his *Conceptions*. Among these, his account of what he called the "self-absorbed" person accurately outlines both the developmental good-bad dichotomy and clinical all-or-none attitudes.

> Objectively, to us, the person concerned is the mother; to the infant, these are two vaguely limited but entirely distinct people. The discrimination of the Good Mother pattern of events and the Bad Mother pattern of events constitutes a primary bifurcation of interpersonal experience evidence of which persists in most people throughout life.
>
> These people have no grey; everything tends to be black or white. Their friends are simply wonderful people. People whom they dislike are just simply impossible. Their "love" is melodramatic to a degree that confounds its object—excepting the object be another self-absorbed person.

The sole psychoanalytic reference I have been able to turn up is an article by an Indian analyst, Girindrashekhar Bose,[3] entitled, "'All or None' Attitude in Sex." The following is a description of the patient's attitude.

> If sex is permissible with one woman at all, why should it not be so with all women including near relatives, like sister and mother and for the matter of that with persons of the same sex as well and with children and old persons; in other words there should be no compromise or restraint in sex if it is to be allowed at all; it should be either all or none; once a person yields to sex there is the chance that he will be carried away by it and will not be able to observe any restraint whatsoever. The idea of restraint does not at all appeal to the patient. He thinks restraint is an impossibility in matters of sex and it is for this reason that he voluntarily took up the ideal of no-sex. Since one pleasure leads to another it is desirable to shun all pleasures in life lest they should lead to sex. The patient is against forming any attachment whether it be with his wife or with his children or friends or any inanimate object.

The author relates these opposite attitudes to active and passive wishes. Accordingly, "If these two opposite portions fail to effect a compromise, an all-or-none attitude toward sex develops" p 94. The problem is connected with conflicting parental identification.

Although I am not conversant with Piaget's concepts, I have included a description furnished me by Dr. Rolf Muuss of Goucher College. Piaget's observation of the cognitive development in the "preoperational" child (ages two to seven years) appears to provide us with a description of a child's normal developmental inability to integrate successive stages, comparable to our all-or-none patient. The child is presented with bar or pencil in a vertical position, and asked to draw or select from multiple-choice illustrations the successive movements as it falls to a horizontal position.

Flavell[4] writing about Piaget, states:

> Preoperational thought, then, is static and immobile. It is a kind of
> thought which can focus impressionistically and sporadically on this or
> that momentary, static condition but cannot adequately link a whole set
> of successive conditions into an integrated totality by taking account of
> the transformations which unify them and render them logically coherent.

Meza[5] recently cited his book, *El Cholerico*, when listing twelve ways
in which borderline patients characteristically expresses anger. Items 6 and
7 would confirm my impression:

> 6. They are unilateral in thinking they are right.
> 7. They insist on an all-or-nothing response.

A psychologist, Lazarus,[6] has referred to our subject as "dichotomous
reasoning," and recommends "cognitive restructuring" in treatment.

Another psychologist, Frankel-Brunswick,[7] refers to what psychologists
call "ambiguity intolerance."

> In these individuals there is, on the surface, a rigid, unambiguous
> adherence to cultural and conventional values, but this is combined with
> an underlying destructiveness directed toward these same values; this
> combination of opposites is in contrast to the establishment of a healthy
> "medium distance" to the culture.
> In a similar manner, an underlying ambivalence toward the parents is
> split into a positive and a negative side and expressed through alternative
> media, e.g., stereotyped and exaggerated admiration in response to direct
> questions, combined with the conception of punitiveness and harshness in
> parents revealed in the indirect material. Medium distance is again lack-
> ing, and feelings are expressed in terms of the ends of a continuum rather
> than of a continuum proper.

Finally, Kernberg,[1] in describing the borderline patient's harsh superego,
states:

> These patients respond with an all-or-nothing superego reaction instead of
> the normal, flexible one. In the example of an unexpected call from the
> boss, such patients would not pay any attention to their superior's friendly
> suggestions. They react only if stronger criticism of them is expressed, but
> then with the experience of being cruelly attacked or persecuted. (p 143)

In describing splitting, he states "The *lack of synthesis of contradictory
self and object images* has numerous pathological consequences" (italics by
Kernberg).

THEORY OF DEVELOPMENTAL ORIGIN OF
ALL-OR-NONE PHENOMENA AND THEIR
RELATION TO SPLITTING

The underlying developmental concepts related to splitting draw very
heavily on the theories of Klein.[8] In addition, these concepts are consistent

with Sullivan's "good" and "bad" self and mother. Summarizing from more recent writings, it is postulated that differentiation between self- and object-representation begins to emerge at around three months of age. These emerging and evanescent self-concepts are separated into a "good" self and "bad" self-representations, with corresponding "good" and "bad" object-representations. There tends to be an inability to integrate these extreme polarized attitudes. Denial and projection of the bad aspects of the self on to the object are used to rid the self of the feeling of badness. As maturation and development proceed, sometime around the sixth or eighth month, there comes an ability to integrate good and bad aspects of the self and good and bad aspects of the object with the resulting ambivalent attitudes toward oneself and others. At that point of integration of conflicting attitudes, there develops the achievement of the Kleinian concept of the "depressive position." During this period, then, we see the infant shifting from the so-called "schizoid position" to the "depressive position." It is postulated that later on the borderline personality makes use of this normal developmental pattern of splitting as a defense—not necessarily that there is a fixation or regression to this period of time in development. Actually the difficulties resulting in subsequent borderline personality disorders probably occur later in the separation–individuation scheme. These developmental concepts fit in nicely with the often observed clinical phenomena whereby schizophrenic, especially paranoid, patients show much splitting, and, as they improve, begin to be ambivalent about themselves and others. Along with the ambivalence, we see the capacity to experience depression in response to loss or separation, rather than paranoid delusional attitudes, confusion, or disorganization.

Certainly we can see how splitting or polarization into all or none would be related to the issue of the lack of fusion of aggression and libido. In Hartman's,[9] terms, the lack of neutralization would render the early infant unable to experience much capacity for the modulation of affect. Clinically this lack of neutralization manifests itself in the severe disorders with the aggressive dimension projected onto the object, and in turn the object's being feared. In addition, there is the fear of omnipotence of one's own aggression. Archaic superego manifestations reflect unneutralized aggression. On the libidinal attachment dimension, there exists the experience of the intense attraction with fear of fusion and merging in relation to the object. One can readily see that, with both of these extremes operating simultaneously or alternately, the ability to integrate affects is reduced. The appearance of signal anxiety would threaten with more primitive unintegrated expression of unneutralized libido and aggression, and, therefore, the reevoking of the early all-or-none polarized attitudes. This potential response to anxiety would account for the emergence of all-or-none phenomena in any person, and therefore cut across diagnostic categories and levels of disorder.

IMPLICATIONS FOR PSYCHOTHERAPEUTIC TECHNIQUE

One can readily see how, since splitting is the antithesis of integration, mutuality, and negotiation, collaborative participation in psychotherapy becomes jeopardized by the tendency toward polarization. A corollary important phenomenon of splitting in the patient is reflected in divisive attitudes among members of the treatment team. It becomes very important for the therapist to be alert to this, and to coordinate the treatment approach, allow for polarized opinions, but at the same time facilitate communication. These patients are frequently regarded as "manipulators" when schisms arise among members of the treatment team. Similarly, the borderline patient's rapid fluctuation in level of functioning makes it very difficult to deal with him in a consistent way, if one relates oneself to the cross-sectional behavior rather than to the longitudinal adjustment. The responsibility levels may change rapidly, according to the patient's fluctuation in behavior. Clinical management is influenced by all or none manifesting as impulsivity, stubbornness, explosive anger, vulnerability to separation, rapid shifts in self-esteem, and difficulty in compromising.

Basic to any psychotherapeutic approach is a recognition of the all-or-none process. Unless the therapist is aware of the phenomenon, he will be unable to interest the patient in its observance. Repeated confrontations about all-or-none attitudes assist the patient in recognizing his failure to use more integrative approaches.

Another factor bringing about change in the patient is the therapist's (and other staff's) ability to approach dichotomous aspects in an integrated way. By not taking unnecessarily rigid positions about fees, schedules, and other negotiable aspects of treatment, the therapist conveys a model of potential for compromise in the resolution of differences. A therapists's counterreaction of inflexibility is easily evoked by these patients' frequent extreme stance. These counterreactions must be quickly discovered, and discussed openly with the patient.

For these patients, it is necessary to point out gains made in the course of treatment. The therapist must make explicit the steps being accomplished as they are achieved. As an example, a patient who had remained confined to a seclusion-room area began to be able to rejoin fellow patients in the living room. Meanwhile, she was lamenting her situation by contrasting it with those of her classmates with whom she had grown up and who were now in college or getting jobs. I would have to point out to her the fact that she had been able to move out of the seclusion area, and this was a gain. It is also important to point out the process involving the all-or-none attitude. Consistent with this finding is the inevitable problem these patients have with "working through." A patient was devastated by the recurrence of symptoms connected with separation anxiety. She thought that this was all over and done with the first time around—only to discover that it had to be dealt with again at approaching discharge. She thought, "How can I be getting well if I still have symptoms?" Even pointing out a gain can lead the patient to an all-or-none response, such as, "Well, then, I don't need any more treatment." This, in turn, must be focused for its all-or-none features.

All staff need to be alert to recognizing the patient's externalization of one-half of his or her conflict in order to avoid ambivalent conflicts. The patient may have to adhere to an extreme position, lest he appear weak and be taken advantage of. Instead of joining in the argument, one must try to put the conflict back to the patient. If the therapist attempts to enlist the patient in an exploration of a variety of options, the patient's response is to seize upon one choice, and insist that it is either that or none at all.

Similarly, one must be aware of the patient's tendency either to work out everything by herself, or expect a therapist to do it all. Here, patients will sometimes conceal things from the therapist in order to avoid discussing aspects of the problems. Coupled with this may be the projection of an all-or-none attitude onto the therapist, who is viewed as arbitrary and unwilling to discuss issues.

Finally, we must teach the patient how to attack problems which initially are viewed as impossibly massive. Here I assist the patient in breaking down the problem into manageable parts. A favorite example of mine is the patient who was unable to face her desk piled high with items requiring attention. She had gotten to the point of throwing the morning mail onto the heap while she quickly walked past, looking the other way. I told her to sort it all out according to cheques that needed to be cashed, utility bills to be paid in order to prevent cutting off of services, postponable correspondence, and mail to "occupant" that could be thrown out. Tackling the problem in this way provided her with a model to apply to other all-or-none situations.

In conclusion, I view all-or-none phenomena—when occurring in borderline and psychotic patients—as a broad category of splitting. Focusing on the process should enable the patient to understand a mechanism of resistance in order to facilitate a more integrative approach.

REFERENCES

1. Kernberg OF: *Borderline Conditions and Pathological Narcissism.* New York, Jason Aronson Inc, 1975.
2. Sullivan HS: *Conceptions of Modern Psychiatry.* Washington, DC, William Alanson White Psychiatric Foundation, 1948, p 38, p 39.
3. Bose G: All-or-None Attitude in Sex. *Samiksa* **1,** 1947. Reprinted in *Yearb Psychoanal* **4:**86–98, 1948, p. 87.

Chapter 17

Paradoxical Interventions

Leverage for Therapeutic Change in Individual and Family Systems

LYMAN C. WYNNE

The creation of a regressive transference in classical psychoanalytic treatment of individuals can be regarded as a form of paradoxical intervention. The paradox is that the regressive instability generates stability. As the patient's associations become more "free," he goes into increasing psychological disequilibrium which then appears to produce, homeostatically, a reduced disequilibrium.

Certain conditions and sequences are essential for this paradoxical result in psychoanalysis. First, the dyadic treatment *system* of analyst and patient must have clear *boundaries*, without intrusions from others, and with departures only at agreed-upon times. Usually this condition is described as limit-setting. Acting out and spilling over of conflictual experience into non-treatment settings impedes the analytic process.

Second, the patient must be willing and able to *change*, to bring new ingredients of experience, through free associations, into the dyadic treatment system, thus amplifying the magnitude, and elaborating the pattern, of conflict and disequilibrium.

LYMAN C. WYNNE • Department of Psychiatry, University of Rochester School of Medicine and Dentistry, Rochester, New York 14642.

Third, the analyst holds *steady* in his analytic role and optimally limits his input to interpretations about the patient's productions. This means that the patient's conflictual tension and disequilibrium will not be eased by complementary behavioral changes in the analyst.

Fourth, if the analytic contract is followed, the pressure is squarely on the patient to be the one that reorganizes and *restructures* himself. The assumption is that the patient can draw upon positive resources (ego functions) that continue during the regressive transference and enable him to work within the framework of the analytic relationship. Both the treatment relationship and the intrapsychic functioning of the patient thus reach a relatively steady state (homeostasis). In conventional terms, this "working through" leads to termination.

The psychoanalytic goal is not, however, simple reversal of the regression. It is not change along one or more dimensions, not, for example, the elimination of tension and conflict. Rather, the intrapsychic restructuring optimally is a creative transformation. It is a new and individually unique "solution," induced because the paradox of analysis actually is insoluble. The analysand stays within treatment boundaries, and tries to be simultaneously more "free" (primary process functioning), and more able to choose his thoughts and actions (secondary process). This problem, however, cannot be resolved so long as he merely tries to adjust to one expectation or the other. Instead, the successful psychoanalysis stimulates a new perspective, new "rules," a structured transformation of the self and of the analytic relationship, not mere adjustment.

The analytic structural change, in theory, is a "second-order" change,[1] not in the size of psychological functions, but in their pattern.[2] This theoretically optimal outcome occurs if the patient undergoes what I have called "the anguish and creative passions of not escaping double binds,"[3] in this instance, of "therapeutic" double binds. (Double binds, I hasten to note, are more complex repetitive patterns than paradoxes; that distinction is beyond the scope of this discussion. See Sluzki and Ransom.)[4]

To be sure, this "classical" analytic paradigm is rarely carried through in actual practice. Either the analyst or the analysand is apt to retreat from the task, perhaps for good and sufficient reasons, but more often, I fear, through a failure to comprehend the necessary conditions and the potential rewards of a creative outcome. Nevertheless, as a treatment paradigm seen from a systems perspective, the classical psychoanalytic method is one form of paradoxical intervention. To my knowledge, it has not heretofore been recognized as paradoxical; but, I submit, it does warrant this designation.

Traditionally, it has been said that schizophrenic and borderline patients are unsuitable for classical analytic treatment. Such patients seem unable to stay within the boundaries of the analytic relationship. Hence, the regression diffuses into nontreatment settings, and the pressure of "need" for equilibrium is dissipated. If classical analysis is attempted, "deviance" is continuously amplified with inadequate homeostatic reequilibration, and the possibility of a paradoxical transformation does not develop.

A small but distinguished group of analysts have treated borderline and schizophrenic patients, following as closely as possible the regressive transference model, modified with a number of so-called parameters to help hold the psychotic transference within the treatment system. For example, in his technique of direct analysis, Rosen[5] quickly used his powerful personality to contain the psychotic problem within the relationship with himself; temporarily, he appeared to achieve remarkable success. Unfortunately, the follow-through was disappointing. More often, and with more success, analysts have relied upon less dramatic methods for more slowly and enduringly establishing boundaries of the therapeutic relationship before the psychotic regressive amplification is encouraged.

In addition, for patients who are deeply psychotic, such treatment needs to be carried out within a supportive milieu, most often in a hospital setting. If the spillover of the regressive difficulties cannot be contained within the dyadic relationship with the analyst, hopefully it can be contained within the hospital milieu. This model for treatment of individual schizophrenics in hospitals, for example at Chestnut Lodge, continues to emphasize that the dyadic relationship is the *primary* system within which the regression takes place. The traditional division of functions between therapist and administrator illustrates the principles that I have described; the administrator and hospital staff are more concerned with the supportive and nonparadoxical contributions to treatment. The social system of the hospital is, moreover, expected not to interfere, so long as the regression remains within the dyadic relationship. In earlier years, at least, the still broader systems of family and community were mostly excluded; hopefully, they too did not interfere with treatment. Most importantly, the family did not take the patient out of the hospital before restabilization and a new equilibrium could be achieved.

I hasten to add that a fully psychotic regressive transference is not sought by most psychotherapists today with individual schizophrenics. Nevertheless, I believe that individual psychotherapy with borderline and schizophrenic patients labors under some of the same handicaps of the more classical regressive transference model. Perhaps the most important difficulty is that the patient's changes, before they have stabilized, tend to overshoot or undershoot, in see-saw swings from disturbing amplification of symptoms to constricted lack of change. This boundary problem makes paradoxical intervention of this kind difficult as long as the patient's ego boundaries remain permeable, fragmented, or disintegrated. That is, there is no personality system to stabilize in a clear way. Later, when recovery has proceeded to some degree, then *selective* use of paradoxical approaches with individuals may be fruitful, for example, as proposed by Frankl.[6]

For the most part, then, therapy that initially is intended to follow the analytic model often veers toward a supportive approach, especially for more disturbed patients. Supportive psychotherapy, in contrast to analysis, is nonparadoxical insofar as the intent from the start is to reduce disequilibrium directly and not seek to modify the personality as a system.

Behavioral therapy is also nonparadoxical, usually with more of an emphasis upon processes and behaviors, each undergoing direct positive change, as in social skill building, and usually without explicit use of a concept of psychological structure or personality as a system. This is less true with a number of recent extensions of behavioral treatment concepts. Family therapy may be either paradoxical or nonparadoxical. My own preference is to use nonparadoxical methods whenever they seem likely to work for a suitable treatment goal; but certain problems, usually characterized by a repetitive treatment failure or impasse, yield remarkably well to a thorough and consistent application of paradoxical principles in the context of a therapeutic system with a sustained and identifiable boundary.
boundary.

When paradoxical interventions are used with families, a systemic transformation is sought, just as in psychoanalysis, but the primary "system" is the family, not the individual personality. In addition, the *direction* of paradoxical intervention in psychoanalysis and in family therapy usually is the opposite: while analysis usually begins by amplifying "deviance," family therapy (in the form I shall describe) usually begins by strengthening and stabilizing aspects of the family homeostasis.

The latter approach, in which homeostasis is positively connoted[7] and supported, may seem strange indeed, because change from a homeostatic impasse is routinely a treatment goal. The immediate and most obvious objection is that the symptoms simply will be perpetuated, and that not only the individual patient's difficulties but also the family's presumably disordered way of functioning would be enduringly sustained. What is the likelihood that change will emerge in family systems that for so many years have been described as highly pathogenic?

First of all, I must stress the fundamental principle that in any enduring system there is a dynamic equilibrium between deviance amplification and deviance reduction. The concept of an open system maintained in a steady state with directional change implies that tendencies to deviance amplification are more or less balanced by counteractive forces. For example, increases in tension are reduced with the negative feedback of counteractive processes. When Walter Cannon dubbed these self-regulating or self-equilibrating properties of the biologic systems with the term homeostasis, he also suggested that the concept might apply to social organization. However, he was especially impressed with the stability of the inner biologic system in the face of constant external change. For example, thermoregulation of warm-blooded animals is a truly impressive example of finely tuned feedback in which the stabilizing processes receive more attention than the change-producing processes. However, in other biologic functions, such as blood pressure and heart-rate regulation, the capacity to deviate significantly under conditions of internal and external stressors is also highly important, with the level of the baseline equilibrium also changing, but more gradually.

In my view, those who have applied systems theory to psychological and social systems have vastly overemphasized the deviance-reducing, negative feedback aspects of these systems, and often overlooked altogether the equally crucial and inevitable change-producing, deviance-amplifying aspects of living systems. Change does not need to be pushed or forced; it occurs "naturally from within." However, psychotherapists, including family therapists, often write and act as if only through their heroic input will change ever be induced in "resistant," "stabilized" patients and families, most of all in schizophrenics and their families.

Before turning to the kinds of paradoxical interventions that are currently used in family therapy, I should acknowledge that most present-day treatment of schizophrenics, both from a pharmacologic and a psychosocial approach, is preoccupied with maintaining the "equilibrium" of the schizophrenic, not in structural or system change of either patient or family. The schizophrenic has been regarded as in a highly tenuous and vulnerable state, subject to decompensation either from overstimulation or understimulation. Overstimulation has been regarded as producing deviance amplification, with fragmentation and disorganization of the individual's personality system. Understimulation has been viewed as leading to the so-called negative (deficit) symptoms of social withdrawal, inertia, flatness of affect, and a chronic residual state, which could be regarded, from a systems standpoint, as the endpoint of excessive deviance-counteracting forces.

From the therapeutic standpoint, these approaches exemplify concern with the principle of equilibrium. Wing,[8] for example, has described therapy with schizophrenics much as if one were helping the patient walk a tightrope from which he is likely to fall to one side or the other. The implication is that the patient has such an extraordinary vulnerability, a permanent handicap, that the therapist is foolhardy, if not irresponsible, who allows or encourages amplification of any of the problems. Understandably, a reduced range and quality of functioning often results with this type of therapy. Whether such extreme caution is necessary depends upon one's concept of the degree of vulnerability of schizophrenics. Such therapy is explicitly nonparadoxical, though the systems principle of a homeostatic equilibrium is clearly utilized. These methods are direct and safe, at least in the sense that they are not likely to induce major criticism from persons outside of the treatment setting, but the possibility of significant systemic change and growth of new potentialities is sacrificed. I have already noted the special hazards of paradoxical intervention using the classical psychoanalytic model.

In contrast, paradoxical therapy with family systems that begins by supporting the "overstabilized" side of the family equilibrium does not carry these hazards. In capsule form, this alternative type of paradoxical intervention involves the strengthening of negative feedback, the homeostatic and stabilizing tendencies within the family system. The paradox lies in the strategy of supporting a lack of change in order to induce change.

The idea of not only tolerating but positively connoting various difficulties of the families of schizophrenics is in accord with my view that these families are not exclusively pathogenic. Their assets and resources for contributing to therapy have been very inadequately recognized. Applied to the family unit, this viewpoint is similar to that expressed by Searles[9] who has eloquently described the positive, reciprocal aspects of the relationship between the schizophrenic and his much-maligned mother.

Additionally, the use of paradoxical interventions with families eliminates the confrontational tone which has been justly criticized as characterizing some forms of family therapy. Blaming, and suggesting that things should be done differently—certainly a form of implicit blaming—is avoided with the paradoxical emphasis upon support of the way things are.

Once the battle for structure, to use Whitaker's term,[10] has been won by the therapist, and his leadership for the family treatment system has been established, then the therapist can prescribe that certain "small" aspects of family functioning should be carefully maintained, in a self-conscious manner, often with special sequences, timing and ritualization. Because family patterns "normally" are maintained out of awareness, the prescriptions of deliberate stabilization of *any* detail puts in motion, inexorably, processes of change that will reverberate throughout the family system.

As Selvini-Palazzoli and her colleagues have emphasized,[7] the participation of *all* family members in the paradoxically prescribed pattern powerfully magnifies the process of change. But, because the therapist has been supporting and confirming a pattern that the family members themselves have regarded as fixed and usually as necessary, the family's tendency to extrude, oppose, or question ideas from outsiders is undercut. After the therapist has become the family's staunch ally, he expresses even more concern than they about the problems and dangers of change. When change does begin, often with dramatic speed, it is initiated and supported by the family members themselves, not pushed or forced by the therapist. Indeed, continuation of the symptom is usually helpful until the shift to a new dynamic balance and a new focus for family functioning has been firmly achieved.

Most families of schizophrenics have had a variety of contacts with hospitals, therapists of various persuasions, clinics, and social agencies. Nevertheless, their social network as a whole usually is remarkably restricted. Many years ago, I described how some of these families try to minimize their constant disequilibrium by acting as if they were a closed system, without the usual "gates" for entry and exit, and without being able to acknowledge internal changes due to growth, aging, etc. I used the metaphor of a family boundary being like a "rubber fence";[11] change ("deviance") is interpreted as nonchange by these families in accord with enduring family myths. For example, schizophrenic symptoms often are viewed as not a change of the patient's "real self," but as something extraneous that takes place outside the family boundary. The family therapist has a preliminary task of sorting out who and what is included in the "family," and establishing a workable location for himself. Family boundary definition, then, should precede the use of paradoxical interventions. Because the social network beyond these families is often restricted, they often appear to have defined themselves as distinct systems. Nevertheless, when the therapist tries to negotiate his role with them, he discovers serious family boundary problems.

Because social skills are often lacking in schizophrenics, and sometimes in other members of their families, the use of nonparadoxical behavioral methods to correct these problems can and should proceed alongside, or as a component of, family therapy. Similarly, medication is compatible with family therapy. However, the family therapist needs to be aware of what these procedures are, and to be alert to their potential impact, directly and indirectly, upon the entire family system.

A CASE EXAMPLE

In the case vignette I shall describe here, the parents, both age 34, and one daughter, age 13, were all enmeshed in turmoil over the symptoms of the identified patient, the wife, who had been diagnosed as having anorexia nervosa. By old-fashioned DSM–II criteria, she also would have been called a latent or borderline schizophrenic, but she would not have met current criteria for "characteristic" schizophrenic delusions and hallucinations. Nevertheless, she had a long history of quite bizarre behavior, odd, if not delusional, ways of reasoning about her behavior, and a complex, circumstantial mode of using language. Her husband and daughter had "adjusted" their own behavior in a manner that was remarkably complementary to hers (and conversely). The family unit was easily identified because the family had just moved to a new section of the country and had, as yet, no new treatment or social contacts.

At the time of referral to me, the husband told me that he was "wearing out," that the daughter was tense, irritable, and becoming like her mother, and that his wife, according to the most recent medical report, would die if she did not receive intensive inpatient treatment. She was, in fact, a woman of five feet, seven inches in height, but weighing 65 pounds. Her normal weight was 135 pounds. She had been amenorrheic for twelve years. Later, a metabolic and nutritional expert told that me he could not understand why she was still alive, because any slight metabolic deviation would have produced renal insufficiency, complicating her severe calcium and potassium deficiency. She had lost all her teeth because of her metabolic imbalance, and had been hospitalized a year before in a state of extreme cachexia. Medical treatment, working at the level of the biologic system, with psychoactive drugs and other means, had enabled her to survive, but it had not enabled her to recover. The most disturbing symptom to her and her family was not her metabolism or weight loss, but her bulimia: she gorged massively three times a day, primarily to induce vomiting, and secondarily to keep her weight down.

My emphasis on her biologic functioning is made in order to point out that, in a systems approach, one need not and should not look only at the family system. Some family therapists, I think, have been on dubious grounds when they have seemed to emphasize *only* the family. In fact, in broader terms of systems thinking, all living systems are open and linked. This includes biologic systems, the system of organization of the individual personality, the family and small primary group systems, as well as larger social networks. Each of these system levels needs to be considered. Because they are open and linked, there is the potentiality of *initiating* change at *any one* of these levels, whether it is pharmacologic, biologic, or at the level of the personality, family, or social network. The problem in therapy is to select one's priorities—the level that will give one the best therapeutic leverage for effective and, hopefully, rapid change.

In response to the referral request, I had planned an initial family consultation, with the understanding that she might be admitted to a behavioral therapy unit, where a life-saving effort with intensive medical treatment could be made if necessary. However, her medical status was stable, though obviously serious. When I asked why they were coming for treatment, the vomiting and weight loss were not mentioned. What she said instead about the "presenting problem" was: "There's a problem of retaliation." I will not go into the psychodynamics and family history, but should note that, before describing anything about the current symptoms, both husband and wife went on to describe the conflict that she had had with her mother, and which he said that he had "inherited." As the story unfolded, what became most apparent was that each member of the family experienced the vomiting as an extremely hostile, aggressive, upsetting act, in which she was "throwing money down the toilet." The enormous amount of food which she consumed and vomited was being "wasted." Her husband instantly pointed out that her father too had been concerned about saving money, indeed he had been a banker. She felt extremely guilty about the hurtfulness that this "waste" imposed upon her husband and daughter, but cyclically, after a few hours of remorse and reduced tension, she would settle back into renewed buildup of tension and anger, followed by gorging and vomiting, ad nauseam.

I was impressed with the husband's involvement, not only in his buying the food but also in his supervising the vomiting, and the daughter, in turn, "mothering" him in his distress. They described how their lives were consumed by this cycle, including time not only for obtaining the food, but also for cleaning up the kitchen and the bathroom where she would seclude herself. Literally, no "ordinary" relationships in the home with one another or with friends had taken place for years. In addition to pharmacologic and medical treatment, she had been in psychoanalytically oriented psychotherapy for three of four years, during which the pattern had stabilized somewhat, but with no fundamental change.

At a point in the consultation when I felt able to identify the cyclical impasse of the family system, I decided to introduce a paradoxical family intervention. Such an intervention initially minimizes change, and insists upon homeostasis and stability; sometimes this may involve "prescribing the symptom." But one does have a choice of "symptoms." I said that her malnourishment, low weight, and inability to bring about change was obviously a very dangerous situation. However, I joined them in identifying the focal problem as the waste and destructiveness associated with her vomiting. I said that it was not possible or desirable to change this problem too quickly, that we should try at least to maintain an equilibrium, to keep things the way they had been, and only work toward change slowly. I said, "I don't want you to do anything differently about the waste of food, but I do want to introduce some minor changes very slowly. I want you to continue to prepare the food in the same quantity as before." I had her give me a list of the food she had prepared the previous day. Some thirty dollars worth of food had been vomited on that day. I stressed that she continue to prepare such food exactly the same, except that she was now to put the food *directly* into the toilet, and skip the step of putting it into her mouth and stomach.

Amazingly, neither she nor her husband regarded this suggestion as surprising, but she did say that there was one problem: the toilet would clog up. We worked out the behavioral plan that she would cut the food up into small pieces at the table so that it could flush down easily. Her husband was bit uneasy about this because he felt that the same amount of food was going to be wasted. I said, "I'm sorry. We have to stick with this problem for now, and we'll have to see later if change can become possible. But for now we have to continue with wasting the same amount of food as before." Then we worked out a plan in which the husband, who already was deeply invested in his wife's eating problem, was to make sure that she continued to prepare the same amount of food as previously, for example, for lunch on the day before, seven pieces of chicken, two and a half quarts of mashed potatoes, a full apple pie, and a quart of ice cream. This all had been vomited in about 20 minutes. He also was to supervise her putting this food in the toilet. She and her husband together were to keep a detailed written record of all the food, and its cost, that was "wasted" down the toilet. I noted, rather casually, that when she was not going to have a gorging/vomiting "session," then she could have a small amount of food of her choice. That was the end of the first session.

They came back in ten days. This lady, who had vomited three times a day for thirteen years, had not vomited at all. What was the mechanism of change? Let me look for clues in the next session. The wife said that this had been the most "dynamic experience," the most "eye-opening experience" she ever had had in her life, and that it was in sharp contrast to the effect of all the interpretations made by her psychotherapist. She regularly had set aside her "insights" about such interpretations, and they never really had affected her behavior. When she saw all that food going down the toilet, food that she had deliberately placed there and had not "involuntarily" vomited, she realized for the first time what she had been doing. I did not need to make any interpretations whatsoever; *she* made them.

However, the husband mentioned some "problems" that had come up during the preceding ten days. For a couple of days she had wanted to continue with the gorging/disgorging, and he had had to enforce my instructions and insist that she throw the food down the toilet. On the day preceding the second interview, another type of relatedness emerged. It was clear from her history that the vomiting and gorging cycles had begun when her husband had been away on an extended job assignment. He had, in fact, been away during her entire pregnancy. Under these circumstances, she had felt lonely, unattractive, rejected, and "retaliative." He, in turn, would soothe her destructive retaliation by becoming accommodating to her. He described himself as keeping the marriage "normal" by buying these huge quantities of food for her to vomit. He described himself as being a "nice guy," "accommodating," and so on, when she was in the kitchen and bathroom. But he would withdraw from the relationship when she came out.

On the day before the second interview, this sequence had included his watching football on television all afternoon and evening and refusing to talk with her. She had not been occupied in the bathroom but was trying to interest him. She felt rejected, and, as in the past, she felt a great surge of motivation to gorge herself. She also, as in the past, felt physically chilled. Now, however, she suddenly realized that if she did gorge herself, the food and vomiting then would make her feel "warm." Her husband insisted that she not gorge but, rather, throw the food down the toilet directly. It was then that she had a creative "solution." Instead of gorging herself, she went and cuddled up on her husband's lap and became warm in a new way. The husband, who had been hoping for such physical advances from her for years, now was nonplussed. He discovered, to his dismay, that he did not know how to respond to her. At this point we could move on to a new stage of therapy; the structure of the family system had changed.

In this second meeting, I warned them that change was taking place too fast, that they were getting out of their accustomed equilibrium too quickly, and that too rapid change might be dangerous. One thing we had to do was reinstate the gorging and vomiting at least twice, but now at a designated time, Tuesday evening and Friday evening, with deliberation and planning (and, therefore, now fully within her ego control). Those two planned but highly stressful instances of vomiting were the last that have occurred in the subsequent months.

The family homeostatic system thus moved to a new kind of problem, to a relational one that would deal directly with the problems of warmth, distance, closeness, and rejection in the family system—problems which also now involved the daughter in a crucial way. With respect to the vomiting–gorging–wasting problem, we shifted to a nonparadoxical behavioral approach suggested by my cotherapist, Dr. Ronald Kokes, in the third session: she could cease "wasting" food down the toilet, so long as there was no gorging or vomiting. If she were to vomit even once, then she would have to resume preparing the large quantities of food and dispose of it down the toilet for two full days. Actually, this never occurred, and she has gradually but steadily gained weight, over 20 pounds in a few months. Meanwhile, the whole family has transformed its way of living and relating—but that is a story for another occasion.

This case illustrates a long-standing, cyclical impasse in which paradoxical systems-oriented intervention was used, but not (I must strongly state) with the random stimulation of oppositionalism or negativism. Instead, it was used with an understanding-in-depth of this family's dynamics, of their family boundaries, and of the possibility of containing the problem within a new family treatment system.

Finally, this approach involves a very valuable research opportunity which deeply impressed me when I observed the Selvini team in Milan. Paradoxical intervention is best used in the form of an explicit hypothesis-testing approach to treatment. Unlike most therapists, Selvini-Palazzoli and her colleagues formulate and actually write down what their hypothesis explicitly is, and what the intervention is expected to produce.[7] Then they observe and describe the changes that follow, and whether or not their predictions are supported and their hypothesis is correct. In accord with Popperian philosophy, they note, and I would agree, that one learns as much or more from the failures as from the successes. Failures narrow the options and alternatives about what is possible. This, then, is a focal, problem-oriented approach to therapy and not a random, scattered attention to all possible difficulties that might be mentioned by family members or inferred by the therapist. In the simple example I have described, there were a number of problems on which one might have focused. By focusing on *minimal* change rather than on maximal change, the system's deviance-amplifying characteristics, within defined boundaries, were utilized. The further change, and the maintenance of change, then were initiated from within the family, and from within the individual family members.

REFERENCES

1. Watzlawick P, Weakland JH, Fisch R: *Change*. New York, WW Norton & Co, 1974.
2. Bateson G: *Mind and Nature*. New York, EP Dutton, 1979.
3. Wynne LC: On the anguish and creative passions of not escaping double binds: a reformulation, in Sluzki CE, Ransom DC (eds): *Double Bind: The Foundation of the Communicational Approach to the Family*. New York, Grune & Stratton, 1976, pp 243–250.
4. Sluzki CE, Ransom DC (eds): *Double Bind: The Foundation of the Communicational Approach to the Family*. New York, Grune & Stratton, 1976.
5. Rosen J: *Direct Psychoanalytic Psychiatry*. New York, Grune & Stratton, 1962.
6. Frankl VE: Paradoxical intention: A logotherapeutic technique. *Am J Psychother* **14**:520–535, 1960.
7. Selvini-Palazzoli M, Cecchin G, Prata G, et al: *Paradox and Counterparadox*. New York, Jason Aronson, 1978.
8. Wing J: Social influences on the course of schizophrenia, in Wynne LC, Cromwell, RL, Matthysse S (eds): *The Nature of Schizophrenia: New Approaches to Research and Treatment*. New York, John Wiley & Sons Inc, 1978, pp 599–616.
9. Searles H: Positive feelings in the relationship between the schizophrenic and his mother. *Int J Psycho-Anal* **39**:569–586, 1958.
10. Napier AY, Whitaker CA: *The Family Crucible*. New York, Harper & Row Publishers Inc, 1978.
11. Wynne LC, Ryckoff IM, Day J, et al: Pseudo-mutuality in the family relations of schizophrenics. *Psychiatry* **21**:205–220, 1958.

Chapter 18

Discussion: The Practice of Psychotherapy with Schizophrenics

DANIEL P. SCHWARTZ

As a discussant, I must convey to you what I regard as the impossibility of my task. Each of these men—Will, Paul, Schulz, and Wynne—has given us a paper. These are windows on—an intriguing glimpse of—the larger corpus of their work. And it would not be too much to say of each of them that—in different areas—using different language and techniques, different conceptual frameworks—they are and have been among the giants who have moved our small science of man and the treatment of schizophrenia along. Of that larger corpus of these papers, I can only say that they continue to enlighten—to suggest.

I say science of man and treatment of schizophrenia advisedly here, because, in fact, we most regularly have those two agendas—and they are often related, but the nature of the methodologies for discovery and proof in each agenda may not be the same. The cost–benefit ratio derived from the work of an Otto Will, of a Ted Lidz, of a Lyman Wynne—as it moves without control group, as it opens our eyes regarding the relationship of the individual's self-respect to his available options for action, as it opens our conceptual capacities to the family's various and central communicative

---

DANIEL P. SCHWARTZ • Austen Riggs Center, Stockbridge, Massachusetts 01262.

influences—that cost–benefit ratio calculation should not be left even to a careful statistical methodologist, let alone an insurance company. Neither should we demean the valuable demands of the Philip Mays, of the Gordon Pauls, who ask of us that we repetitively *attempt* to gather our data, or formulate our hypothesis in sentences which are capable of generating specifiable procedures of verification.

Dr. Will today asks us to be reminded of the *tasks* of human development, of adolescence—tasks of formation of an identity, of the nature of the self, of modulation of the pain of being alone, of tolerating intimacy. He notes the psychosis-precipitating effect of a human relationship in a person prone to schizophrenia. He notes the urgency such a person contends with by virtue of the introduction of previously dissociated fragments of the self, of options for action in life's seemingly narrowing space. He points—the therapist's measure is his willing capacity to hold that pained other's dreaded self in his words and silence, in his capacity to understand. The therapist's measure (perhaps the mothers, the teachers too) in his holding still and steady, while he fights for that person's "oncoming future."

Schulz—out of his work on self–object differentiation—perhaps as one form, one precocious, costly attempt at individuation—examines the human capacity to require and present the self in its responses—fierce and fixed as an "all-or-nothing" phenomenon. That clarifies something for me, as an observer, and those reminders of this "all-or-nothing's" responsive functions and forms, its maladaptive presence, and destructive invitations to others to respond in kind, are welcome. They test the modulation, the maturity, the knowledge of the therapist and hospital staff.

Wynne describes a family and a therapy in terms of systems theory. There must be boundary maintenance and regulation; there must be capacities to link one system with another; there must be within the system internal differentiation of the components, and deviance (change) must be accompanied by its reaction with associated mechanisms for amplification and deviance reduction. The technique of "paradoxical intervention," he notes, in family therapy, holds and values the apparent deviance in the family in order to allow the family to respond to that fixity of *equilibria* by evolving adaptive homeostatic deviance reduction (change). He invites us to consider the conscious promotion of a transference regression in classical psychoanalytic treatment, or the often unwelcomed transference psychosis in the individual psychotherapy of schizophrenic patients, as a "reverse" paradoxical intervention, in which, as the therapists hold the boundaries steady, a regression occurs. This "temporary" amplified deviance (change) is to be resolved hopefully through interpretation. In his comparison of these two different situations of paradoxical intervention—family therapy with disturbed families—is found helpful and reverse paradoxical intention in psychotherapy is accompanied by considerable dangers. At the least, that "systems" view is fascinating.

Paul deals with those patients most impaired by this disorder, schizophrenia. He notes the several conditions for survival, develops measures which track the frequencies of such behaviors reliably—notes which are required for and which interfere with such a survival event, modifies the contingencies of these response patterns, and with apparently remarkable helpfulness and clarity, using instrumental conditioning principles and techniques, alters the rates of occurrence of these behaviors, and thereby facilitates those patients' capacity to move toward the least restrictive setting available.

There is, in each of these men's work, remarkable clarity and effectiveness. I would like to, but I will not (mostly) quibble with success. One could ask Dr. Will to clarify—since intimacy and loneliness precipitate a schizophrenic experience, and a therapist attempts to make himself available to the patient for the purposes of human attachment—which is an intimate act and arouses loneliness in the patient. How does one know whether this will cause or cure? One notes in thinking of the "all-or-nothing" phenomena that Dr. Schulz has clarified that totalistic response systems ("all-or-nothing"?) and concomitant conceptualizations are regular portions of each new developmental epoch from birth, to "eighth-month anxiety," to early stages of symbiosis and individuation, to adolescence, and marriage—and present themselves as some characteristics even of group formation (pseudospeciation?). One suspects that he is attempting to separate "all-or-nothing" phenomena described in his work from other defensive organization of the ego, whose rigidities are variously determined by forces ranging from narcissistic defenses, and paranoid attempts at organization, to hysterical and holistic regressive phenomena. And I think that one could consider it questionable whether "splitting," as it is used by either Kernberg or the Kleinians—with its implications of early organized and unintegrated intrapsychic organizations of partial self–object and impulse (according to good and bad polarities), is demonstrably on a continuum with other "all-or-none" phenomena described. Or are these two split "all-or-none" organizations side by side?

Wynne's characterization of the regressively disorganizing effects of nonsupportive, individual psychotherapy seems absolutely correct, from the point of view of the effect of the actions on the structure of a therapy, viewed as a closed dyadic system. Ida McAlpine, Merton Gill, and I, among others, have had a good deal of interest in that therapy–action structure, and its discussion must involve those therapeutic actions called inquiry, or clarification, which, however unwittingly, violate and therefore disrupt previously established values within the patient—systems of inner organization of actions-personally established inner guides. For example, the therapeutic assumption that the patient *has* a body, or *has* a clear perceptual capacity, is not at all always congruent with the patient's view, where often this idea of having a body, or repeating to one's self what one has observed, has been previously denied or held in check. For that patient, that assumption introduces "deviance"—and that's disorganizing! But equally interesting would be a discussion of "Paradoxical Intention properly used"—its seemingly magical, deceptive, contemptuous (toward the patient) properties—its relatedness to hypnosis, and its collusion in a variety of symbiotic manipulative relationships—its long-range effects upon patients' and families' "trust"—its unwitting communications to the family about their relationships to their therapists, and more.

Dr. Paul's book, from which his paper is drawn, leads one to ask for details of the use of aversive conditioning—and his concerns about its misuse—its limits? Its necessities? What is involved in using a "vapor spray" and a "totting horn" to make the seclusion room (a "time-out" room), "not too comfortable" for assaultive patients? Questions of nonteam evaluators interviewing the patients who recovered in regard to their inner response to the conditioning program, and their sense of relatedness to the "social instrumental learning staff" as compared with the milieu staff, would be very helpful.

Well, you can see the paradox—I'm incapable of quibbling. Instead, let me suggest what similarities may be apparent from a psychoanalytic view of these different contributors' approaches. How might one understand their relation to current problems and thinking in analytic investigation? Finally, what might some of the complexities of data about intrapsychic structure be that would add to our discussion?

First, the similarities. All these men regard the patient as amenable to psychological influence. Each defines a task—Dr. Will searches for attachment, Dr. Schulz for modulated foci, Dr. Wynne for valued stabilities of family action which appear maladaptive. Dr. Paul requires the delineation of the conditions of "elicitation," "reward," and "discriminative stimuli" relative to his various response frequencies.

The task definition in individual, family, and group approaches apparently and appropriately divides us—(there is often a disjunction between a focus upon the processes of attachment, and the nature of boundary functions of a family). For an analyst, each of these investigators—Will, Schulz, Wynne, and Paul—each in his appropriately different language and area, is engaged in an inquiry about ego functions. Their inquiry is about ego functions and their relation to action toward themselves, toward others, and the condition of their exercise. What actions, Will asks, are implied on the therapist's part and on the patient's part for attachment to occur? What allows one to modulate that "all-or-none" reaction; what are the determinants of the ego's actions in organized and holistic rigidities, asks Schulz. What kinds of interventions relative to the family will give them permission to free their behaviors from frozen stereotyped family maladaptions—Wynne? What are the contingencies of nakedness and assault, and not saying hello, as responses that are still available for reinforcement and work in schizophrenia? What degree of variance is there still available in the custodially warehoused and tormented ill?, asks Paul.

And, at least for an analyst, these commonalities—of each of these men's work—are important to redefine in our own language of ego concepts, considering the potentialities of behavior, not as an all-or-none phenomenon, but as a plastic repertory, with range and limit, whose totalistic rigidities and available flexible playfulness need explication.

Finally, what does intrapsychic data's complexity ask of all these scientists that they count—what motivation, however small, should they note and measure; what structure and variance might they usefully note—if they are to deal with the richness of man, with the complexities of schizophrenia?

Let me suggest what these might be by closing with a clinical example. An attractive and intelligent young man is persistently delusional. His face he sees and regards delusionally as grotesquely disfigured. He is compelled to spend much time secretly examining its monstrous quality in the mirror, and hides from human contact. In the hospital a girl smiles at him, likes him. He has a dream and speaks of both to his therapist. The dream is that his face, covered with disfiguring grotesque acnelike lesions, has blood spurting out of each deformed area. He awakes frightened. He says that he is pleased and frightened by the girl's interest. As he backs away from the encounters, he thinks to himself that he is shy. He describes to himself, to his analyst, his thoughts. They suggest, yes, he is afraid she won't like him, he'd better leave. But more than that—if he were to stay—she would discover that (he would discover) he would disappoint her. Her image of him would be betrayed—she would not see him as all good, so smart, so cool. He backs away, his therapist notes, from his own morality; "unfaithful betrayer," he regards himself. He carries in his mind a private "Scarlet Letter." It says, "betrayer at hand." The patient becomes anxious in the hour. It is difficult for him to think or speak. But he is reminded of experiences in the course of his growth when he was and felt betrayed, experiences where he did in fact betray others sexually and emotionally. A loved sibling leaves him and his family traumatically at a crucial age—he is "betrayed;" a loved mother appears about to be driven out of her own home—"betrayed." He, the patient, vengefully and shamefully, with avoided grief, violates and betrays a family celebration by his unexpected and abrupt absence. He reminds his therapist that, after the occurrence of his disorganization and the appearance of his delusions, he could not leave his own room at home for more than a year. His delusion was to him a mark of shame which all could see. He himself apparently could see and suffer—though not fully understand—his own punitive and protective morality, his therapist remarks. The day before his delusions appeared, the patient said that he had been reading the bible for a class—Leviticus, Chapter 20. There, God says, "I will set My face against the man, and cut him off from among his people." The portion refers here to that person who would violate the taboos of sexuality, the boundaries of gender, relation, and generation by his lust. And if one reads, God says, "He that hath made naked our fountains shall be cut off from their people." The patient then says, "You know, I haven't told you that two years before my breakdown (when adolescent developmental issues were pressing), I came home drunk one night and tried to scald my leg under the shower. The water wasn't hot enough, so I boiled some up, walked into my mother's bedroom, and said 'do you want some of this (poured on her)?'; she said, 'no,' and I poured the boiling water over my chest. There was a pause in the hour, and he said, puzzled and sad, 'it was somehow to make myself clean.'"

The next day, the patient, sulking, face turned half away in anger, the therapist acknowledging an appointment about to be missed, were both intertwined in interactions which appeared inextricably to involve them in limited but real mutual betrayal.

I mean only to remind us of the lawfulness within the person, within the hour, within the therapist's and patient's behaviors. The congruence of dream and hidden intrapsychic structures of value and morality, of historical individual past, family and social systems all operative—and mark out the lawful movement of the participants toward the future within each therapeutic occasion.

I mean only to remind us that the nature of life's tasks and the ego's functions are indeed complex. Those of us who are fortunate enough and burdened enough with the pursuit of these data, note and study these stabilities and change, note their relation to rules governing tasks and ranges of behavior relative to other systems, systems with their "faults" and histories—all are involved in the contingencies which limit and arrange the excitement of life and the evolution of a valued sense of self. These all intrapsychic and interpersonal and systemic and personal variables need to be measured and understood.

Chapter 19

General Discussion

QUESTIONS FROM AUDIENCE

QUESTION FOR DR WYNNE: How does the theoretical position and treatment approach that you presented resemble and/or contrast with Murray Bowen's systems approach to family therapy and schizophrenia?

DR WYNNE: My impression is that Murray Bowen works predominantly in a stabilizing non-paradoxical fashion to reduce the swings of symptomatic disturbance. When I use non-paradoxical approaches, our emphasis on health and resources is quite similar. Broadly speaking, such therapy "coaches" toward building of social skills, just as social learning approaches also do, but each with different specific techniques. Bowen works primarily with the parents in order to achieve results with the child, whereas I usually include children in the meetings. However, despite the physical absence of the children, Bowen is thinking about the family as a unit, and the linkage between the marital subsystem and others in the total extended family. In that sense, there is some overlap in our conceptualizations, but I think much more conceptual and theoretical work is needed to compare different versions of systems theory. My version is derived from general systems theory as described by von Bertalanffy and others. Bowen's version gives special emphasis to the historical roots of the family.

QUESTION FOR DR. PAUL: Cognitive disorganization may be reflected or not reflected in readily observable behavior. Have you considered measures of ability versus inability to think rationally before and after treatment? Thinking ability may have considerable predictive power for the long-run adaptive capacities of the patient.

DR. PAUL: Yes, we certainly have thought about it. But as far as a pre-post design for the particular group we were working with, the typical kinds of examinations for thinking or nonobservable processes were not usable, since over 75% of patients were either mute or totally incoherent. We have done several studies on the relationship between the cognitive distortion measures from the observational assessment systems with other measures, and there does turn out to be a good deal of cross-instrument consistency between the observable behaviors and other assessment procedures. As I mentioned, the cognitive factors are one thing that is cross-situational. If you measure cognitive functioning in the office, treat it in the office, get changes in the office, it is likely to generalize to other situations. That is, once you get the cognitive ability in an office setting, then that's unlikely to go away.

Could I give a response to Dr. Schwartz? He said to me that he thought he was slipping a little dirty one in there, mentioning some things from the book out of context. I thought so, too. But since it has been mentioned, I do want to address it. The questions regarded details of the aversive conditioning, "vapor spray," "tooting horns," and seclusion rooms.

Let me say first of all that I welcome discussions about these factors because, I think in any institutional setting—particularly with the severely disabled—assaultive behavior and other intolerable behaviors are going to occur. They must be dealt with, and if we don't approach them head-on, openly, without guilt, and handle them systematically and carefully, the staff are going to do aversive things that are worse than any of us would consider. That, for starters, is my basic position.

I also feel very strongly—and we have data to back it up—that there are reasonable ways of dealing with intolerable behaviors that interfere with other people's rights and cause tissue damage to self or others. These behaviors cannot be tolerated. They cannot be allowed to continue. By having a totally integrated constructive program with rules of progression as to when contingencies apply and when they don't apply, about 93% of the activities that go on will, in fact, by actual measure, be positive activities. Thus, when aversive procedures have to be applied, they wind up being a very small component, but an important component of a total program. We compared the social learning program which explicitly did use aversive procedures—and I'll tell you a little bit more about those in a moment—with the other programs. Approximately 7% of total interactive activities could be considered at all aversive in the social learning program. In the milieu program, which had absolutely no contingencies with the exception of contingencies for assaults, approximately 12% to 14% of interactions were aversive, and in the traditional hospital programs, where there was supposed to be nothing aversive, 20% of the interactions were aversive, by actual measurement. This was discovered by having observers actually in there recording.

The "vapor spray" and the "tooting horn," lest you get concerned that there is a terrible mad-scientist kind of operation going on in the social learning program, were used only occasionally, and in a sequence. First of all, we actively ignored problem behaviors, while focusing on adaptive activity; second, time-out in seclusion was given for fixed periods of time if the previous procedures were inadequate. But some people would commit an intolerable act in order to get into seclusion to sleep. After severe problems of that sort had been going on for about a week, there would be an additional review by the staff. For those patients, we could prescribe an aerosol horn to be tooted intermittently through the window, or, on occasion, a cold water mist (the "vapor spray") could be sprayed to keep patients from sleeping while they were in seclusion. That served the purpose. This didn't occur for all of the patients who went into seclusion. Mostly the procedures involved just using time-out within the focus of a constructive program. These contingencies made the verbal interventions much more effective. Again, by actual measure, you could terminate maladaptive behavior in the social learning program where you had these about how I quietly maneuvered things with the pipe-smoking by the sounds of the puffing on the pipe. I haven't smoked in quite a while.

The point I have in mind, however, is simply this. I am aware of many ways in which I, as a psychotherapist, direct the course of events, and I do it in ways that are quite frequently pointed out to me by patients who say that now I am withdrawn, which means I don't like something, or that I show an interest when they seem to be getting on the track that I consider to be correct, and so on. I don't have any great objection to the idea that there is purpose in what I do as a therapist—that there is direction.

The thing that seems to me to be important is that I know at least a little something about the purpose and direction. The idea that one can have a goal in mind, and that he can engage in behaviors that might move toward that goal, seems to me fair enough. It seems to me also necessary that he have some idea about the significance of his behaviors, being able to notice their effects. He must know that what he does is not neutral. It's the denial of any intent to intervene or to control that I consider to be unfortunate. That kind of unconscious maneuvering is not helpful.

QUESTION FOR DR. SCHULZ: Is there a relationship between progress by increments and repetition of insights as discussed by Dr. Stanton, and the reluctance of a patient to talk about change or changes taking place for fear that the change will no longer be his or hers?

DR. SCHULZ: The whole question of the patient's resistance to change, I think, is a fascinating one, and it is of course multiply determined. The all-or-none aspect of it may for a particular patient be a feature of that phenomenon, but there are other features, too. The whole issue of the sense of loss, of giving up symptomatology, of the grief work in leaving an identity as a patient, the whole issue of the fears of what lies ahead outside that one might now be involved in, issues of competition, of whether one will be accepted or not if one risks trying, if the patient puts himself on the line, the risk of intimacy on the outside, the concern about fusion that might result if one becomes involved with others, these are just some of the multiple factors that enter into the question of anxiety about change in patients. With any particular patient, the therapist may have to deal with a number of these things over a period of time. The working-through process I find is especially a problem with patients who want instantly to be well in their terms; that is, they cannot stand to wait.

QUESTION FOR DR. WYNNE: Why should the paradoxical approach necessarily lead to a reduction in the susceptibility to future illness more than a direct approach?

DR. WYNNE: If the paradoxical approach is successful in changing the rules that govern cyclical sequences, then the family has moved on to another type of system, a system that has new principles governing it. An enduring impasse with a high vulnerability to relapse has been interrupted, after which the family members usually are more available for contact with direct and nonparadoxical approaches. Social skills building, for example, may then be introduced more easily. It seems to me that these approaches are not at all at odds with one another. I use them together, but first one must identify and establish the conditions under which paradoxical interventions are likely to be effective. That includes defining boundaries for the family system, and defining who it is that is involved. Building up social skills directly may help define the role of family members, so that contradictory elements become easier to identify. A paradoxical intervention to dislodge an impasse may then be carried out in a comprehensive treatment program.

One of the problems of many approaches to the individual is that the therapist fails to become aware of the contributions of other people to the individual and his difficulties. In the example that I gave, an individual therapist with the wife would not easily see how the husband was playing into and helping perpetuate the cycle. In general, I believe that if

available contingencies. Verbal interventions started out being 94% effective, and ov
time went on 97% effectiveness in the social learning program. Straight verbal instructio
in the milieu program for terminating maladaptive behavior of this sort started out abo
75% effective, and went down from there to less than 55% effectiveness. So, having tl
contingencies available and carefully used made the verbal procedures much more effe
tive, without having to use the aversive procedures.

QUESTION TO PANEL: How does one reconcile dynamic processes with direct modification
problematic behavior?

DR. SCHULZ: I think that theme runs throughout the conference, and I myself do not have tl
problem about shifting framework from intrapsychic to behavioral. It seems to me th
intrapsychic things manifest themselves in behavior. That's what we can see in some for
or another. That's what we are looking at. What we postulate as lying behind behavi
may be an intrapsychic framework to make sense out of that behavior. But I really dor
see the problem, for instance, in placing self-representation or object-representation in
behavioral context.

DR. WYNNE: Moving this question from individual behavior to the family, I think that t
psychodynamic issues that you brought up, Clarence (Schulz), about all-or-no
phenomena, are in a way rather similar to what I was talking about in terms of t
dynamic equilibria in family systems, with oscillations between extreme stasis, whi
might be called the "none side," and extreme amplification, which might be called the "
side." Both individual personality systems and family systems do tend to swing cyclica
from one extreme to another; in effect, the "coin" is turned over without really changi
the system properties. If one steps from the intrapsychic sphere to a family syste
perspective, you can link these changes back to the same behaviors, including communic
tion. Then you won't fall into the trap of making disconnected theoretical propositions.

DR. PAUL: I would agree. I think it's a problem of the level of the terminology that's bei
used. I think any of the concepts, whatever the theory, are eventually going to refer
behavior that is either observable or verbalizable. It's going to be cognitive behavi
affective behavior, or motoric behavior, and whatever the concepts are, the organizi
concepts then go the next step up. I was originally trained as an ego-analy
psychotherapist. You may not believe it now, but I used to talk more in the language th
has been used elsewhere in this conference, and sometimes still do. I think I understa
what most of the people are talking about, but we need to be more descriptive. I think
need to be careful about discriminating when we are talking about abstract concepts ar
hypotheses about why a person acts in a particular way, and when we are trying to I
descriptive and concrete about what a person is doing, to make sure that we don't confu
the two.

DR. WILL: I don't have anything to say about this subject in terms of actual theory, because
am not a theoretician. I rather vaguely recall some 15 years ago, I think 1964, an artic
entitled something like "The Psychotherapist as the Influencing Machine." I was intrigu
by the article, and at the time I was offended by it. But I had cause to think about it son
more when, years ago, there was published a report of a recorded interview, in which
unfortunately was the therapist. I smoked a pipe at that time, and I remember th
someone listened to these recordings and talked to me about them. He pointed out that
seemed to be directing the course of the conversation by certain grunts that I made, so
stopped grunting but kept on smoking. Then there was a fellow who went over recordin
of mine later on, I think it was at Stanford, and he made a rather painful observatic

one can step out of the exclusively individual-oriented approach and look at the context, it is often possible to induce enduring changes more effectively, and to reduce susceptibility to further episodes.

Much behavioral work of the kind that Dr. Paul has described makes use of the family these days. In a number of settings, behavioral therapy is increasingly family-oriented; this overlaps with what I have been talking about, especially if there is an effort to listen and to explore and collect data about the functioning of the family system, as well as about the presenting patient. Then these approaches can move from one level to another. Social learning techniques can be powerfully effective, as Dr. Paul showed, without explicit paradoxical treatments.

The family and social network approaches may have some advantages, if one needs to move out of an impasse. A tip-off as to whether you need something different is whether you are stuck therapeutically. If nonparadoxical approaches work, all power to them. I use them myself, but I like to have alternatives as well.

Part IV

New Directions

Chapter 20

The Developing Guidelines to the
Psychotherapy of Schizophrenia

THEODORE LIDZ

The past decade has not been felicitous for the psychotherapy of schizophrenic disorders. Indeed, it is being taught in so few places that there is danger that the light will go out, and that the knowledge and skills that had gradually been accumulated will be lost. The reasons are not difficult to find. The major hope for overcoming this great destroyer of the mind and spirit has been placed in psychopharmacology and in advances in our knowledge of the neurochemistry of the brain. Studies of adopted-away children have supposedly produced incontrovertible evidence that we are dealing with a disorder whose etiology is basically genetic. Economics and politics have led to the dispersion of schizophrenic patients into dilapidated hotels and boarding houses, straitjacketed by drugs so that they create little problem for society. Experiments with so-called long-term intensive psychotherapy, carried out for all of six months, and other studies of the results of the work of relatively untrained therapists, have been used to indicate that though psychotherapy may be helpful, it is hardly worth the time and expense. But now times may be changing. Neuroleptic drugs, though use-

THEODORE LIDZ • Department of Psychiatry, School of Medicine, Yale University, 25 Park Street, New Haven, Connecticut 06519.

ful when properly administered, have not provided an answer, and, when used in heavy dosages for long periods of time, they may impede chances for improvement or recovery. The mounting incidence of tardive dyskinesias is forcing a reconsideration of prolonged pharmacotherapy. The social conscience of people begins to cry out against the community placement of chronically psychotic persons numbed by neuroleptic medications, when it is simply hiding and neglecting them in run-down hotels, apartments, and cheaply run nursing homes. It is becoming apparent, as several papers by my colleagues and myself will soon demonstrate, that any genetic influence shown by the Danish-American adoption studies is neither very stong, nor proven beyond reasonable doubt. Further, the studies of Bleuler,[1] and those of Ciompi and Müller,[2] have shown that, if they are given a reasonable chance, schizophrenic patients will usually gradually improve over the years, and do not suffer from a progressively deteriorating condition. Then, too, the very large number of persons who have wished to attend this conference indicates that there is still, or once again, considerable interest in the difficult art of the psychotherapy of schizophrenic patients.

The failure of controlled studies of psychotherapy to demonstrate any notable improvement has not discouraged some of us. Most of those who engage in the psychotherapy of schizophrenics believe they are still in the process of learning and improving their art. Still more important, those who have followed the transformation of patients who have been withdrawn, disorganized, and delusional into well-functioning persons, know that psychotherapy can accomplish, and has accomplished, what no other treatment has even approached. This woman who had been delusional, fearful, and antagonistic for several years, and through several hospitalizations in excellent institutions, is now a tenured professor in a leading university. This man whose condition was deemed hopeless after spending two years in a hospital repeating fixed delusions, obtained his degree in metallurgy, has married, and has been making a large income traveling to remote parts of the world as a metallurgical advisor and salesman. This young woman who became psychotic shortly after starting college was transferred to the Yale Psychiatric Institute after her condition continued to deteriorate during several months in another private hospital. She has now not only resumed her university education, but progresses toward becoming an outstanding artist and is far more capable of leading an independent and well-organized life than before she became ill. We may not be able to provide statistical evidence of the efficacy of psychotherapy of schizophrenic patients, but such experiences have been very convincing; and the participation in the virtual rebirth of a lost individual is among the most gratifying experiences a therapist can have.

Despite the partial eclipse of the psychotherapy of schizophrenic disorders during the past two decades, the great increase in the understanding of the nature and etiology of these conditions has altered and considerably improved our psychotherapy. Psychotherapy no longer consists of efforts to bestow unconditional love to undo the hypothesized maternal rejection, or of giving symbols of nurture and love in the manner of Sechahaye,[3] or of making intuitive direct interpretations in the style of Rosen,[4] or of early and constant interpretations of the patients' projective identifications as carried out by Rosenfeld[5] and others of the Kleinian school, or of permitting the patient to live through the psychosis with minimal interference, in the belief or the hope that the patient will emerge more imaginative and complete than before the psychosis, as Laing has taught.[6]

The psychotherapy of schizophrenic patients has had to free itself from some of its dependence upon psychoanalysis. Analytic technique with its relative passivity, waiting, and the maintenance of anonymity by the analyst is not simply of little value, but often countertherapeutic. Schizophrenic patients not only require the therapist to be committed and consistent, but capable of involvement as a real person who is sufficiently certain of his own boundaries to be secure from overinvolvement and from needing the narcissistic supplies provided by the patients' love or gratitude. Whereas analytic theory has helped the understanding of schizophrenic patients greatly, it has also misguided by it teachings that the schizophrenic's difficulties derive primarily from deficiencies in the mother–child relationship in the first two or three years of life, or from innate defects in the libidinal or aggressive drives; and that narcissistic fixations prevent the establishment of a transference relationship, as well as by its pessimistic avoidance of involvement with such narcissistic conditions. Whereas a personal analysis is usually a very important experience for a therapist to enable him to hear unconscious processes, to understand the vicissitudes of oedipal strivings, to be secure of his own boundaries and needs, etc., psychoanalytic training has often been detrimental to those young therapists who, seeking the approbation of their analytic teachers or copying their technique, behave as analysts with patients unsuited for psychoanalysis. The psychotherapy of schizophrenic patients is not something that everyone can learn and undertake, not even many highly skilled analysts, for it requires an ease in relating to others, security of boundaries, a tolerance to hear the unthinkable, and a freedom to be oneself without fear of losing oneself in the intense commitment required.

What then are some of the advances in our knowledge of schizophrenic disorders that help guide our therapy? What are some of the new understandings of the therapeutic process that permit our efforts to be more successful?

As I have stated previously,[7] I believe that the understanding of the family milieu in which schizophrenic patients grow up has been a major factor in providing direction and focus to our therapy. Indeed, this symposium would not have been held in my honor, if the studies of the families of schizophrenic patients carried out under the direction of Dr. Fleck and myself[8] had not formed something of a watershed in the understanding and treatment of schizophrenic disorders. I can here only indicate how the various studies of the transactions in families of schizophrenic patients have clarified the nature and etiology of schizophrenic conditions, and provided definite guidelines for therapeutic efforts.

Schizophrenia is essentially a disorder of mid- and late adolescence, even though the actual onset often comes somewhat later in life. Adolescence is a critical period when individuals undergo a marked change in their relationships to their parents and should virtually complete the lengthy process of separation from them to achieve individuation as reasonably well-integrated, self-sufficient, and self-directed persons capable of relating intimately with someone outside the family. It is a time when parental directives become self-directives, modified by the ways of other idealized figures. Persons who become schizophrenic have been unable to surmount such developmental tasks, not simply as a result of maternal rejection or oversolicitude in early childhood, or from some innate incapacity that interferes with developing stable object relationships, but because of the seriously disturbed and distorting family transactions that continued throughout the patient's formative years which failed to provide the essentials for a child's development and individuation by the end of adolescence or early in adult life. The basic difficulties would seem to derive from the egocentricity of a parent, or both parents, who could not relate to the child as having feelings, perceptions, and wishes discrete from the parent's, but rather needed the child to remain an adjunct, who could complete and give meaning to the parent's life. Some patients have grown up within families that were so seriously disturbed, lacking in essentials, and which communicated so vaguely or aberrantly that they were never able properly to emerge from the family nexis as independent children or adolescents, and may be considered *developmental* schizophrenic patients, akin to process or poor premorbid schizophrenics in other terminologies. Others develop with a fair degree of adequacy, but are unable to attain firm ego identities as integrated personalities no longer deeply dependent upon parental guidance and protection. When unable to surmount the developmental tasks of late adolescence, they not only regress to an anaclitic or symbiotic dependency, but also cognitively to preoperational egocentric magical forms of thinking in which the filtering functions of categorical cognition is lost. These patients may be termed *regressive* schizophrenics, akin to reactive or good premorbid schizophrenia in other terminologies. Developmental and regressive schizophrenia are not, however, separate entities, but polar paradigms, and most schizophrenic patients fall somewhere between these polarities.

The studies of numerous schizophrenic patients and their families that have now been carried out permit a therapist to become aware of the critical characteristics of the aberrant family environments in which schizophrenic patients grow up, and the types of developmental problems such families create in their offspring.

In one type of family, the mother cannot properly differentiate her needs, perceptions, and emotions from those of her child, whom she expects to remain a part of her and provide a sense of completion to her life, and the mother's ways of relating to and rearing children are not countered by the father, who is passive and ineffectual within the family. Sons raised in such families may not overcome the initial symbiotic bond to the mother, have problems with their gender identity, fear their incestuous impulses when they enter adolescence, and lack an adequate male figure with whom to identify. In families in which the parents are caught in an irreconcilable conflict competing for the loyalty of the child and undercutting one another's worth, the child can be caught in a bind as satisfying the directives or wishes of one parent provokes rejection by the other, and the irreconcilable parents are apt to become irreconcilable introjects preventing the development of an integrated personality. The parents not only repeatedly place their child in "double binding" situations, but convey numerous irrationalities, and communicate in vague ways that prevent their offspring from attaining firm and coherent categories to enable them to think coherently about family matters and personal relationships.

When a therapist recognizes that a major reason patients become schizophrenic is because they had never properly overcome the symbiotic relationship to a parent to become persons with clear and firm self-boundaries capable of directing their own lives, the therapist gains many guidelines for relating to such patients. The patient who had been involved in completing a parent's life or salvaging the parents' marriage had never been recognized as a discrete individual, confirmed by the parents as a person with different feelings and perceptions than theirs and with a life of his own. The patient had felt smothered, engulfed, and deprived of individuality by a parent, and became bewildered and overwhelmed when he voluntarily or involuntarily attempted to become independent. Although the difficulties in separating from the mother started in very early childhood, a critical period when separation and individuation become necessary for further development starts in midadolescence and becomes essential in late adolescence. I wish to emphasize again that the difficulties at these times are not simply resultants of the early parent–child relationship, but in a large measure have become insurmountable because of concurrent intrafamilial transactions that require therapeutic attention.

Indeed, a central task for the therapist lies in releasing the patient from the bondage of completing a parent's life, or bridging the schism between his parents, to enable him to invest his energies in becoming a person in his own right. In particular, the therapist seeks opportunities and openings to help the patient free himself from the need to perceive and feel the way his parents have required him to, and instead have him begin to trust his own feelings and perceptions as guides to living. It requires the therapist to confirm the patient's worth as an individual through considering the patient's feelings and perceptions as potentially meaningful. This usually means that the patient must begin to recognize that his parents, whom the patient considered knew the way and why of living, had rather aberrant ways of perceiving, relating and living. When this is accomplished, if it can be, the patient has moved a long way toward emergence from the psychosis.

Only a few of the various specific leads and guidelines for therapy that come from such understanding of the typical predicaments that beset schizophrenic patients can be considered here. Perhaps most important is that the therapist can be certain that these patients are facing very real problems in their current life situation, rather than, as has often been thought, difficulties due to their aberrant fantasies, to their innately strong hostile or sexual drives, or to intrapsychic resultants of early childhood neglect or trauma, and that these ongoing problems will be related directly to the long-standing problems in the intrafamilial transactions. It is on these very real and tangible problems that the therapist seeks to focus as soon as feasible. It is here, rather than on the interpretation of delusional material, or on the patient's projective identifications, or with other intrapsychic processes that one starts.

There are several critical junctures in development at which schizophrenic disorders are likely to appear. When the onset occurs shortly after puberty, the patient is apt to be so deeply enmeshed in a symbiotic relationship with the mother that he or she cannot relate beyond the family, and the symbiotic bond leads the new sexual impulsions into incestuous channels, a direction fostered by a parent's incestuous proclivities together with the absence of another parent capable of standing between the patient and the seductive parent. The frequent onset shortly after leaving home for college or to enter the armed forces relates to the parents' inability to consider that their child can manage on his own—much as in school phobia—and to the intense anaclitic needs of the young person without sufficient integration, resources, and capacities to relate to and communicate with strangers. Another common time of onset is when the parents divorce, or are seriously considering divorce. The patient then feels hopeless of ever becoming free of the obligation to complete the life of a parent, becomes panic-stricken because the divorce fans the incestuous fantasies fostered by the nature of the parent–child interaction, and may not only feel torn between the parents, but also hostile over being deserted.

The therapeutic effort is directed as soon as feasible toward bringing the patient to consider the life situations from which he has been fleeing into unreality, and not to foster his flight from them. As intriguing as the patient's bizarre communications, delusional contents, or polymorphous perverse fantasies may be, the therapist is apt to be tapping a bottomless well that enriches the therapist, but does not much benefit the patient unless the material is used to clarify current real dilemmas. Delusions are restitutive measures, and they are needed by the patient until the serious impasses in his life have been examined and understood, if not overcome; and they are rarely, if ever, overcome by uncovering their unconscious meanings. However, it is virtually impossible for the patient to face the life situations that precipitated the psychosis until he can again trust someone—the therapist—not to desert him in his great need, and can believe that the therapist will not reject him when he learns the nature of his impulses and fantasies, that he will be able to survive the patient's hostility, and will support the patient in his despair.

I keep in mind a patient's remark when her therapist sought to have her face the impact of the turmoil that preceded her parents' divorce. The patient said, "You must be even crazier than I am, if you think I'm going to let myself experience that despair again." The remark is critical, and the close relationship between schizophrenia and depression and despair must be recognized. The underlying depression is essentially anaclitic—a feeling of intolerable emptiness, that may be a means of warding off murderous impulses, but which also reflects the insecurity and despair because the needed person has turned away from the patient. There is need for therapeutic caution, for the patient may become more delusional as he attempts to face the life situations confronting him; but such flare-ups can usually be contained if a good therapeutic relationship has been established.

Awareness of the anaclitic core of the psychosis and the intensity of the patient's anaclitic or symbiotic needs has provided a number of guidelines for therapy. The therapist can anticipate that, just when he feels encouraged by indications that the patient is beginning to trust him and is forming a meaningful relationship with him, the patient may flee—from the treatment situation, from the hospital, or into a more regressed condition. The therapist may then become so discouraged that he gives up in actuality, through losing his commitment to the patient, or by deciding to rely upon pharmacotherapy. If, however, the therapist realizes that the patient, because of his fear that his growing attachment will again leave him vulnerable to disillusionment and despair, is unconsciously testing the therapist's commitment, a major hurdle can be overcome, and a firmer relationship almost always follows. Similarly, awareness of the patient's intense dependency and fear of the emptiness when independent lets the therapist anticipate that each time the patient progresses to take a step toward increased independence an upsurge of anxious emptiness occurs—as when a hospitalized patient moves to a section with less supervision, or gains permission to go out unaccompanied, or anticipates discharge from the hospital. The regressive flare-up of symptoms, and perhaps the efforts to find protective closeness of fusion by sexual acting out, can set back the therapeutic process unless anticipated and made the focus of the psychotherapy, and unless the therapist can temporarily provide an increase in support. The appreciation of the anaclitic core of these patients' problems also permits us to understand the admixtures of schizophrenic reactions with amphetamine and LSD psychoses, anorexia, and nymphomania that have changed the phenomenology of adolescent schizophrenic disorders so greatly in recent years.

An understanding of the family situations of schizophrenic patients can help overcome a common major impediment to successful treatment—the parents' premature and often abrupt removal of the patient from the hospital or from psychotherapy. Here the parents rather than the patient need help, and a therapist who feels that his contact with parents must be minimal requires a collaborator who copes with parents' concerns. The symbiotic mother is very likely to believe that the patient cannot survive without her care, and may suffer from such intolerable anxiety that she will take the patient home unless someone undertands her predicament and helps alleviate her anxiety. A second cause of parental disruption of therapy has to do with a parent's fear that the patient's attachment to the therapist will disrupt the child's dependent relationship with the parent. A third occurs when the patient begins to show overt hostility to a parent or parents, which is rather naturally taken as an indication of a worsening of his condition, rather than a move towards improvement. Then, too, the parents may need to have a sick child at home to serve as a scapegoat, the apparent source of the family unhappiness, to mask the parents' incompatability.

It is important for therapists to realize that, even though the patient had attained some degree of independence, when regressed, needy and insecure, he will, like a preoperational or preoedipal child, believe that a parental figure can supply all of his needs, and that if this person fails to do so, he is being rejecting and malevolent. He will seek to endow the therapist with the omniscience and omnipotence that the small child believes his parents possess. He builds up expectations that a therapist can never fulfill, and then will perceive the therapist as bad, and turn from him in disillusionment or in hatred. In brief, the schizophrenic patient does not suffer from ambivalence, as Bleuler[9] believed, but rather, like the small child, is incapable of ambivalence, and tends to split a person into a good or a bad object. An important aspect of therapy is fostering the capacity for ambivalence;

that is, to recognize that the same person can be malevolent and benevolent, helpful and hurtful, thoughtful and thoughtless, and so forth, in order to help the patient stabilize his object relationships. A related task lies in helping the patient overcome the egocentric orientation that opens the way for delusional thinking by using the transference to help him recognize that others, including the therapist, may view events from a different orientation than the patient.

From the very beginning, the therapist attempts to make it clear that he is not an omniscient or all-powerful savior who can direct the patient's life, protect from anxiety, and fill all of the emptiness forever. Rather, he is a trained person who can examine situations, feelings, and beliefs together with the patient whose needs and opinions he respects, thus confirming the patient's individuality. He hopes that together they can find a workable way of life for the patient. By helping the patient sort out problems and possible ways of coping with them, the therapist helps him learn to make decisions—a critical aspect of ego functioning—but the decisions are to be made by the patient, not for the patient, except in emergencies. Interpretation, particularly textbook interpretation, has little place, and runs counter to such needs. Bestowing love, particularly an intrusive love that permits the patient little room for escape from the therapist's benevolent protectiveness, is too likely to seem a replay of what had occurred in the patient's family, and can drive the patient into panic, or even into suicide, as the only way of escape.

One of the very substantial advances has been the advent of family therapy, which may take many forms. Those who have conducted conjoint family therapy with the families of schizophrenic patients soon become aware of how closely intertwined the distorted personalities and relationships are within these families, and that often little movement can be expected in the patient's therapy unless there are also shifts in the family's equilibrium or disequilibrium. However, particularly with older patients, family-oriented therapy need not be conjoint family therapy, but rather a major focusing of the therapy on how the disturbed family transactions have affected the patient. Because of the patient's need to preserve an image of his parents, but also often because the aberrant family environment is not recognized as being abnormal by the patient, unless the therapist is alert to the fact that serious family problems exist, as they always do with such patients, they may never be brought into the therapy by the patient.

Quite aside from the need to cope with the family and the family problems, it has become apparent that not all that needs to be accomplished in therapy can be achieved by individual psychotherapy alone—particularly with those patients who are closer to the developmental than the regressive side of schizophrenic disorders. Improving socialization, the development of cognitive skills, inculcating various adaptive techniques, as well as making it possible for the parents to relate differently to the patient, all require help from other therapists. It is for this reason that we continue to require hospitals or residential treatment centers to achieve the very marked personality changes essential to a good and stable therapeutic result.

In this relatively brief presentation of an extremely complex topic, I have primarily sought to designate that experience in carrying out therapy and supervising the psychotherapy of schizophrenic patients has been sharpening and improving the skills needed to help schizophrenic patients emerge from their psychoses. Increasingly, directives for the coherent treatment of schizophrenic patients are emerging.

Experience, however, must be transformed into a theory of the nature of schizophrenic disorders, in order to permit generalization. The study of the families of patients has been a major factor in helping to produce a more coherent theory, as well as therapy. I believe we are now well on our way toward achieving a theory that will further unify our understanding of schizophrenic patients, and will provide still clearer guidelines for therapeutic efforts. Some critics deplore spending the enormous time and effort required to treat a single schizophrenic psychotherapeutically; but a major reason why it is essential to pursue the intensive and prolonged psychotherapy of schizophrenic patients lies herein—to gain the intimate understanding that will permit more incisive and decisive therapeutic approaches that will, in turn, permit the effective treatment of ever larger numbers of schizophrenic patients.

REFERENCES

1. Bleuler M: *The Schizophrenic Disorders*. New Haven, Yale University Press, 1978.
2. Ciompi L, Müller C: *Lebensweg und Alter der Schizophrenen*. Berlin, Springer-Verlag, 1976.
3. Sechahaye M: *Symbolic Realization*. New York, International Universities Press, 1951.
4. Rosen J: The treatment of schizophrenic psychosis by direct analytic therapy. *Psychiatr Q* **21**:3–25, 1947.
5. Rosenfeld HA: *Psychotic States: A Psychoanalytic Approach*. New York, International Universities Press, 1965.
6. Evans R: *R. D. Laing: The Man and His Ideas*. New York, EP Dutton, 1976.
7. Lidz T: The influence of family studies on the treatment of schizophrenia. *Psychiatry* **32**:237–251, 1969.
8. Lidz T, Fleck S, Cornelison A: *Schizophrenia and the Family*. New York, International Universities Press, 1965.
9. Bleuler, E: *Dementia Praecox or the Group of Schizophrenias*. New York, International Universities Press, 1950.

Chapter 21

Medication and Psychotherapy in Outpatients Vulnerable to Psychosis

MALCOLM BAKER BOWERS, JR., and DAVID GEORGE GREENFELD

INTRODUCTION

The literature dealing with the individual treatment of schizophrenia and related conditions has been derived almost exclusively from work with inpatients. Indeed, before the 1950s, psychotic patients were treated primarily in hospitals. Our field owes a lasting debt to the patience and intuitive genius of the individuals who developed this literature, including Theodore and Ruth Lidz, and others who are contributors at this conference. Working in the days before neuroleptic drugs, and sometimes intentionally without them, these workers described the powerful role of persistent, concerned human contact in the treatment of psychotic disorders.

With the advent of neuroleptic drugs, many patients are able to live outside the hospital because of improved symptom control, but often their condition is, in Klerman's phrase, "better but not well," The remaining morbidity is often evident in just those areas of human development which

MALCOLM BAKER BOWERS, JR., and DAVID GEORGE GREENFELD • Department of Psychiatry, School of Medicine, Yale University, 25 Park Street, New Haven, Connecticut 06519.

have always been the province of the psychotherapies. Yet, to date, we have little information regarding the combined use of medication and psychotherapy in outpatients vulnerable to psychosis.[1-3]

One of the most spirited attempts to examine the relationship between the use of medication and psychotherapy occurred at McGill University in the late 1950s, and was published under the title *The Dynamics of Psychiatric Drug Therapy*, edited by G. J. Sarwer-Foner. Psychopharmacology was an infant discipline. Yet the intimations of an interactional model were present at that meeting, a model which we feel has increasing relevance for today's practice. For example, one component of the emerging model was the idea that neuroleptic drugs, when effective, acted upon a central nervous system characterized by an endogenous vulnerability to a psychotic state. Freyhan,[4] representing this view stated:

> We must keep in mind . . . that we are not giving drugs to treat conflicts or the complexities of the unconscious mind. This must remain the domain of psychotherapy. If there are certain psychopathological symptoms which make psychotherapy impossible and drug therapy is instituted in order to facilitate psychotherapy, then drug therapy must aim at the modification of particular target symptoms. In this case, drug treatment is limited to specific goals which should be clearly distinguished from the broader aims of psychotherapy.

Another component of that newly emerging model emphasized the role of the behavioral interaction between doctor and patient. Sarwer-Foner,[5] in support of this view argued:

> In . . . by far the larger group of patients, the physiological effects, (of the drug), though present, . . . are interpreted by the patients according to their individual patterns of coping with their impulses and colored by their contacts with the physician. If . . . the drug is administered as another variable in a setting for psychotherapy . . . then this drug is incorporated as . . . indicating either the physician's benevolence, malevolence or other of the affective meanings that influence a patient's interpretation of his surrounding realities and the way he reacts to them.

We have used the historical perspective provided by this conference held twenty years ago as a starting point for evaluating and clarifying the model implicit in our own current clinical work. We have used medication and have worked psychotherapeutically with certain outpatients for over ten years. For the general psychiatric clinician, there is really no choice. These patients require continuing care, and one uses one's training to assist them. Our training has been both in psychotherapeutic work and in the use of medication. We are not here arguing for one type of treatment over another, or for the absolute efficacy of our approach, say, against some other form of treatment, or even compared to an untreated group. We are simply interested in making explicit the model which has emerged from discussion and reflection upon our clinical experience. Our primary data source has been our clinical notes describing our sessions with our patients. In research language, this report could be termed "hypothesis-generating." In addition to describing our experience, we will call attention to certain issues which may be useful in planning prospective studies.

PATIENT GROUP

This report will thus be a composite, retrospective, descriptive account of our experience with the individual outpatient treatment of a group of patients vulnerable to psychosis. The reference group consists of 21 patients, 13 men and eight women, ages 18–56, mean age 27.8 at the beginning of treatment with one of us. Seventeen were single, four were married at the beginning of therapy. The following diagnostic groups were formed using, Research Diagnostic Criteria (RDC) criteria: schizophrenia, nine (seven definite, two probable), schizoaffective illness, seven (six definite, one probable), and other functional psychosis, five. Six patients had never been hospitalized before treatment with us began. Ten patients had been hospitalized one time, three patients twice, one three times, and one four times. Each patient was followed in individual outpatient treatment by one of us for periods varying from six months to ten years (average 2.5 years).

Although treatment efficacy is not the focus of this paper, some information regarding patient status during treatment may be useful as a general indication of concurrent function. During the course of our treatment, there were no successful suicides or serious suicide attempts. Five patients were hospitalized once during this period. One patient was treated in a long-term hospital setting; another patient had to be hospitalized for chronic care, and treatment by us was not continued. Seven patients were fully self-supporting during treatment, and three contributed partial support. Five patients were full-time students, two were students half-time and employed half-time. Two functioned as housewives, but were not otherwise employed.

PHASES OF TREATMENT

Psychotherapeutic work is the phrase we prefer to describe the context in which the entire treatment takes place. We use this term in a broad sense, to connote both the formation of and the activity within the doctor–patient relationship. Within this context, neuroleptic medication has a specific therapeutic role. It provides a means for the control of the psychotic state, and, where appropriate, for prophylaxis against its recurrence. We have found that the control of psychotic symptoms is usually a precondition for effective outpatient treatment of patients vulnerable to psychosis. Medication and psychotherapy interact in complex ways throughout the course of treatment. This interaction adds a level of complexity to an already challenging task, and may consume considerable amounts of treatment time.

In reviewing our experience, we have tentatively identified four phases of treatment: (1) the development of the therapeutic alliance, (2) the assessment of vulnerability to psychosis, (3) the pursuit of developmental goals, and (4) the attainment of increasing control and autonomy within the therapeutic relationship. These might properly be called interdependent tasks of treatment, for they are not phases in the strictly linear sense. Each demands attention throughout the course of treatment, and an impasse in any one of these tasks may compromise progress in the others. Nevertheless, when we review the content of our therapeutic activity, we find that these tasks typically form a sequence of central concerns, each commmanding successively a major portion of psychotherapeutic effort and time.

Phase 1: The Development of the Therapeutic Alliance

Since outpatient psychotherapy requires the voluntary participation of the patient in his treatment, the quality and character of the therapeutic alliance is of paramount importance, and constitutes the initial focus of the therapy. Patients vulnerable to psychosis commonly have great difficulty in forming stable, trusting human relationships, making it particularly difficult for them to engage in a specialized collaborative relationship necessary for the mastery of symptoms and problems. An effective therapeutic alliance is necessary to protect the stability of the treatment and to insure a collaborative context for therapeutic work.

A detailed discussion of the technical maneuvers useful in enhancing the therapeutic alliance is beyond the scope of this paper. Patients present a wide variety of familiar concerns and resistances to engagement in treatment. Tact, patience, and restraint were attitudes which seemed to us most effective in facilitating the establishment of a working alliance. Many of our patients were initially guarded, suspicious, and aloof. These patients were particularly sensitive to issues of autonomy and control, and frequently had serious concerns about the therapist's motivation and intentions. When neuroleptic medication is an integral part of the treatment, the therapist is confronted with a technical dilemma with regard to such patients. Since the suppression of psychotic symptoms frequently facilitates the development of the therapeutic alliance, it is tempting to prescribe medication in the hope of speeding progress toward this goal. On the other hand, effective treatment with neuroleptic medication requires the active collaboration of the patient.

In our experience, achieving this goal frequently requires a willingness on the part of the therapist first to reach with the patient some degree of common understanding about the nature of his symptoms and the role of the proposed medication. The tangibility of medication makes it a frequent focus for a variety of the patient's fantasies and fears. The patient's perception of the purposes and actions of a proposed medication may be distorted by the psychotic symptoms it is intended to treat. A careful exploration of these fantasies and distortions may be necessary before medication can be introduced into the treatment. When these tasks are neglected, the patient may refuse medication, or, what is perhaps worse, he may accept a prescription, but take the medication intermittently or not at all. The resulting deception not only compromises the pharmacotherapy, but has an adverse effect upon the therapeutic alliance itself.

We have found that medication is most effectively approached, like all therapeutic issues, with full and open discussion leading to negotiated agreement with the patient. In general, we have *not* found it necessary that a patient fully confront his illness in order to enlist his compliance with a medication regimen. Some partial acknowledgement of illness and symptoms may permit the patient to agree with his therapist that medication serves a useful function. When possible, we have found it is far better for the patient to feel free to discuss his compliance or the lack of it openly in the therapy, rather than to feel obligated to be deceptive about it. In such an atmosphere, the patient's concerns and fantasies about the medication can be explored, and irrational obstacles to the use of medication can be removed.

Other patients were initially terrified, demanding, and dependent. These patients tended to rely heavily, if not exclusively, upon medication, not only to control symptoms, but also to allay their terror of the psychotic experience. These patients tended to be severely limited in the range of their emotional responses and in their willingness to explore troubled areas in their lives. In our experience, the early stages of treatment with these patients involved giving them considerable reassurance and support, in order to provide a period of stability. Subsequent attempts to reduce the dosage of medication often caused the patient considerable anxiety, and provided an opportunity to discuss with the patient his magical expectations and overvaluation of the role of medication in his treatment.

Some side effects, such as severe akathisia, may make compliance with medication virtually impossible.[6] The therapist must know enough to make the necessary changes in medication in such instances, and not attempt to psychologize noncompliance. In other cases, medication may reduce or eliminate some symptoms which are gratifying or in the service of denial of illness.[7] A trusting alliance may enable a patient to risk the reduction of such symptoms. For many patients, questions about medication and its effects may be the focus for larger concerns about relapse, prognosis, and problems in the relationship with the therapist. The active exploration of these concerns may be necessary, not only to insure medication compliance, but also to help define other important areas for therapeutic work.

Phase 2: The Assessment of Vulnerability to Psychosis

In this context, we view vulnerability as a clinical concept which includes a degree of endogenous vulnerability of uncertain etiology. An assessment of the threshold of this endogenous vulnerability is initially made by a careful evaluation of the severity of precipitants in previous psychotic episodes, and of the patient's response to medication. As treatment proceeds, this assessment is refined and modified through attention to the quality of the treatment alliance, the patient's response to and compliance with a medication regimen, and to the tendency for return of psychotic symptoms under various stress conditions. These include the stresses of developmental challenge, work, and loss or change in family or other close relationships. Neuroleptic medication and stress apparently affect vulnerability in reciprocal fashion.[8,9] Vulnerability is thus not a static variable, as the following case illustrates.

> A 25-year-old man, previously hospitalized twice for a psychotic illness, had been in outpatient treatment for eight months, and was being maintained on 5 mg per day of haloperidol. He was symptom-free, living apart from his family and working as a volunteer. His therapy had progressed to the point that he wanted to pursue a sexual relationship. In this context his symptoms recurred, necessitating a retreat from this developmental task and a marked increase in his medication for control of psychotic symptoms. On two separate occasions several months apart his symptoms "broke through" a maintenance dose of medication as he attempted this specific developmental step.

Thus, vulnerability can be affected by medication compliance, and by the patient's ability to manipulate adaptively the developmental challenges he confronts.

The patient also begins treatment with his own assessment of his vulnerability to psychosis, an assessment often considerably at variance with that of his therapist. The patient may respond to his illness with intense terror or denial. He may view his psychotic episode as a random aberration, with little awareness of prodromal symptoms or precipitating stress. He may retrospectively exaggerate, minimize, or distort his recollection of his psychotic experience, in ways that increase his vulnerability, or, alternatively, render him a globally constricted psychological invalid.[10]

The patient's attitude toward antipsychotic medication is often a reflection of his evolving assessment of his vulnerability, as the following example illustrates.

A second-year college student was first hospitalized for three weeks at the age of 21 for a psychotic episode precipitated by hallucinogenic drug abuse. He refused treatment after discharge, and returned to school. Six months after graduation from college, he was again hospitalized for two weeks for a recurrence of psychotic symptoms. On this occasion, he denied hallucinogenic drug abuse. He refused longer hospitalization, but agreed to begin outpatient treatment with one of us. Although he became invested in the therapy, he insisted that the medication was unnecessary, and gradually discontinued it, despite his therapist's recommendation to the contrary. Approximately ten weeks after discontinuing medication, he was again hospitalized for the recurrence of psychotic symptoms. During the three subsequent years of his treatment, his medication compliance remained excellent. The resulting stability permitted the focus of treatment to shift to his psychosocial concerns and developmental problems. During the last year of treatment, medication was reduced, and finally discontinued after the patient successfully completed several months in graduate school.

Thus, the patient's capacity to acknowledge and understand his illness and its precipitants may significantly affect the degree of his overall vulnerability to psychosis, since these factors are likely to influence his medication compliance and his ability to manipulate adaptively developmental challenges and other stresses he confronts.

Phase 3: The Pursuit of Developmental Goals

When a workable degree of shared understanding of vulnerability has been achieved, the focus of therapy can begin to shift toward the definition and pursuit of reasonable developmental goals. Even when the patient is in remission with respect to psychotic symptoms, he is faced with the need to struggle toward mastery of persistent "trait" deficits.[11] Our patients have required therapeutic help in facing a variety of developmental tasks, including emancipation from their families of origin, developing the capacity for intimacy, selecting and pursuing realistic vocational objectives, and learning to tolerate comfortably changes in the intensity and quality of their emotional experience. Having endured a psychotic decompensation, the patient must also come to terms with the fact that this experience has occurred, and explore its personal implications and meanings for him—an additional and painfully difficult therapeutic task.

Since patients vary greatly in their ability and willingness to struggle with these problems, we have concluded that the therapist must flexibly tailor his level of activity and style of intervention to the needs of the individual patient. In some instances it has been possible to move toward a typical dynamically oriented exploratory stance, as illustrated by the following example:

A 25-year old graduate student was hospitalized for a psychotic episode precipitated by the breakup of a long-standing relationship with his girl friend. After living together for several years, the patient's girl friend developed a central nervous system disease which left her with a marked organic deficit. After considerable agonizing, the patient finally broke off the relationship, and several months later he suffered a psychotic decompensation. The patient worked hard in therapy, and medication compliance was uniformly good. By the end of one year of treatment, medication had been discontinued altogether, and the patient had begun an active exploration of the content of the psychotic experience and of the developmental issues surrounding it. This highly motivated patient was able to take the initiative in conducting his therapy, and permitted the therapist to take a neutral exploratory stance. As the therapy progressed, he was able to return to school, and later formed a more satisfying relationship with a different woman.

At the opposite pole of the spectrum are patients whose high levels of vulnerability, limited intelligence, and severe "trait" deficits render them profoundly demoralized, and make a traditional exploratory therapeutic stance ineffective. With these patients, we have used a more directive, supportive style, often actively structuring the content of therapeutic interviews. We have given instruction and advice—not about major life choices, but about current problems and decisions in living. We have occasionally intervened as advocates for the patient with family members or employers when this seemed necessary. We have urged delay and patience when we felt that expectations were excessive. We have generally felt free to applaud clear advances, and to acknowledge signs of progress. Similarly, we have found it useful to express a reasonable sympathy for the inevitable setbacks that occur in the course of treatment.

Throughout this process, we have found ourselves keeping an eye open for the emergence of symptoms, both old and new. It has not always been an easy matter to separate emerging symptoms from "trait" deficits. For example, the gradual development of a retarded depressive picture or hypokinesia in a patient taking neuroleptic medication may be mistaken for a "process" course.[12] Lack of initiative, social withdrawal, and diminished capacity for emotional expression may be misinterpreted as a poor prognostic sign. By contrast, rapidly developing social initiative and energy may be misconstrued as true therapeutic progress, when in reality it heralds relapse. Patients also often have difficulty distinguishing recurrent psychotic symptoms. They may mistake appropriate anxiety and emotional arousal for prodromal symptoms of psychosis. Similarly, they may misinterpret euphoria and excitement as signs of improvement, when in fact they represent impending relapse. In our experience, rapid and dramatic improvement is suspect, and we have found that most lasting improvements occur slowly, after considerable effort. In general, our instincts have been to set a slow to moderate pace for outpatients, and we ourselves have tended to make changes gradually, and only after thoughtful discussion.

Phase 4: The Attainment of Relative Autonomy

In the final phase of the treatment we have undertaken, the patient gradually assumes increasing autonomy within the treatment alliance and in his personal affairs. We have felt that nurturance of tolerable and manageable autonomy is a guiding principle throughout treatment. For the minority of patients who no longer need neuroleptic medication and whose therapeutic progress has been substantial, true termination may be possible. The majority of our patients, however, fell short of this goal, but were able to manage increasingly without intensive treatment. Psychotherapeutic meetings were gradually scheduled at greater intervals, until the patient was able to assume responsibility for initiating sporadic contacts as necessary. Where medication was necessary for prophylaxis against recurrent psychotic symptoms, patients were gradually taught to regulate their own medication, based upon their understanding of vulnerability and prodromal symptoms.

The majority of our patients remain limited to some degree by persisting "trait" deficits and residual vulnerability to psychosis, requiring at least intermittent use of prophylactic medication. The therapist and patient must, in each instance, decide which are reasonable and realistic treatment goals, and when intensive therapeutic effort has reached the point of diminishing returns. This is often a difficult decision, and we have usually arrived at it gradually, and in concert with our patients. Although we have felt free to share with patients our views about realistic goals, we have been reluctant to impose these views on our patients. When a particular patient has reached a functional plateau and declares himself satisfied with this level of progress, we have usually been willing to let well enough alone. On the other hand, when a patient insists he wishes to risk struggling to achieve a higher level of function, we have attempted to support and assist in this effort.

POSSIBLE IMPLICATIONS FOR FUTURE STUDIES

Our experience thus suggests to us that the endogenous vulnerability to psychotic illness can be influenced by human interaction. During individual outpatient treatment, this influence can be exerted on two levels. At the primary level, a variety of psychosocial stresses can apparently lower the threshold to recurrent psychosis. An effective therapeutic relationship can assess the details of the interaction between stress and vulnerability, and can facilitate behaviors which aim to promote growth yet avoid relapse. At the secondary level, neuroleptic drugs can protect against the morbid interaction of stress and endogenous vulnerability, and an effective therapeutic relationship can maximize intelligent medication compliance. Therefore, the nature of the therapeutic alliance seems to us a critical variable related to outcome in these patients.[13] Another important variable is the degree of endogenous vulnerability. Presently we have no direct measure of endogenous vulnerability. However, in our experience, patterns of response to medication have provided useful clues to the estimation of vulnerability in the clinical setting we have described.[14-16] As a result of our experience, therefore, we suggest that some thought be given to the assessment of the therapeutic alliance, and to drug response as an index of vulnerability, as possible correlates of outcome in future studies of medication plus individual psychotherapy in outpatients vulnerable to psychosis.

REFERENCES

1. Havens LL: Problems with the use of drugs in the psychotherapy of psychotic patients. *Psychiatry* **26**:289–296, 1963.
2. Havens LL: Some difficulties in giving schizophrenic and borderline patients medication. *Psychiatry* **31**:44–50, 1968.
3. Group for the Advancement of Psychiatry: *Pharmacotherapy and Psychotherapy: Paradoxes, Problems and Progress*, Volume IX, report No 93. New York: Group for the Advancement of Psychiatry, March 1975.
4. Freyhan FA: Neuroleptic effects: Facts and fiction, in Sarwer-Foner GJ (ed): *The Dynamics of Psychiatric Drug Therapy*. Springfield Ill, Charles C Thomas Publisher, 1960. p 113.
5. Sarwer-Foner GJ, Koranyi EK: Transference effects, the attitude of treating physician, and countertransference in the use of the neuroleptic drugs in psychiatry, in Sarwer-Foner GJ (ed): *The Dynamics of Psychiatric Drug Therapy*. Springfield Ill, Charles C Thomas Publisher, 1960 p 395.
6. Van Putten T: Why do schizophrenic patients refuse to take their drugs? *Arch Gen Psychiatry* **31**:67–72, 1974.
7. Van Putten T, Crumpton E, Yale C: Drug refusal in schizophrenia and the wish to be crazy. *Arch Gen Psychiatry* **33**:1443–1446, 1976.
8. Birley JLT, Brown GW: Crises and life changes preceding the onset of relapse of acute schizophrenia: Clinical aspects. *Br J Psychiatry* **116**:327–333, 1970.
9. Brown GW, Birley JLT, Wing JK: Influence of family life on the course of schizophrenic disorders: A replication. *Br J Psychiatry* **121**:241–258, 1972.
10. Bowers MB Jr: Psychosis and human growth. *Hum Context* **3**:134–145, 1971.
11. Bowers MB Jr: Clinical components of psychotic disorders: Their relationship to treatment. *Schizophr Bull* **3**:600–607, 1977.
12. Van Putten T, May PRA: "Akinetic depression" in schizophrenia. *Arch Gen Psychiatry* **35**:1101–1107, 1978.
13. Tuma, AH, May PRA, Yale C, et al: Therapist characteristics and the outcome of treatment in schizophrenia. *Arch Gen Psychiatry* **35**:81–85, 1978.

14. Van Putten T, May PRA: Subjective response as a predictor of outcome in pharmacotherapy. *Arch Gen Psychiatry* **35**:477–482, 1978.
15. Bowers, MB Jr: Psychosis precipitated by psychotomimetic drugs: A follow-up study. *Arch Gen Psychiatry* **34**:832–835, 1977.
16. Rappaport M, Hopkins HK, Hall K, et al: Are there schizophrenics for whom drugs may be unnecessary or contraindicated? *Int Pharmacopsychiatry* **13**:100–111, 1978.

Chapter 22

The Role for Psychodynamic Psychiatry in the Treatment of Schizophrenic Patients

WILLIAM T. CARPENTER, JR.
and DOUGLAS W. HEINRICHS

INTRODUCTION

Intensive interpersonal therapy of schizophrenia, based on principles of psychotherapeutic or phenomenologic exploration, interests many, but has been the purview of only a few. Most psychiatrists (psychoanalysts or not) are not extensively engaged in psychotherapy of patients with psychotic illnesses. Most patients with schizophrenia are treated in circumstances where skilled interpersonal approaches are not provided as a therapeutic option, let alone as an integral aspect of clinical care. This was actually true before antipsychotic medication was the preeminent consideration in treatment, but a major shift in attitude within our profession now places the psychotherapy of schizophrenia in an extremely precarious position.

During the postwar period, including the early 1960s, influential departments of psychiatry in this country were psychodynamically oriented, and psychoanalytically based treatment and theories of psychopathology

WILLIAM T. CARPENTER, JR., and DOUGLAS W. HEINRICHS • Maryland Psychiatric Research Center, Department of Psychiatry, School of Medicine, University of Maryland, P.O. Box 3235, Baltimore, Maryland 21228.

were taught—at times to the exclusion of other relevant concepts. Those receiving psychiatric education during those years were taught the importance of the doctor–patient relationship, the extraordinary emotional power in the dyad of healer and sufferer, and the importance of using psychotherapeutic techniques in the treatment of patients. New approaches to treatment with psychotropic drugs and behavioral techniques were viewed with suspicion, although the former soon took hold as a routine aspect of clinical care of schizophrenic patients. It was believed then that it would be unethical to treat schizophrenic patients without psychotherapy.[1] However, even during this period actual practice was inconsistent with therapeutic philosophy. Once psychiatrists left their hospital-based training programs, many did not continue to assume responsibility for the care of psychotic patients. For many years, psychoanalysis was the pinnacle of clinical behavioral sciences, but you could pass over most institutes' rosters of training analysts with a divining rod and not find a handful who would welcome the referral of a schizophrenic patient.

The experience of patients was even more disquieting. The typical schizophrenic patient was poor, and faced a fragmented health care system. If enduring clinical care was provided, it was in the public sector. Institutions serving the patient were understaffed, both quantitatively and qualitatively; custodial care often replaced treatment, and resolute social workers, vocational counselors, activity therapists, and others were relegated to "ancillary" status in the most pejorative sense.

The situation for most schizophrenic patients has now changed. Pharmacotherapy is ubiquitous, and, fortunately, is no longer held in low esteem. Treatments designated ancillary are often the only viable interpersonal approaches. Psychiatrists have been reluctant to take these treatments seriously, and intellectual and financial support has come increasingly from the field of "human resources," rather than medicine, as patients are more likely to be in the community (ill or not), whereas hospital populations have shrunk. The change in psychiatry's attitude towards the treatment of schizophrenia is seen in the fact that it is now considered unethical not to administer medication to schizophrenic patients. Interpersonal treatment is no longer viewed as the ideal, or even necessary. Antipsychotic medication may make the patient more available for psychotherapy, but this concept is touted in drug advertisements more than in the clinic and hospital practice. This negative view of present clinical standards is at odds with principles of care articulated by many psychiatric educators and clinical directors, but we think it difficult to reject this judgment, if one has reviewed the treatment experiences of any sizable number of schizophrenic patients.

These introductory remarks are not meant to sully the contributions of those bold clinicians who have spent long and difficult years persevering in the exploration of the psyche with schizophrenic patients, nor of those psy-

whereas the psychotherapist's strength is attention to more subtle intrapsychic and interpersonal functioning, we can understand why problems are created by the lack of collaboration in investigating treatment modalities. The pharmacotherapist has not carefully assessed those variables which best reflect the course and outcome of schizophrenia, and has overgeneralized from the narrow base provided by examining psychotic relapse and hospital readmission rates. The psychotherapist has had the potential to contribute substantially to the development of sophisticated clinical methods, but these contributions have all too often been criticisms after the fact, rather than collaboration in study designs.

It is not simply competing therapeutic philosophies that are at issue here. We believe that psychodynamic psychiatry's extensive reliance on abstract theory and theoretically based clinical inference has an isolating effect which impedes collaboration. This is not a criticism of theory, for complex human phenomena cannot be understood with reductionistic concepts. However, practical application of psychoanalytic knowledge is easily imagined, and theory can be articulated in a manner which invites collaboration. It is unnecessary to relegate cross-disciplinary collaboration to some future synthesis which brings Freud's "Project" to fruition.

SOME CONSEQUENCES OF DECREASING EMPHASIS ON THE PSYCHOTHERAPY OF SCHIZOPHRENIA

Direct and indirect consequences have followed the withdrawal of the psychodynamic psychiatrist from the treatment of schizophrenic patients. A few such effects on clinical care will be adumbrated before discussing those relating to clinical research.

Clinical Issues

• Fewer psychiatric educators are prepared to teach the importance of a thorough evaluation of the person with psychopathology, and the psychiatrist-in-training is less likely to model himself after clinicians competent in psychiatric phenomenology. Today's emphasis on quick diagnosis based on highly specificable psychopathologic manifestations followed by (in fact, usually preceded by) the major treatment decision (i.e., administration of psychotropic drugs) belies the complexity of our clinical material. Schizophrenic patients quickly pass through hospitals without a responsible attempt to understand their experiences, their concepts and attitudes concerning their illness and therapy, what social and familial factors are supporting or undermining their mental functioning, the role of family and others, what strengths can be fostered, and other considerations crucial to intelligent clinical care.

• At times the health care system maximizes countertherapeutic forces. We confront our psychotic patients with an array of services to be found with various people in separate facilities. The schizophrenic patient's motivation, capacity to persevere, or even his difficulty in establishing relationships is not taken into account. Continuity of care now implies linkage of services, rather than enduring commitment between patient and clinician. A deep and abiding personal interest in our patients has shifted to an emphasis on rapid processing techniques.

• Nonmedical mental health professionals no longer find the physician understanding of the interpersonal basis of their work or helpful in elucidating hidden or subtle aspects of psychopathology which may require the attention of specialized workers. The mental health team often prefers the psychiatrist to restrict his efforts to diagnosis and pharmacotherapy. Treatment team leadership capable of integrating social, psychological, and biological data relevant to schizophrenia, and translating this synthesis into treatment planning, is a forsaken ideal.

• Treatment goals do not include the possibility of gains beyond restoration to the previous level of functioning. psychotherapists have a bias towards increasing health, as well as reducing illness. Psychotic episodes are remarkably informative personal crises, but the opportunity for conflict resolution and enhanced adaptation is missed by the clinician with a single-minded determination to eradicate symptoms and reduce hospital stay.

Research Issues

The body of knowledge relevant to the effect of any treatment on the course of schizophrenia has been seriously compromised by the failure of psychoanalysts and psychodynamically interested psychiatrists to participate vigorously in developing research methods. Three consequences have been: (a) the paucity of systematic, empirical research on psychotherapy of schizophrenia conducted by knowledgeable psychotherapists with designs suitable for testing hypothesized effects; (b) the unanswered challenge of several very influential studies comparing psychotherapy and pharmacotherapy which demonstrated drug benefit and failed to demonstrate any meaningful psychotherapeutic benefit; and (c) scores of drug/placebo studies which have been uninformative on many critical aspects of drug/illness interaction.

The criticism of current methods can be succinctly presented, since these issues have been discussed in the literature.[1-8] Treatment research in schizophrenia has not adequately accounted for those variables most likely to reflect the core course of illness. That which is easiest to specify and measure has been emphasized, while that which reflects subtle intrapsychic and interpersonal functioning has been largely ignored. We know a great deal about antipsychotic drug effects on symptom reduction during psychotic periods. We know much less about drug effects on overt features of role performance, and virtually nothing about drug effects on quality of functioning. As important as hospital status and symptom status are, these variables have a demonstrably modest association with other aspects of functioning, and represent only a partial information base on which to predicate treatment efforts.[9-11] In addition to inadequacies in evaluation of treatment effect, designs for testing psychosocial therapy have been justly criticized for methods of patient selection, therapist selection, setting and time-frame for conducting treatment, and insufficient effort focused on change criteria most likely to reflect psychotherapeutic efficacy. This, combined with the avoidance of clinical trials by psychotherapists, has resulted in the present situation, where it cannot be determined whether failure to demonstrate efficacy of psychotherapy is based on the weakness of the treatment, or weakness of study design.

NEW DIRECTIONS IN CLINICAL RESEARCH

This view of treatment research in schizophrenia suggests that the most fundamental and important new direction for psychotherapy of schizophrenia will be a turn to clinical research methods in an attempt to elucidate the effect of treatment. If this is energetically pursued, the 1980s will be richly informative regarding the strengths and limitations of psychotherapy of schizophrenic patients, and the interaction between drug and psychosocial treatments. The psychotherapeutic community may inculcate the principles of clinical science, replacing indoctrination with healthy skepticism.

New directions in clinical investigative methods can be expected. Psychotherapists will eschew the present tendency to measure *only* highly specifiable phenomena, such as hospital readmission or hallucinations. They will develop systematic and reliable assessment techniques for more complex and subtle manifestations of schizophrenic illness. The course of the illness will be charted in its impact on the person, rather than simply by tracking psychotic symptoms. Identifying those clinical features central to schizophrenia which can be consistently defined and reliably assessed will provide a basis for assessing the effect of various therapies on aspects of schizophrenia such as deteriorating social relationships, impaired initiative and spontaneity, the restricted range and flexibility of the ideational field, and the inability to experience ordinary pleasure and gratification. Investigators should be attentive to the patient's strengths as well as his weaknesses, and will seek to understand the role of treatments in maintaining intact functions as well as in reducing deficits. Such clinical methods* will provide appropriate data with which to test psychotherapeutic efficacy, and will enable pharmacologic and other treatments to be evaluated from a broad phenomenologic base, rather than a specious descriptive base.

The psychotherapeutically oriented clinical researcher will also provide a more appropriate time perspective to clinical studies than is presently encouraged by the focus on symptom status and rapid discharge. For many patients, schizophrenia is a lifelong illness; yet current therapeutic trends stress those aspects of the illness which can be readily altered, ignoring all others. Third-party influences curtail treatment to rapid, "pragmatic" approaches, and keeping a psychotic patient out of the hospital seems more important than restoring health. If there is to be a future role of interpersonal treatment and enduring therapeutic relationships for the schizophrenic patient, it depends on the demonstration, through carefully designed clinical investigations, that interpersonal strategies introduce demonstrable therapeutic effects, as well as humane care, to the treatment of schizophrenic patients.

NEW DIRECTIONS IN THEORY APPLICATION

With involvement of psychodynamic investigators in clinical research, an unproductive dichotomization is likely to continue, unless accompanied by a basic advance in our theoretical model. On the purely theoretical level, biologic and psychologic thinkers may consider etiologic hypotheses about a wide range of schizophrenic experience, as illustrated in Figure 1. However, at the pragmatic level of treatment strategies, biologic and psychologic

---

* The feasibility of developing more sensible and sensitive clinical methods can be illustrated by briefly describing the "Quality of Life Scale" being developed for treatment and outcome studies at the Maryland Psychiatric Research Center. A semistructured interview of 30–60 minutes duration is used to probe 22 areas of experience and functioning. The first nine items relate to richness, intimacy, and satisfaction in interpersonal relations. The next four consider the utilization of occupational skills, and the degree of fulfillment derived from them. Seven areas focus primarily on the richness and vitality of intrapsychic life, including the level of purposefulness, motivation, curiosity, capacity for pleasure, rapport, and empathy. Two items address personal hygiene and appearance, and the extent of commonplace possessions and activities. Although it considers complex and pervasive dimensions of living apart from specific psychotic symptoms, this scale does not presuppose or require adherence to any particular psychologic theory of mental functioning or etiological hypothesis of schizophrenia. Rather, the investigator is asked to assess the patient's capacity to function and the quality of his experience, and systematically record these relevant clinical judgments. Formal presentation of this scale will follow further clinical and psychometric evaluation, but preliminary use indicates that clinicians can make reliable judgments on difficult-to-specify aspects of psychopathology ordinarily omitted from clinical methods.

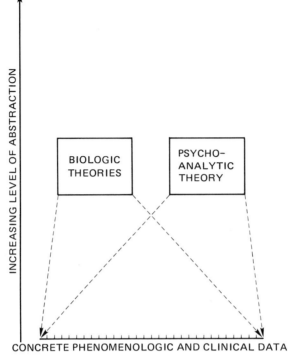

FIGURE 1.   Relationship of biologic and psychodynamic theories to clinical data.

therapists each are inclined to claim, with varying degrees of evidence, to be capable of explaining and treating different segments of schizophrenic psychopathology (Figure 2). Psychopharmacologists relate florid psychotic symptoms to biochemical mechanisms, and treat them with antipsychotic drugs. Psychotherapists use psychologic constructs to explain dimensions of intrapsychic and interpersonal dysfunction, and treat them with psychotherapy.

This position does an injustice to both the complexity and the basic unity of the illness. Most facets of schizophrenic psychopathology are susceptible to influence by both biologic and interpersonal interventions. This is not to deny that certain dimensions are more profoundly influenced by one or the other. In the control of florid symptoms of acute decompensation, neuroleptics now have primacy, and it is likely that future advances in this area will be pharmacologic. Psychosocial treatments are more readily applied to issues of social and occupational functioning and the capacity for intimacy and gratification. Yet most clinicians are familiar with rapid psy-

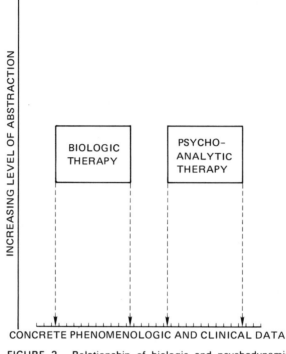

FIGURE 2. Relationship of biologic and psychodynamic therapies to clinical data.

chotic symptom reduction in response to environmental change, as well as enhanced interpersonal functioning following antipsychotic drugs. Thus, both biologic and psychologic theories need to consider the impact of their respective interventions on the full range of schizophrenic psychopathology. However, an important conceptual problem exists, in that each model must be able to characterize and understand the influence of the other on its own treatment effects, and on common observational data. The problem is rooted in the fact that both biologic and psychologic theories tend to use explanatory concepts that are illsuited for understanding the impact of categorically different interventions. The role of insight, personal relatedness, and environmental change cannot presently be grasped by neurochemical formulations. The efficacy of neuroleptics is difficult to understand in terms of psychodynamic or interpersonal theories.

Today's biologically oriented investigators better appreciate the complexity of mental functioning, and are more open to interdisciplinary dialogue, than many psychotherapeutic workers appreciate. It is ill-advised to seek only new theory which can unify biologic and metapsychologic paradigms in the fulfillment of Freud's ambitions of the "Project for a Scientific Psychology."[12] Apart from the fact that this development is undoubtedly far in the future, this attitude usually assumes that the unification is essentially of theoretical interest, beyond current problems and methods.

Although a theoretical resolution of this dualism is not to be deprecated, the practical requirements of intelligently combining biologic and psychologic strategies for maximal therapeutic impact presses for a synthetic paradigm useful now. Such a need can be fulfilled by a system based on explanatory concepts of fewer levels of inference from observable data than current biochemical or psychodynamic theories, yet comprehensive enough to be applicable to both. Rather than replacing these paradigms, such a framework would provide a "final common pathway" for understanding treatment effect for both biologic and psychologic interventions and their interaction.

The development of such an explanatory model mediating between biologic and psychologic formulations and concrete clinical data is a challenging theoretical task essential for the comprehensive understanding and treatment of schizophrenia in the 1980s. Figure 3 illustrates this position. At this point, we can only indicate a few concepts likely to be part of such a theoretical construct.

Stress can be such a unifying concept, implying both a physiologic state of the organism and a subjectively experienced apperception. Clinicians agree that stress has a disorganizing potential for the schizophrenic. It should also be appreciated that stress avoidance can lead to an undersirable constriction of the person's functioning and experience. Some have suggested that the withdrawal and amotivational states seen in schizophrenics represent a self-imposed constriction of this sort, as defense against disorganizing stress. Biologic and psychologic interventions can be assessed in terms of their impact on this common dimension. The disorganizing impact of stress can be reduced with neuroleptics. Insight-oriented therapy can help the patient reformulate his experience to allow modes of response that can lead to increased mastery and resolution. This seems most important for unavoidable stress, and for stress resulting from destructive interpretations and distorted meanings imposed by the patient on his experience. At times, environmental stressors can be altered (e.g., vocational training can increase job security; family intervention can sometimes alter stress-inducing patterns of interaction; foster homes can stabilize practical problems of living). Numerous interventions are possible at the stress–functioning interface. Organizing concepts which integrate the broad data base relevant to this interface are necessary, while narrow approaches will be misleading (e.g., schizophrenics should not be urged to seek employment because the stress causes relapse).

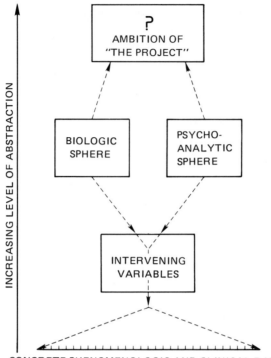

FIGURE 3. Position of intervening variables in relating biologic and psychodynamic spheres to each other and to clinical data.

Sensory stimulation and information processing are concepts that lend themselves to a similar formulation. There is some evidence that schizophrenics are impaired in their ability to process and filter sensory input. Over-stimulation can lead to symptomatic exacerbation, and understimulation to deficits in functioning. Neuroleptics may have a corrective impact on sensory processing dysfunctions, and protect against overstimulation. Interpersonal interventions and environmental manipulations can increase or decrease stimulation for the patient, and can support or disrupt integrative functioning. The related concept of physiologic arousal readily illustrates the interactions between social, psychological, and biological variables. State of CNS arousal is related to genetic factors, and can be altered biochemically (e.g., amphetamine), psychologically (e.g., sexual fantasy), and socially (e.g., seeing a horror movie with friends at a Sunday matinee, rather than alone in your basement on Saturday night). Altered states of arousal can impede psychic functioning, and restoration to optimal arousal can be approached environmentally, interpersonally, and pharmacologically.*

These concepts attempt to integrate intervening variables affecting mental states and personality functioning, paralleling the approach in some high risk studies where concepts of vulnerability are heuristically important. The examples we provide have several interesting similarities with each other and with vulnerability concepts. First, they all conform to the "inverted U" relationship with level of functioning, as represented in Figure 4. For each of these variables, extremes lead to deteriorated functioning and/or exacerbation of symptoms. Maximal functioning occurs in intermediate ranges. Second, all types of interventions can be assessed in terms of effect on the same intervening variable (i.e., increasing or reducing stress, provoking or reducing arousal, raising or lowering sensory input). Third, the variable impact of similar interventions at different times can be understood by appreciating the changing locus of the patient on the continuum of the intervening variable. Thus, treatment designed to reduce arousal would be expected to improve functioning when a person is hyperaroused, but worsen functioning when he is hypoaroused. Fourth, such explanatory concepts encourage testing of the impact of cumulative interventions of mixed types (e.g., pharmacologic and psychosocial), rather than either/or designs (e.g., psychotherapy versus drug treatment).

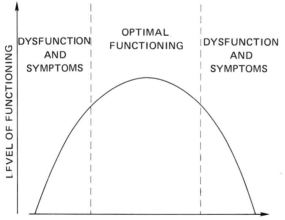

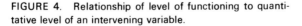

FIGURE 4.   Relationship of level of functioning to quantitative level of an intervening variable.

* Several recent reviews have discussed arousal, attention, and information-processing paradigms, including a Rochester-based conference published in the *Journal of Psychiatric Research* (Vol 14, Nos 1–4, 1978), and a collection of discussions in the *Schizophrenia Bulletin* (Vol 3, No 1, 1977).

A NOTABLE EXCEPTION

Family theory and therapy have been less afflicted with the problems we have reviewed, and have made greater progress toward synthesizing concepts. Starting from highly complex and abstract models and systems theory, concepts characterizing interactional modes, patterns of alliance and power, and communicational dysfunction became articulated. These concepts were carefully defined from clinical observations, and thus can be recognized and understood without requiring allegiance to specific etiologic models or metapsychological theory. This increased the likelihood of consensual validation, hence, these concepts have had a profound impact on a broad range of family therapists—from the most theoretically oriented to the most pragmatic and eclectic. The proximity of concept to clinical data allows clinical experience to modify the concepts, and clinical investigators to test theoretical tenets and therapeutic hypotheses. The following can be cited as sanguine consequences.

1.   Family theorists and family therapists continue to influence each other, a process which results in fresh ideas and new clinical approaches.

2.   Family theorists and investigators have, by and large, maintained a keen interest in developments in genetics, human biology, pharmacology, developmental psychology, and group and societal processess. What they think and do is actually influenced by experimental and clinical data, and attitudes are inclusive rather than exclusive. Combining genetic, psychophysiologic, and family variables in the study of vulnerability is an example.

3.   Workers in the family field have been willing to articulate clinical approaches of potential applicability to the modal schizophrenic patient (i.e., chronically ill, unemployed), and have not limited their interest to a highly selected subgroup of schizophrenic patients (i.e., articulate patients of high social standing).

An example of the last point is found in the work on expressed emotion in families of schizophrenics reported from England by Brown,[13,14] and later by Vaughn and Leff.[15] These workers note high relapse rates in schizophrenic patients living with highly critical, hostile, and overinvolved relatives. In such cases, antipsychotic drugs play a decisive role in reducing relapse, and decreasing contact with the censuring relative may be protective. In the low-expressive families, medication appears to play no role in preventing relapse, a remarkable finding deserving greater study, since the majority of their patients came from low-expressive households. This will interest the pharmacotherapist, since the risks of long-term drug use are substantial, and are justified only in circumstances where appreciable benefit can be expected. The psychophysiologist is already interested in attempting to ascertain the impact of interpersonal environment on ANS arousal.

The above studies are subject to criticism beyond the scope of this paper, but two deficits remind us of the crucial role of the psychiatric phenomenologist. No information is provided or sought relevant to the patient's vulnerability to high expressed emotion, to what form the hostile interaction takes, or to what coping mechanisms are effective or ineffective, It is as though the individual patient is irrelevant, except as a passive receptor. Similarly, the impact of expressed emotion on the patient is measured in narrow terms of readmission/relapse, rather than reflecting broadly on the course of schizophrenia. In fairness, this lack of attention to the individual and the individual/family interaction is atypical of family research, where most investigators have been drawn from, or influenced by, psychoanalysis.

Expressed emotion, in short, has many qualities (noted above) that make it a good candidate for intervening variable research. Various interventions can be assessed in terms of increasing or decreasing its impact, and changes in the amount of expressed emotion confronting the patient at various times can be determined. It is sufficiently close to observable data that specific hypotheses about its consequences can be tested. The powerful demonstrations of its impact promise to make it highly influential in therapeutic practice and treatment policy. Yet, the failure to temper the concept with a careful phenomenologic apprectiaion of the individual and the actual role of family interactions may result in its mechanistic and uncritical application. For instance, in this country, with the pressure for quick decisions and rapid discharge, clinicians may be willing to base major recommendations on unifactorial and superficial considerations. A variable such as familial expression of emotion and attitude could be misused as an isolated guide for both drug and environmental treatment decisions.

IMPLICATIONS FOR PRACTICE

It is our belief that the advances in research and theory put forward in this paper will signficantly alter the practice of psychotherapy with schizophrenic patients.

There will be less emphasis on psychotherapy as a relatively pure treatment strategy. Rather, the psychodynamic psychiatrist will be involved in providing a multifaceted and integrated treatment program. Decision making will be based on a range of psychologic, biologic, and social variables. Final common pathway and intervening variable concepts will facilitate an intelligent prediction of the impact of each treatment singly, or in combination. Careful understanding of the individual patient will include an assessment of his current capacity to respond to, and utilize, each intervention. Thus, while a psychotically disorganized patient may not have the cognitive competence to process and utilize certain verbal interventions that might otherwise reduce anxiety, medication or environmental strategies may be efficacious in achieving the same desired effect. During another phase of illness, psychological insight may prove effective as the main therapeutic thrust, or in combination with other modalities. All too often the psychotherpist offers an inflexible treatment modality to the limited number of patients with the financial resources to afford, and the psychological capacity to profit from, his help. All others are diverted to workers providing "inferior" therapies. By offering a multifaceted and flexible treatment, the psychotherapeutically oriented physician will work with patients with a wider range of capacities and socioeconomic backgrounds.

By applying his special skills to the full range of treatments, the psychodynamic psychiatrist can have an impact on all treatments. A humaneness and respect for the individual patient's experience will enhance the quality of pharmacologic and social interventions. His emphasis on the value of an enduring doctor–patient relationship will encourage the organization of treatment into consistent, personal involvement of therapists with patients over long periods of time.

The use of intervening variables can relate various theories and treatments derived from them to specific functional aspects of the patient. Consequently, we expect the psychotherapist to be increasingly concerned with concrete therapeutic goals. Assessment of success in therapy will not be limited to global and abstract appraisals of structural change. More attention will be paid to specific targets of treatment, such as occupational functioning, social skills, and the capacity to meet the practical demands of life—the concrete building blocks of loving and working. Psychotherapists will be more attentive to giving basic education about the illness to the patient and his family, providing opportunities to develop vocational and social skills, and guiding the patient in improving his physical and material surroundings.

By applying various treatment strategies to a broad range of patients, the psychotherapeutically oriented psychiatrist will be in a position to develop criteria to identify that subgroup of schizophrenics for whom an intensive, insight-oriented therapy is the treatment of choice. As a result of such focusing, the more traditional model of psychotherapy may be utilized in a more productive manner.

This pattern of clinical practice will create an especially vital role for the psychiatrist. He has the requisite background to integrate data from sociology, psychology, biochemistry, physiology, genetics, and pharmacology. As polemics about therapeutic modalities lessen, and interest in integrated, multifaceted treatment approaches grows, the psychiatrist will have the intellectually challenging and demanding responsibility for the phenomenologic evaluation of the patient, for the application of complex data to the differential diagnosis of psychosis, for the assessment of strengths and weaknesses in a wide array of functioning areas, and for the application of therapeutic techniques which will include pharmacologic, interpersonal, and environmental dimensions.

REFERENCES

1. Feinsilver DB, Gunderson JG: Psychotherapy for schizophrenics: Is it indicated? A review of the relevant literature.*Schizophr Bull* **6**:11–23, 1972.
2. Carpenter WT, McGlashan TH, Strauss JS: The treatment of acute schizophrenia without drugs. *Am J Psychiatry* **134**:14–20, 1977.
3. Carpenter WT: Comments on the confluence of psychiatric phenomenology, interpersonal therapies, and clinical research methods in schizophrenia, in Muller C (ed): International Congress Series, No 464. *Psychotherapy of Schizophrenia: Proceedings, Sixth International Symposium on the Psychotherapy of Schizophrenis.* Lausanne, September, 1978, Amsterdam, Excerpta Medica, 1980.
4. Group for the Advancement of Psychiatry: *Pharmacotherapy and Psychotherapy: Paradoxes, Problems and Progress.* New York, Mental Health Materials Center Inc, 1975.
5. Gunderson JG: Drugs and psychosocial treatment of schizophrenia revisted. *JCE Psychiat* 25–40, 1977.
6. May PRA: Psychotherapy research in schizophrenia: Another view of present reality. *Schizophr Bull* **9**:126–132, 1974.
7. May PRA: Schizophrenia: Evaluation of treatment methods, in Freedman AM, Kaplan HI, Sadock BJ (eds): *Comprehensive Textbook of Psychiatry.* Baltimore, Williams & Wilkins Co, 1975, pp 955–982.
8. Mosher LR, Keith SJ: Research on the psychosocial treatment of schizophrenia: A summary report. *Am J Psychiatry* **136**:623–631, 1979.
9. Strauss SJ, Carpenter WT: The prediction of outcome in schizophrenia: I. Characteristics of outcome. *Arch Gen Psychiatry* **27**:739–746, 1972.
10. Strauss SJ, Carpenter WT: The prediction of outcome in schizophrenia: III. Five-year outcome and its predictors: A report from the International Pilot Study of Schizophrenia. *Arch Gen Psychiatry* **34**:159–163, 1977.
11. Schwartz CC, Myers JK, Astrachan BM: Concordance of multiple assessments of the outcome of schizophrenia: On defining the dependent variable in outcome studies. *Arch Gen Psychiatry* **32**:1221–1227, 1975.
12. Freud S: A project for a scientific psychology, in Strachey J (ed): *The Standard Edition of the Complete Psychological Works of Sigmund Freud.* London, Hogarth Press, 1966, vol 1, pp 283–398.
13. Brown GW, Monck EM, Carstairs GM, et al: Influence of family life on the course of schizophrenic illness. *Br J Prev So Med* **16**:55–68, 1962.
14. Brown GW, Birley JLT, Wing JK: Influence of family life on the course of schizophrenic disorders: A replication. *Br J Psychiatry* **121**:241–258, 1972.
15. Vaughn CE, Leff JP: The influence of family and social factors on the course of psychiatric illness: A comparison of schizophrenic and depressed neurotic patients. *Br J Psychiatry*, **129**—125–137, 1976.

Chapter 23

The Quality of Outcome from Psychotherapy of Schizophrenia

JOHN G. GUNDERSON
and BEVERLY GOMES-SCHWARTZ

INTRODUCTION

This paper explores the problems of measuring outcome from intensive exploratory psychotherapy with schizophrenic persons. Four dimensions of outcome which may be specific to such treatment are proposed in conjunction with a semistructured interview for reliably evaluating these dimensions. Preliminary results indicating the potential validity of this interview will be presented, and their implications will be discussed.

Among the variety of outcome measures which have been employed in previous efforts to evaluate the effects of psychotherapy with schizophrenic persons, the most common are recidivism rates, sign and symptom change, and indices of social functioning.[1] Such indices of outcome have been useful in documenting changes brought about by psychopharmacological, milieu,

JOHN G. GUNDERSON • Director of Psychotherapy, McLean Hospital, Belmont, Massachusetts and Associate Professor of Psychiatry, Harvard Medical School, Brookline, Massachusetts.   BEVERLY GOMES-SCHWARTZ • Assistant Psychologist, McLean Hospital, Belmont, Massachusetts and Instructor of Psychology, Department of Psychiatry, Harvard Medical School, Brookline, Massachusetts. This research was supported by PHS Grant #25246-03 of the National Institute of Mental Health.

and group therapy.[2,3] Yet the relevance of these measures of signs and symptoms or overt behaviors to the effects of an exploratory psychotherapy in which the stated goal is to enrich the patient's understanding of himself is not obvious. Indeed, it seems possible that diminution of bizarre or socially unacceptable behavior and intrapsychic change could be relatively independent dimensions of psychotherapy outcome.[4,5] The patient undertaking an exploratory therapy naturally expects that, by understanding himself better the quality of his life may be enhanced. It is difficult to know, however, how such changes may be discerned, let alone measured. With the exception of occasional intriguing hints, the literature has largely ignored the nature of successful outcome from psychoanalytically oriented therapy.

Although there have been some efforts by Semrad,[6] Bellak,[7] and Schulz[8] to develop measures of the types of changes exploratory psychotherapy is intended to bring about, these measures have had serious psychometric problems, and have not been tested prospectively. The only scale used prospectively in past research that attempts to measure outcome variables which might be specifically affected by exploratory psychotherapy is the Camarillo Dynamic Assessment Scale.[9] This scale includes ratings of insight, affective contact, anxiety, ego strength, the extent to which the environment suffers, motivation, object relations, and sense of personal identity. Both the breadth of this instrument's intended applicability (i.e., for all types of psychopathology), and the unreliability of its scoring[10] diminish the value of this scale in studies of psychotherapy of schizophrenia.

Because of this lack of appropriate and reliable outcome measures, one of us (Gunderson) specified a series of hypotheses about changes which might be more specific for schizophrenic patients treated with intensive psychotherapy, and subsequently developed an interview schedule (The Psychotherapy Outcome Interview, see appendix) for assessing these hypotheses. These hypotheses arose out of clinical and research experience with schizophrenic patients treated with long-term individual psychotherapy. The hypothesized psychological changes fall into the following four dimensions: *Longitudinal Awareness*, *Insightfulness*, *Object Relatedness*, and *Subjective Experience*. After describing these four dimensions as they were developed into a semistructured interview, we will then look at some preliminary efforts to evaluate whether and in what sequence intensive psychotherapy brings about changes along these dimensions in schizophrenic patients.

THE PSYCHOTHERAPY OUTCOME INTERVIEW

The Psychotherapy Outcome Interview was developed to systematically address areas of change in schizophrenic patients. This interview consists of nine sections, which assess aspects of the four dimensions. Longitudinal Awareness is assessed through sections on continuity of past and present, and realistic overview. Insightfulness includes sections tapping externalization, self-observation, and anticipation. Object Relatedness includes both object love/differentiation, and object need/trust. Subjective Experience is gauged by sections on ambivalence and affective flexibility. Each of the nine sections consists of a series of inquiries, concluding with an overall summarizing statement which, states in positive terms the outcome goal. For example, affective flexibility is judged according to the criterion: "The patient experiences a wide range of affect, including irritation and guilt, on a regular basis." Each of these nine statements is rated on a scale from 1 (not present) to 7 (optimally).*

The first dimension, *Longitudinal Awareness*, involves insight about the origins, consequences, and continuity of one's psychopathology throughout his life. This includes how childhood experiences and relationships with parents helped to form one's personality, and how this personality in turn has left one vulnerable to subsequent psychoses. This dimension includes an evaluation of the degree to which patients' psychoses have become integrated into the continuity of their lives, as opposed to sealed off. These concepts were first introduced here at Yale by Soskis & Bowers,[11] and have more recently been the subject of a series of papers by McGlashan and co-workers.[12,13]

A second aspect of Longitudinal Awareness includes the degree to which the schizophrenic patient realistically appreciates the implications of his psychopathology. This involves the knowledge that he has major psychological limitations, and, more importantly, the degree to which this knowledge alters and informs his plans for the future, i.e., has made him feel his fate is self-determined. Each patient is asked whether his present knowledge about himself could have allowed him to live his past life differently.

The second dimension of outcome which may be specifically related to a successful exploratory psychotherapy for a schizophrenic patient is the capacity to be insightful within current and ongoing life experience, i.e., *Insightfulness*. One aspect of Insightfulness is related to the common tendency among schizophrenic persons to externalize (i.e., to explain subjective experience by external situational determinants). The tendency to externalize can be seen in the extent to which patients view themselves, or others, as disadvantaged, misunderstood, and mistreated, and in the degree to which this perception is attributed to the malicious intentions of their parents or others. Since the followup interviews are within a period of time

---

* Scale ratings on the Interview are 0 to 6. These are converted for convenience in data recording and analysis.

in which the recurrence of more openly paranoid symptoms are common, inquiries are also made about ideas of reference, and the degree to which, when these symptoms recur, the patient has some distance about the cause and purpose of the symptoms.

Stanton[14] has described how a schizophrenic patient's capacity to observe himself with some curiosity, detachment, and analytic skill is an important ego activity. In the self-observation section of the interview, patients are asked about their awareness of themselves in a variety of meaningful situations. For example, whether they are aware of how they communicate things to bring about hoped-for responses from others (shock, concern, amusement, etc.), or whether they can think about themselves or have fantasies, even while engaged in other activities, such as talking or sexual intercourse.

A third aspect of Insightfulness is the degree to which self-knowledge allows the person to anticipate potentially difficult situations. This capacity for anticipation ideally requires some knowledge of the relationship of one's major conflicts to life circumstances. Patients frequently will first come to recognize certain internal signals as warnings of impending psychological difficulty, and only later will they tie these to the social or interpersonal situations in which the warning symptoms emerge.

A third major dimension of outcome which was hypothesized to be specific for intensive individual psychotherapy involves *Object Relatedness*. Part of this dimension is related to the variables Schulz[15] sought to measure in his self–object differentiation scale. To improve reliability on this dimension in the Psychotherapy Outcome Interview, more global assessments on fewer aspects of object relations were attempted. We evaluate whether there is an ability to recognize discriminable aspects of other people, and the degree to which the patient is able to distinguish himself from others. For example, a patient who lacked this capacity described himself as being "mellow, thoughtful, and kind," and shortly thereafter described his father, to whom he said he was closest, as "mellow, thoughtful, and benign." This lack of discrimination in describing one's self *vis à vis* an important other is taken as evidence of a rather gross failure of self–object differentiation.*

In assessing Object Relatedness, particular attention is paid to issues which might be more specific to the changes one would anticipate in the first few years of work with a schizophrenic person. For example, the issues of trust, and the ability to feel comfortable depending on another person, are particularly important for a recovering schizophrenic person during this time framework. This is because many schizophrenic people are profoundly

---

* An important and closely related concept which is not directly addressed is the patient's level of self-identity, and the stability of this identity. A means of evaluating this is still in the process of being developed.

isolated, and frightened of becoming dependent. Another issue concerns the intimacy of the relationships which patients form. This includes the degree to which a recovering schizophrenic patient is able to share with others ideas or experiences which they had previously considered as shameful (e.g., their sexuality), or as betrayals (e.g., discussing family secrets).

The fourth major dimension of outcome, *Subjective Experience*, concerns how patients experience their daily life, and is closely related to what is sometimes referred to as the quality of life. Subjective Experience involves evaluation of a capacity for ambivalence. This includes being able to maintain complicated perceptions of one's own situation and social circumstances, tolerating uncertainty and ambiguity (rather than resorting to all-or-none thinking), and, most important, recognizing and accepting one's own helplessness. Another aspect of ambivalence is the degree to which the person is interested in current social, political, or moral issues, and is, moreover, willing to take an identifiable position on any of these issues. Usually, the schizophrenic person shows no interest in such things, or has extreme or idiosyncratic views, which are not openly discussed.

The other section included in our assessment of Subjective Experience is a measure of the range and flexibility of affect. Particular attention is paid to the capacity for sadism, concern, and humor—the latter especially with respect to one's self. Particularly glaring is the schizophrenic person's inability to accept wishes to hurt anyone else, even to the point of refusing to be in circumstances where getting something for himself might involve compromising someone else (e.g., competitive situations).

In their entirety, these outcome variables reflect changes toward greater humility, conflict, and uncertainty—but also less egocentricity, and greater flexibility. The interview takes about one hour, and though patients find many of the questions difficult, it is thought-provoking, and not unpleasant. No one has refused, or even complained about completing or returning for repeat interviews at later followup periods. Interviewers appreciate the open-endedness of the probes, and the clinical depth that the interview encourages.

PRELIMINARY RESULTS

As indicated in Table I, the reliability on the Psychotherapy Outcome Interview variables is uniformly high. Thus, reliability ratings are only slightly enhanced by using the mean scores from two raters, or by combining the sections to establish scores for the four dimensions. Despite disparities in clinical experience and in familiarity with the interview concepts, good reliability was easily established between raters after only a few interviews.

TABLE I.   Interrater Reliability[a]

Interview scores	Reliability of single rater	Composite reliability
Longitudinal awareness	.89	.94
Continuity past & present	.79	.88
Realistic overview	.79	.88
Insightfulness	.93	.96
Externalization	.89	.94
Self-observation	.84	.91
Anticipation	.79	.88
Object relatedness	.94	.97
Object love/differentiation	.88	.94
Object need/trust	.95	.97
Subjective experience	.93	.96
Ambivalence	.76	.86
Affective flexibility	.87	.93
Total	.95	.97

[a] Reliability coefficients calculated with Finn's r formulas $n = 14$ patients.

To assess the validity of the interview as a measure of the effects hypothesized to be unique to intensive exploratory psychotherapy, we compared three groups of schizophrenic patients who have received intensive psychotherapy with groups who received equally long but nonexploratory supportive psychotherapy. Most patients were young adults—at least when they started psychotherapy—and had been in treatment with experienced therapists for varying lengths of time—from six months to more than 20 years. All patients with two years or less of treatment met World Health Organization criteria for schizophrenia,[16] and were randomly assigned to treatment as part of an ongoing study of psychotherapy (NIMH Grant #MH25246, A. H. Stanton, Principal Investigator). However, for the purposes of this pilot study, long-term schizophrenic patients who had not been randomly assigned or screened with research diagnostic criteria were included, to gain greater knowledge of the long-range effects of the treatments. Although efforts were made to keep the raters blind to the treatment condition of the patients, this proved largely unfeasible.

Table II shows that greater differences between the therapy conditions emerged with time, and in each instance the statistically significant differences favored those receiving intensive psychotherapy. This was most obvious for the dimension of Longitudinal Awareness and its component section, continuity of past and present. Only on the dimensions of Object Relatedness and its component section, object need/trust, was there any indication of greater discrepancy favoring the intensively treated patients

TABLE II. Differences Between Intensive and Nonintensive Treatment Groups

Interview scores	6 month Means			1-2 years Means			>2½ years Means		
	INT[b] (n = 11)	NON (n = 12)	p[a]	INT (n = 8)	NON (n = 8)	p	INT (n = 10)	NON (n = 8)	p
Longitudinal awareness	4.23	3.44		4.44	3.03	.05	4.83	3.28	.04
Continuity past & present	4.18	2.67	.05	4.50	2.67	.03	5.00	2.94	.01
Realistic overview	4.27	4.21		4.38	3.38		4.65	3.63	
Insightfulness	3.30	3.06		3.96	3.42		4.30	3.35	
Externalization	3.09	3.04		4.56	4.00		4.20	3.69	
Self-observation	3.27	3.21		4.31	3.31		4.45	3.38	
Anticipation	3.60	2.92		3.00	2.94		4.25	3.00	.06
Object relatedness	3.77	3.10		3.84	2.91	.08	3.75	2.81	
Object love/differentiation	4.10	3.29		3.44	2.56		3.70	2.69	
Object need/trust	3.55	2.92		4.25	3.25		3.80	2.94	
Subjective experience	3.09	2.71		3.47	3.13		4.10	2.91	
Ambivalence	2.64	2.67		2.31	3.13		3.75	3.13	
Affective flexibility	3.55	2.75		4.63	3.13	.05	4.45	2.69	.02
TOTAL	3.58	3.07		3.93	3.15		4.25	3.12	.06

[a] probability two-tailed t-test.
[b] INT = Intensive Therapy, NON = Nonintensive therapy.

TABLE III. Means and Significant Effects for Treatment Groups by Length of Treatment Analyses of Variance

Interview scores		Means[a]			Significant Effects	
		6 month	1–2 years	>2½ years	Group[b]	Length[c]
Longitudinal	INT	4.17	4.25	4.83	.006	
awareness	NON	2.96	3.03	3.28		
Continuity	INT	4.00	4.00	5.00	.001	
past & present	NON	2.43	2.69	2.94		
Realistic	INT	4.33	4.50	4.65	.06	
overview	NON	3.50	3.38	3.63		
Insightfulness	INT	3.33	3.61	4.30		
	NON	3.19	3.42	3.35		
Externalization	INT	3.17	4.42	4.20		
	NON	2.93	4.00	3.69		
Self-observation	INT	3.00	4.08	4.45		
	NON	3.21	3.31	3.38		
Anticipation	INT	3.83	2.33	4.25		
	NON	3.43	2.94	3.00		
Object	INT	3.25	3.63	3.75		
relatedness	NON	2.96	2.91	2.81		
Object love	INT	3.50	3.25	3.70		
differentiation	NON	3.21	2.56	2.69		
Object need	INT	3.00	4.00	3.80		
trust	NON	2.71	3.25	2.94		
Subjective	INT	2.25	3.13	4.10		.07
experience	NON	2.29	3.13	2.91		
Ambivalence	INT	1.83	2.08	3.75		
	NON	2.43	3.13	3.13		
Affective	INT	2.67	4.17	4.45		
flexibility	NON	2.14	3.13	2.69	.02	.04
TOTAL	INT	3.26	3.65	4.25	.08	
	NON	2.89	3.15	3.12		

[a] n's for groups at 6 mths, 1–2 yrs and >2½ yrs = INT (6, 6, 10); NON (7, 8, 8).
[b] F (1, 39).
[c] F (2, 39).

with between one and two years of therapy, as opposed to those with longer treatment histories.

Table III shows the results of an analysis of variance in which the effects of length of treatment by treatment group were tested.* Subjective Experience and its component, affective flexibility, show the greatest tendency for continued growth in both treatment conditions over time. Moreover, this direction of change was found for most variables as a function of duration of the treatment. Examination of the mean scores for intensively treated patients shows that, though the ratings on each of the four dimensions increased slowly but surely over time, even among the group of long-term intensively treated patients there remained considerable room for improvement. These increases contrast with the mean scores for the nonintensively treated schizophrenic patients, which showed very little pattern for improvement over time. When the length of treatment was held constant and the effects of the type of therapy were examined by ANOVA, the same variables which were found significant by t-tests once again emerged as most responsive to intensive therapy treatment. Again, the overall total score on the interview showed a positive trend for intensive therapy.

To test how the variables employed in this study correlate with other types of outcome measures, the scores were compared with scores on the Psychiatric Status Schedule (PSS) and the Camarillo for those patients where such data was available. Only Subjective Experience showed a tendency to correlate with a measure of behavioral symptomatic disturbance from the PSS. All dimensions, including each individual section, correlated more highly with scores from the Camarillo.

DISCUSSION

The preliminary nature of these results must be emphasized in view of the mixture of samples, the generally small sample sizes, the lack of complete psychometric testing of the instrument, and the fact that the raters weren't always blind to the treatment condition of the patients. Nevertheless, some of the results reported here, and some of the clinical observations gained from doing these follow-ups, are noteworthy.

One clinical observation is that the emphasis upon external life situations may help some supportively treated patients to be especially clear

* In this analysis, only the results from the latest Psychotherapy Outcome Interview were included, for those patients who had been interviewed at several times in the process of their therapy. Hence, the numbers are smaller than those for t-tests where the results of repeated interviews were included.

about the external circumstances that precipitated their regressions. In contrast, it occasionally seemed that some intensively treated patients were surprisingly naive in this area, perhaps due to the emphasis on intrapsychic determinants.

A second clinical impression concerns some surprising limitations which occur despite high ratings on several dimensions. For example, it is possible for patients to appear well acquainted with much of what was involved in their becoming psychotic, and yet to believe that this knowledge might have limited preventive impact. On the dimension of Insightfulness we observed a patient who demonstrated a well-developed capacity to observe herself as she performed according to the expectations of others in a variety of social situations. Yet, she was using her self-observations to distance herself from meaningful engagement with her object world. Hence, she could concurrently complain that her alienation from others remained untouched by her psychotherapy experience. These examples show how patients can score highly on an outcome dimension specific to intensive therapy, but without meaningful psychological "growth."

The results which are available are consistently supportive of the potential validity and usefulness of the Psychotherapy Outcome Interview as a means of assessing changes from intensive psychotherapy. Given the traditional difficulty attaining reliable measures of intrapsychic function, the high reliability of the ratings are impressive, and attest to the value of the interview procedure. Nearly all of the interview's sections showed that patients who received intensive psychotherapy were functioning at a higher level than those who did not. Differences on several of the variables achieved statistical significance, despite the low number of subjects. The validity of the interview is also supported by impressive correlations between the dimensions and another measure of intrapsychic change, the Camarillo. However, we have not tested whether the various sections reflect independent aspects of change, or whether the dimensions have construct validity. Larger samples are required before the interview can be adequately evaluated on these issues.

An important but unsurprising observation illustrated by our results is that psychological changes of the type that intensive therapy is intended to bring about seem to occur slowly and gradually. Hence, at the time of the initial six-month evaluation, differences between patients treated intensively and those treated nonintensively were only beginning to appear. This may explain why in May's study[17] patients who received only six months of nonintensive therapy showed only one advantage over those who received drugs without psychotherapy. That advantage was on the insight scale of the Camarillo, and is consistent with our finding that insight into the origins of one's psychopathology is the first area affected by dynamic psychotherapy. Those patients who received the longest intensive treatment (at least 2½ years) evidenced considerably more advantages over their nonintensively treated counterparts than did those with six months of intensive therapy. Yet, even the group who received 2½ or more years of intensive therapy were functioning far from optimally in these areas of outcome. However, two patients from this group with the longest treatment histories did attain close to optimal levels on many dimensions. This suggests the potential for continued growth with further psychotherapy, as has been suggested by Rubins;[18] but our samples do not yet allow us to evaluate this very interesting possibility. Because of the unknown biases which determined the treatment given this sample and the referral of these patients for this study, we can only say that the results are consistent with the hypothesis that intensive therapy favorably affected these higher scores. It remains a viable but still untested hypothesis that schizophrenic patients who are able to achieve high scores in some or many of these dimensions of outcome may be relatively invulnerable to recurrent psychoses.[19]

The current data suggest some intriguing possibilities about differential patterns and rates of change. The earliest and strongest area of difference between groups was in the section on Continuity of Past and Present. This may reflect that an early focus on psychotherapeutic attention amongst our experienced therapists was developing a sense of historical perspective, and specifically investigating why the patients became psychotic when they did. It is, in any event, in line with the findings of McGlashan and others[12,13] that patterns of integrating or sealing off one's psychosis can become established rather early in the course of treatment. The area of Subjective Experience showed the greatest tendency to improve steadily with time in treatment—even when patients in nonintensive therapy were included. This may be an encouraging sign for schizophrenic patients in general who remain in long-term treatment. Our least encouraging trend is in the area of Object Relatedness. The overall scores remain particularly low in this dimension. This may reflect that most of the intensively treated patients were hesitant to talk very directly about the nature and importance of their ongoing relationship to the therapist. Changes in trust and intimacy may be present in that relationship before being evident elsewhere in the patients' lives. It is also possible that this very important dimension is the last to show change or, of course, it may be the dimension where change is least likely to occur. This latter possibility would be particularly disappointing, since intensive therapy is expected to provide a model of a human relationship which can be generalized into a greater capacity for trust and intimacy.

In summary, we have presented a set of hypotheses about the nature of outcome which may be specific for intensive exploratory psychotherapy with schizophrenic patients. These hypotheses were tested by means of a semi-structured Psychotherapy Outcome Interview. Our results demonstrated the reliability of this interview, and support its validity as a measure of change from intensive psychotherapy. Some preliminary analyses indicate that the changes which occur from intensive psychotherapy occur slowly and gradually, and that the various dimensions of outcome may change in a patterned sequence.

Despite the generally hopeful nature of this report, we believe that the expectation that a controlled outcome study can convincingly answer the persisting questions about the value of psychotherapy for schizophrenia is premature, naive, and probably harmful. What can realistically be expected at this time is that a controlled outcome study will further refine hypotheses about such issues as proper patient selection, qualities of good therapists, particularly useful techniques, and time frameworks, and will help to develop better means of recognizing and measuring the ways in which patients change when this occurs. This, in turn, can pave the way for future and increasingly definitive outcome studies. This paper has offered an incremental addition to the understanding and measurement of outcome. It thus helps to fill, partially, one obstinate hole in the leaky dam which the Lidzs have worked so untiringly to buttress.

REFERENCES

1. Feinsilver DB, Gunderson JG: Psychotherapy for schizophrenics: Is it indicated? (A review of the relevant literature), in Gunderson JG, Mosher LR (eds): *Psychotherapy of Schizophrenia.* New York, Jason Aronson, 1975, pp 403–430.
2. Gunderson JG: Drugs and psychosocial treatment of schizophrenia revisited. J.C.E. Psychiatry **38**(12):25–40, 1977.
3. Gomes B: Psychotherapy outcome with schizophrenics: A review of the literature. Paper presented at the Sixth Annual Meeting of the Society for Psychotherapy Research, Boston, June 1975.
4. Rubins JL, Rucker MS: On evaluating the effectiveness of psychoanalytic therapy for the acute schizophrenias. *Am J Psychoanal* **34**:241–256, 1974.
5. Strupp HH, Hadley SW: A tripartite model of mental health and therapeutic outcomes: With special reference to negative effects in psychotherapy. *Am Psychol,* **32**:187–196, 1977.
6. Semrad EV, Grinspoon L, Feinberg SE: Toward the development of the ego profile scale. *Arch Gen Psychiatry* **28**:70–73, 1973.
7. Bellak L, Hurvich N, Gediman HK: *Ego Functions in Schizophrenics, Neurotics and Normals: A Systematic Study of Conceptual, Diagnostic and Therapeutic Aspects.* New York, John Wiley & Sons, 1973.
8. Schulz C: Self and object differentiation as a measure of change in psychotherapy, in Gunderson JG, Mosher LR (eds): *Psychotherapy of Schizophrenia.* New York, Jason Aronson, 1975, pp 305–316.
9. May PRA, Dixon WJ: The Camarillo Dynamic Assessment Scales. *Bull Menninger Clin,* **33**:1–35, 1969.
10. Wexler M: Comment on the five treatment comparative study, in Gunderson JG, Mosher LR (eds): *Psychotherapy for Schizophrenia.* New York, Jason Aronson, 1975, pp 431–433.
11. Soskis DA, Bowers MB: The schizophrenic experience: A followup study of attitude and post hospital adjustment. *J Nerv Ment Dis* **149**:443–449, 1969.

12. McGlashan TH, Levy ST, Carpenter WT: Integration and sealing over. *Arch Gen Psychiatry* **32**:1269–1272, 1975.

13. McGlashan TH, Docherty JP, Siris S: Integrative and sealing-over recoveries from schizophrenia: Distinguishing case studies. Psychiatry J Study Interpers Processes **39**: 325–338, 1976.

14. Stanton AH: The significance of ego interpretative states in insight-directed psychotherapy (Harry Stack Sullivan Colloquium). *Psychiatry* **41**:129–140, 1978.

15. Schulz C: Self and object differentiation as a measure of change in psychotherapy, in Gunderson JG, Mosher LR (eds): *Psychotherapy of Schizophrenia*. New York, Jason Aronson, 1975, pp 305–316.

16. Carpenter WT Jr, Strauss JS, Bartko JJ; Flexible system for the diagnosis of schizophrenia: Report from the WHO international pilot study of schizophrenia. *Science* **182**:1275–1278, 1973.

17. May PRA: *Treatment of Schizophrenia: A Comparative Study of Five Treatment Methods*. New York, Science House, 1968.

18. Rubins JL: Five-year results of psychoanalytic therapy and day care for acute schizophrenic patients. *Am J Psychoanal* **36**:3–26, 1976.

19. Gunderson JG: The value of psychotherapy of schizophrenia: A Semrad memorial. *McLean Hosp J* **III**:131–145, 1978.

Appendix

Revised 4/79

THE PSYCHOTHERAPY OUTCOME INTERVIEW

J. Gunderson, M.D. (4/78)

I. CONTINUITY OF PAST & PRESENT

1. How would you describe yourself? (What kind of person would you say you are?)
2. Do you have some idea how that quality developed?
3. Did your childhood experience contribute? How?
4. Did your relationship to your parents contribute? How?
5. Do you feel that your current problems existed before you became psychotic?
6. What is there about you which may have predisposed you to become psychotic?

THE PATIENT RECOGNIZES THAT HIS PAST, INCLUDING HIS PSYCHOSIS, IS A COHERENT EVOLUTION INTO THE PRESENT.

6—optimally
5—markedly
4—distinctly
3—moderately
2—mildly
1—a little
0—not at all

(Do not rate on basis of whether the patient has a theory about the etiology of his illness.)

II. OBJECT LOVE & DIFFERENTIATION

1. Who do you feel closest to? What is he/she like?
2. Are there problems in that relationship? What sort? What do you do together?
3. What is it like for you to love someone? Have you used the word "love?"

270

4. Is there anyone who you know loves you?
   What do you think he/she loves about you?
5. Who do you feel knows you the best?
   Can you tell them about your troubles or about aspects of your life you feel ashamed of?

THE PATIENT CAN BE CLOSE TO AND
ACKNOWLEDGE APPRECIATION FOR
AND BY SPECIFIC OTHERS.

6—optimally
5—markedly
4—distinctly
3—moderately
2—mildly
1—a little
0—not at all

III. OBJECT NEED: TRUST

1. Do you feel a need for people?
   Could you live without anyone around?
   Does your ability to function depend on anyone?
2. Do you experience loneliness or a longing for more companionship?
3. Does anyone take care of you in any way?
   What is that like for you?
   How do you feel about being dependent on others?
4. Are there any particular ways in which you feel comfortable depending on others?
   Are you able to depend on anyone for this?
5. Is there a particular person (or persons) that you have learned you can depend upon that you previously felt you couldn't?
6. Do you generally expect people to let you down? Do you watch carefully to avoid getting hurt?

THE PATIENT RECOGNIZES A NEED
FOR PEOPLE AND FEELS COMFORT-
ABLE DEPENDING UPON THEM TO
MEET HIS FELT NEEDS.

6—optimally
5—markedly
4—distinctly
3—moderately
2—mildly
1—a little
0—not at all

(Do not judge on basis of age-appropriateness of felt needs.)

IV. EXTERNALIZATION: PROJECTION AS A DEFENSE

1. Do you tend to feel sorry for people, animals?
    Do you tend to favor the underdog?
2. Do you often feel misunderstood, mistreated?
    How do you understand this tendency?
3. Do you feel your parents are to blame for many of your
    difficulties?
    Could they have done it differently?
    Why do you think they treated you the way they did?
4. Do you sometimes feel people are watching you—or talking
    about you in the streets or in a restaurant?
    How do you respond to this?
    How do you understand this belief?
5. Do you sometimes feel that public events or events in
    newspapers, on TV, have special relevance to you?
    How do you understand this?
6. Do you sometimes feel that your problems could be greatly
    diminished by a change of your environment?
    Do you try to effect this change?

DESPITE A TENDENCY TO SEE IN-
TERNAL CONFLICTS EXTERNALLY
THE PATIENT RECOGNIZES THIS AND
INFREQUENTLY ACTS UPON THIS
PERCEPTION.

6—optimally
5—markedly
4—distinctly
3—moderately
2—mildly
1—a little
0—not at all

(A patient who shows little tendency to
    externalize should be given a high score.)

V. SELF-OBSERVATION

1. Do you ever feel detached—as if you were observing yourself do
    things?
    Things which you know aren't in your interest?
    Why?
2. Have you noticed that your mind can be on one subject even as
    you talk about something else?
    What is that like for you?
3. Do you sometimes feel that what you say is contrived for its
    effect?

4. How recently have you noticed something regarding yourself that you had previously not known?
5. Are you aware of the sexual fantasies which you have, even while engaged in intercourse?

THE PATIENT FREQUENTLY OBSERVES HIM/HERSELF EVEN WHILE ENGAGED IN VARIOUS BEHAVIORS.

6—optimally
5—markedly
4—distinctly
3—moderately
2—mildly
1—a little
0—not at all

VI. ANTICIPATION

1. When have you felt most vulnerable to becoming psychotic?
2. What sorts of situations are especially troublesome for you?
3. Do you make any efforts to avoid or master these situations?
4. What is your understanding of why these situations trouble you?

THE PATIENT CAN RECOGNIZE PAR-TICULARLY STRESSFUL CIRCUM-STANCES AND MAKES EFFORTS TO AVOID OR MASTER THESE.

6—optimally
5—markedly
4—distinctly
3—moderately
2—mildly
1—a little
0—not at all

VII. AMBIVALENCE

1. Do you experience helplessness?
   What is that like for you?
2. Are there issues (personal, political, or moral) which you have strong opinions about?
   Has this opinion changed?
   Do you discuss it with anyone having other opinions?
3. What is your attitude about:
   (a) *gun control*
   (b) *TV violence*
   (c) *Nixon*
   (d) *your inpatient administrator*
   (e) *homosexuality*
   (f) *rape*

4. Do you tend to see things as:
   (a) all or nothing
   (b) good or evil
   (c) now or never

THE PATIENT SHOWS A CAPACITY & TOLERANCE FOR UNCERTAINTY, NOT KNOWING, AND HELPLESSNESS.	6—optimally 5—markedly 4—distinctly 3—moderately 2—mildly 1—a little 0—not at all

VIII. REALISTIC OVERVIEW

1. Do you sometimes feel that you've been a failure?
2. Are there periods in your life which seem wasted?
   Would you want to do it over again differently?
   Do you feel you could if you knew then what you know now?
3. Have your plans for your future changed?
   Do you anticipate problems in reaching your goals?
   Does the future seem more difficult than it used to?

THE PATIENT RECOGNIZES HIS LIMITATIONS AS HAVING DEPRIVED HIM OF SATISFACTION IN THE PAST AND AS LIKELY TO INFLUENCE HIS FUTURE.	6—optimally 5—markedly 4—distinctly 3—moderately 2—mildly 1—a little 0—not at all

IX. AFFECTIVE FLEXIBILITY

1. Are you a person with a lot of feelings?
   Do you feel more now than you used to?
   How do you explain that?
2. Are you aware that you sometimes hurt other people's feelings?
   What's that like for you?
   Do you ever knowingly hurt someone else?
   How come?
3. Do other people effect your feelings?
   Do you ever get angry with others?
   How do you respond to that?

Are you more (argumentative, sarcastic, moody, grumpy) than you used to be?

4. How is your sense of humor?
    Do you find it hard to laugh?
    Do you ever laugh at yourself?

5. Do you feel concerned about other people?
    Do you worry about patients you've met during your hospitalization?

6. Do you experience any feelings now which are new—or, at least, unrecognized by you before?

THE PATIENT EXPERIENCES A WIDE-RANGE OF AFFECTS, INCLUDING IRRITATION AND GUILT ON A REGULAR, DAILY BASIS.

6—optimally
5—markedly
4—distinctly
3—moderately
2—mildly
1—a little
0—not at all

Chapter 24

Toward Comprehensive Understanding and Treatment of Schizophrenia

JOHN S. STRAUSS, JOHN P. DOCHERTY, and T. WAYNE DOWNEY

A 24-year-old, white, single woman, Ms. N., is brought to the hospital because of recurrent auditory hallucinations and marked agitation. She has been hospitalized for these symptoms on three previous occasions. The voices have been present intermittently for about six years. Sometimes they call her names, sometimes they comment on her thoughts and actions. She thinks they may be caused by some group trying to control her, but is not sure who it is, or won't say. When the hallucinations are severe, she often becomes agitated with bizarre ritual pacing. She is not elated or depressed.

Ms. N. lives with her rather controlling, somewhat isolated mother, has no friends, and works occasionally helping to clean and do odd jobs in some small neighborhood stores. In the past, she had worked for two years as a salesperson in a women's clothing store, and was apparently quite capable.

She has recently been treated with Haldol, but stopped this medication two weeks ago because she was tired of taking it. Ms. N. is admitted to the psychiatric service of the hospital.

JOHN S. STRAUSS, JOHN P. DOCHERTY, and T. WAYNE DOWNEY • Department of Psychiatry, School of Medicine, Yale University, 25 Park Street, New Haven, Connecticut 06519.

What happens next depends largely on where the hospitalization takes place and what kind of hospital it is. From the approach to assessment, to the entire treatment plan, including whether the mother is involved in the treatment, whether medications and/or psychotherapy are begun, and how long the hospitalization lasts, will depend more upon the particular orientation of the hospital staff and the availability of resources than upon the existence of a commonly accepted, definitive treatment for schizophrenia, the diagnosis given to Ms. N.'s disorder.

In simpler times, when the infectious-disease model dominated the field of psychiatry generally and the notion of dementia praecox or schizophrenia in particular, the goal was to make a diagnosis, and, having identified the disease, to search for the magic bullet that would provide the cure. Now, however, there are many theories and many treatments.

Those many theories can be considered as defined primarily by two basic dimensions. The first of these is the type of information—either observed behavior or mental processes—chosen as a primary focus for assessment and treatment. This dimension reflects the continuing division in psychiatry and psychology between rationalist schools, searching for underlying structures or processes, and empiricist schools, attempting to attend primarily only to that which is directly observable. The second dimension is the time frame of the conceptualization—cross-sectional or longitudinal. Using this framework, it is possible, in Figure 1, to place the main views about schizophrenia, such as the theories of Schneider, existentialist psychiatry, Kraepelin (and currently the St. Louis group), and psychodynamic orientations readily into the four categories constituted by the two basic dimensions.

Although it is possible to pick a theory according to one's background, geographic location, personal preference, or the current style, such a choice does not resolve the question of how to treat Ms. N. There is not one treatment for schizophrenia, or even one treatment per theory, but a wide range of treatment approaches from which to choose. Individual and family

| | Area of Attention | |
Time Frame	Observable Behavior	Mental Processes
Cross-sectional	Schneider	Existentialist
Longitudinal	Kraepelin	Psychodynamic

FIGURE 1. Theories of psychopathology.

psychotherapy, psychotropic medications, long or short hospitalization, a variety of occupational and creative therapies, and other less standard approaches all have been proposed, and most are currently in active use.

While Ms. N. awaits a treatment decision, it is important to note that it is now possible to go beyond selecting a theory for understanding and treating schizophrenia on the basis of clinical intuition or bias alone. A considerable amount of systematically collected information is becoming available, strongly implicating certain key factors as determining the onset of schizophrenia and its course. Working specifically with these factors in treatment might greatly increase treatment effectiveness.

1.   Studies of *stressful life events* have indicated that such happenings are important both at the time of onset of schizophrenia and preceding its recurrence.[1,2] Findings are somewhat controversial, because some studies have suggested that no such relationships exist.[3] The most recent investigations, however, appear to confirm the importance of life events in schizophrenia onset and recurrence, suggesting that negative findings in the past may have resulted from methodologic limitations, ignoring the important meanings of certain types of life events for schizophrenic patients.[4,5] In spite of findings that life events have possible causal relationships in regard to onset and recurrence of schizophrenic symptoms, it is amazing how often information about such events is totally ignored in describing schizophrenic patients, as it was in our case description.

2.   The existence of *biological determinants* in schizophrenia has now been demonstrated. The data for a genetic contribution to schizophrenia are some of the best information on etiology available, though the genetic impact apparently is limited in degree, and the nature of the effect is not clear.[6] Biochemical studies implicating the dopamine system and possibly other neurotransmitter mechanisms have generated suggestive data regarding neuroregulatory dysfunction in schizophrenia.[7] Psychophysiological data suggest that the route for these biological impacts may be through dysfunctions of stimulus management and information processing.[8]

3.   *Social relationships dysfunction*, either in family contacts or in other settings, has been repeatedly demonstrated as important prognostically, etiologically, and in determining recurrence. Level of premorbid social relationships remains consistently one of the best predictors of outcome in schizophrenia, suggesting a close association between this function and processes determining recovery.[9] Communication deviance in families of schizophrenics has been strongly implicated as an important family characteristic in the etiology of this disorder.[10] High levels of "expressed emotion" (actually intrusiveness and negative feelings) in the family have been implicated in replicated studies as factors contributing to relapse.[11]

4.   Finally, *work function*, though it fits least neatly into a narrow version of the medical model, has also been repeatedly demonstrated as a key

prognostic variable in schizophrenia.[12] In some recent pilot studies carried out by our group at Yale Psychiatric Institute,[13] work also appears to have an important organizing effect and impact on self-esteem, assisting in the process of recovery.

The systematic studies indicating the impact of these four areas have all focused on observable behavior, and thus contribute primarily to those theories in the left column of Figure 1. This fact reflects the impact and value of recent systematic studies in psychiatry that have used reliable measures of observable characteristics. It also reflects the considerable difficulties that have been encountered generating comparable systematic data relevant to mental mechanisms and the right column of Figure 1.

Now, how can the variables contributing to schizophrenia and its course be viewed together, in order to devise an optimal treatment plan having an impact on them? To depict the factors contributing to schizophrenia, we have constructed Figure 2.

In the upper left, the symptoms box indicates those characteristics for which patients most often come to treatment, and which are generally considered central in arriving at a diagnosis. It does not take a great leap of imagination to suggest that certain psychological processes must immediately underlie such symptoms. In schizophrenia, these processes include aberrations of perceptual, cognitive, and affective functioning, and, at a somewhat more speculative level, aberrations in what Sullivan called the self system.[14] Including relatively hard data in this concept, we view it as

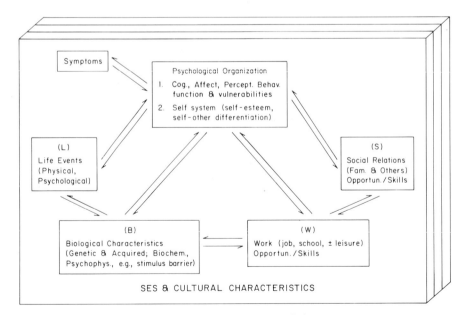

FIGURE 2.   A model for psychopathology.

involving problems of self–other differentiation, as indicated by Schneider's first-rank symptoms,[15] as well as by the work of Schulz[16] and others, and low self-esteem as suggested by many anecdotal reports, and in the more systematic studies by Grinker[17] and Harder, et al.[18] The four areas having an impact on these psychological processes—life events, biological characteristics, work, and social relations—are indicated in the surrounding boxes.

Ms. N., whom we have diagnosed as schizophrenic, is still awaiting treatment as we elaborate in diagram form the probable contributory factors in her disorder and take a sideways glance at the considerable armamentarium of possible treatments, many of which are probably helpful, and none of which has been demonstrated as definitive. But we must continue a bit further. With the many contributing factors in schizophrenia, many available treatments, and incomplete knowledge and efficacy at all levels, we are forced in dealing with reality to develop a mode for integrating the information we do have in an optimal way. Clearly, at least a preliminary theoretical structure is necessary for that purpose.

We would like to suggest that available data can be used to construct, somewhat tentatively, an orientation for such a theory, to help provide a guide for treatment programs. The work of Brown et al.[3] and others[11,19] has provided one important and extensive set of data, beginning to bring together information on life events, medication effects, and family living situation, to help establish the view that one of the major problems in schizophrenia is stimulus management, and that environmental factors influencing this are important in treatment planning. This view implies that some characteristic, possibly biological, limits the range of stimuli within which schizophrenic individuals can operate effectively. Either too little or too much stimulation is viewed as harmful. Thus, according to this orientation, which would be situated in the left column of Figure 1, living situation, life events, and medication need to be considered with this stimulus-range limitation in mind. The data are impressive, and can be combined to form one part of what we believe should be a two-part data-based preliminary theory of schizophrenia and its treatment.

Some evidence for the second part of the theory has also been generated from the work of Brown et al., as well as from other sources. As noted earlier, recent advances in understanding the factors contributing to schizophrenia have involved relatively few systematic studies relating to mental mechanisms, including such concepts as meaning and self-concept, those characteristics on the right hand column of Figure 1. In fact, for many schools of thought, this column in relation to schizophrenia has been all but forgotten. Unfortunately, psychoanalytic theory, a major potential resource for this kind of information, in spite of providing a comprehensive model for attempting to explain phenomena and for suggesting clinical techniques, has had very limited predictive value, in contrast to theories related to the more systematic studies described above. However, several sources of information suggest that limiting concepts of schizophrenia to purely behavioral characteristics is an unnecessary, and inaccurate, truncation of available data.

As noted earlier, Brown et al. and others have found that schizophrenics living in families with high levels of "expressed emotion" were most likely to have relapses. The term "expressed emotion" fits with the investigators' views about stimulus level in schizophrenia. However, the term is somewhat inaccurate. Not merely any emotion, but negative or intrusive expressed emotions are important in contributing to schizophrenic relapse. Rather than fit the findings only to stimulus-level theory, we believe that these data suggest that meaning, not merely stimulus level, is important in schizophrenia. In fact, considering these findings entirely as stimulus quantity is reminiscent of some of the major problems in a similar view of stimulus by stimulus–response theories of psychology popular in the past.[20] As life-events studies are carried out with increasing precision, it is becoming clear that, for them too, not only the presence of events, but their meaning for the individual, may be crucial.[5,21]

Thus, research on observable behaviors is leading to the need to deal with meaning—and its historical and developmental determinants for the individual. For etiology, as with issues of symptom and syndrome definition, diagnosis and prognosis,[12,22] descriptive data suggest, not that we must choose between Kraepelinian "objective" and psychodynamic "mental process" approaches to psychiatry, but that both orientations have valid contributions, perhaps best understood in a systems context.

The studies described above suggest the importance of a subjective aspect, perhaps best viewed in terms of a self-system, in schizophrenia. The importance of that system is also indicated, as noted earlier, in Schneider's first-rank symptoms—mostly delusions and hallucinations of specific content—emphasizing that the boundary between self and others is broken. Innumerable clinical-anecdotal reports provide further weight regarding the importance of the self-system viewed in these terms, an area assumed critical by psychodynamically oriented psychiatrists, but practically ignored by the great majority of psychiatrists, who do not share that orientation.

Thus, the two components of a theory for understanding and treating schizophrenia based on systematic data are that this disorder involves primarily difficulties with stimulus management, and problems with subjective experience perhaps best considered as the self-system. The links between these two characteristics need to be studied further to understand their roles more completely. However, Ms. N. is still waiting, so the data available now must be used to establish basic treatment principles. There are two such principles:

1. The treatment program should help in modulating stimulus levels to fit within the capacities of the individual. Unlike some theorizing in this area, it seems to us that these capacities shift and increase as the person

passes through various phases of the recovery process.[23] Nevertheless, the level of stimulation manageable at any time needs to be assessed as carefully as possible, and medications, psychotherapies, therapeutic milieu, living situation, and demands to function must be considered in light of potential difficulties in this area. Unnecessarily low expectations may, perhaps as with nonschizophrenics, tend to limit the person's function and ability to lead a full life. Excessive demands may put more burden on the individual than he can tolerate or cope with effectively.

Although medications and adjusting environmental situations are major components of stimulus regulation, another important component is the individual's competence in dealing with environmental demands. Many persons, especially perhaps schizophrenics, and most especially those individuals who have had schizophrenic disorders over extended periods, have limited skills in handling even the simplest social relations and work situations. Many patients that we see do not know how to cook or take a bus, have never worked effectively, do not know how to deal with store clerks, talk with potential friends, or carry out the many other activities necessary for effective living. To discharge such patients into the community on medication or even psychotherapy alone puts them under a tremendous stress, which we believe is highly likely to contribute to recurrence or chronicity of disorder.[24] There is a distinct need for therapy integrating a view toward stimulus management and a goal of increasing competence in daily living skills.

2. The second treatment principle is related primarily to the self-system. Although it is possible that issues related to the self-system may resolve spontaneously or with the many types of treatment available adjusting the stimulus level, such an approach seems less than optimal. The self-system can probably be reached most effectively through a continuing personal therapeutic relationship. A psychotherapeutic relationship can assist the individual to understand his abilities and limitations; to expand his functioning; to develop the cognitive structure to integrate his past and present experiences in handling conflicts and stress, and developing autonomy; and to learn to relate and to deal with fears of success or failure. Such a relationship can also facilitate the process of psychological integration, by working with the patient to coordinate his living and treatment experiences during the recovery process.

Frequently, family therapy assists with the goal of helping development of the self-system, especially self–other differentiation, as well as helping modulate the environment. Social skills training and work, besides affecting stimulus management, also have an important impact on the self-system in terms both of self-esteem and of developing autonomy.

The two areas of dysfunction and treatment in schizophrenia may have specific temporal relationships. For example, as the work of Hogarty, et al.,[25,26] and others[27] shows, the impact of the two different aspects of treatment may be demonstrated at different phases of the recovery process, suggesting further practical and theoretical implications.

In schizophrenia, the needs for stimulus modulation and development of the self-system may provide the best data-oriented basis for organizing treatment. Clearly, the treatment modalities available can be structured around these goals in varying ways, and shifted somewhat during the phases of recovery, to meet the developing capacities and needs of the individual. In these ways, attention can be paid both to outer behavior, and to inner mental mechanisms, as they relate to schizophrenic disorders. Although these concepts are still tentative, we believe they may point the way to utilizing currently available treatments for schizophrenia in a way that is most effective.

It is clear by now that a treatment plan for Ms. N. cannot be developed in this report. To do so requires far more data than have been provided in the brief clinical description given earlier. Derived from the basic treatment principles suggested here is the implication that the clinical pragmatics of optimal treatment for the individual patient call for a broad attention to detailed information. What we have tried to provide is a framework for organizing such information, and for considering the many treatment modalities available, in order to develop a maximally effective comprehensive approach to the treatment of schizophrenic patients.

REFERENCES

1. Brown GW, Birley JLT: Crisis and life changes and the onset of schizophrenia. *J Health Soc Beha* **9**:203–214, 1968.
2. Birley JLT, Brown G: Crises and life changes preceding the onset or relapse of schizophrenia: Clinical aspects. *Br J Psychiatry* **116**:327–333, 1970.
3. Brown GW, Birley JLT, Wing JK: Influence of family life on the course of schizophrenic disorders: A replication. *Br J Psychiatry* **121**:241–258, 1972.
4. Morrison JR, Hudgens RW, Barchha RC: Life events and psychiatric illness. *Br. J Psychiatry* **117**:635, 1970.
5. Myers JK, Lindenthal JJ, Pepper MP: Life events and psychiatric impairment. *J Nerv Ment Dis* **152**:149–157, 1971.
6. Gottesman II, Shields J: A critical review of recent adoption, twin and family studies of schizophrenia: Behavioral genetics perspectives. *Schizophr Bull* **2**:360–401, 1976.
7. Meltzer HY, Stahl MS: The dopamine hypothesis of schizophrenia: A review. *Schizophr Bull* **2**:19–76, 1976.
8. Neuchterlein KH: Refocusing on attentional dysfunctions in schizophrenia. *Schizophr Bull* **3**:457–469, 1977.
9. Strauss JS, Kokes RF, Klorman R, et al: Premorbid adjustment in schizophrenia: Concepts, measures and implications. *Schizophr Bull* **3**:182–244, 1977.
10. Wynne LC, Singer MT: Thought disorder and family relations of schizophrenics: IV. Results and implications. *Arch Gen Psychiatry* **12**:201–212, 1965.
11. Vaughn CE, Leff JP: The influence of family and social factors on the course of psychiatric illness: A comparison of schizophrenic and depressed neurotic patients. *Br J Psychiatry* **129**:125–137, 1976.

12. Strauss JS, Carpenter WT: Prediction of outcome in schizophrenia: III. Five-year outcome and its predictors. *Arch Gen Psychiatry* **34:**159–163, 1977.
13. Strauss JS, Ostroff R: Work and psychiatric symptoms. Paper presented at the McLean Symposium: Psychotherapeutic Approaches in the Mental Hospital, Belmont, Mass., June, 1979.
14. Sullivan HS: *Conceptions of Modern Psychiatry.* New York, WW Norton, 1940.
15. Schneider K: *Clinical Psychopathology.* Hamilton MW (trans), New York, Grune & Stratton, 1959.
16. Schulz CG: Present status of the self–object differentiation scale (SOD). Paper presented at the Sixth International Symposium on the Psychotherapy of Schizophrenia, Lausanne, September 1978.
17. Grinker RR Sr, Holzman PS: Schizophrenic pathology in young adults. *Arch Gen Psychiatry* **29:**168–175, 1973.
18. Harder DW, Strauss JS, Kokes RF, et al: Self-derogation and psychopathology. Paper presented at the 86th Annual Convention of the American Psychological Association, Toronto, August, 1978.
19. Wing JK: *Schizophrenia: Towards a New Synthesis.* New York, Academic Press, 1978.
20. Paivio A: Neomentalism. *Can J Psychol/Rev Can Psychol* **29:**263–291, 1975.
21. Paykel ES, Myers JK, Dienelt MN, et al: Life events and depression: A controlled study. *Arch Gen Psychiatry* **21:**753–760, 1969.
22. Strauss JS, Gabriel KR, Kokes RF, et al: Do psychiatric patients fit their diagnoses? Patterns of symptomatology as described with the biplot. *J Nerv Ment Dis* **167:**105–113, 1979.
23. Docherty JP, VanKammen DP, Siris SG, et al: Stages of onset of schizophrenic psychosis. *Am J Psychiatry* **135:**420–426, 1978.
24. Serban G: Stress in schizophrenics and normals. *Br J Psychiatry* **126:**397–407, 1975.
25. Hogarty GE, Goldberg SC, Schooler NR, et al: Drug and sociotherapy in the aftercare of schizophrenic patients: II. Two-year relapse rates. *Arch Gen Psychiatry* **31:**603–608, 1974.
26. Hogarty GE, Goldberg SC, Schooler NR, et al: Drug and sociotherapy in the aftercare of schizophrenic patients: III. Adjustment of nonrelapsed patients. *Arch Gen Psychiatry* **31:**609–618, 1974.
27. Sappington J: Perception of threatening stimuli in process and reactive schizophrenics. *J Consult Clin Psychol* **41:**48–50, 1973.

Chapter 25

Discussion: New Directions

MORRIS B. PARLOFF

It is my happy chore to discuss today the five elegant papers we have just heard, each purporting to identify new directions in the psychotherapy of schizophrenia. I believe that the title, New Directions, was very wisely chosen, for it does not presume to assign directionality to the shifts and changes we have witnessed in the field. In psychotherapy, as in the broader field of treatment, it is rarely possible to state with certainty whether we are moving forward, backward, sideward, or merely windward.

I shall not attempt systematically to comment on each of the papers independently. Instead, I have grouped the presentations under two major headings: (1) Changes in Treatment of Schizophrenia; and (2) Changes in Research on Schizophrenia. I shall refer to the papers as they bear on new directions in these areas.

CHANGES IN THE TREATMENT OF SCHIZOPHRENIA

One of the clearest of changes is the recognition that psychotherapy is no longer the "only game in town" for the treatment of schizophrenia. The

MORRIS B. PARLOFF • Parklawn Building, 5600 Fishers Lane, Rockville, Maryland 20852.

earlier, central role of psychotherapy has been diminished as the therapist's repertoire has been augmented by pharmacotherapy and by behavior therapy. Each of these modalities claims effectiveness, and both claim to have produced important changes in relatively short periods of time. Earlier today, for example, we heard from Gordon Paul that some techniques of behavior therapy were extraordinarily effective in teaching social skills to profoundly disturbed and "regressed" patients.

It appears that all speakers are now willing to concede that psychotherapy should no longer be the sole form of treatment offered schizophrenics, but instead should be combined with a broad spectrum of other modalities and specific interventions. Strauss reminds us that, since the category of schizophrenia includes a heterogeneous array of patients, it is likely that different forms and combinations of treatments may be needed. Moreover, different therapies may be appropriately used sequentially to meet the changing needs of patients over the period of their treatment.

Despite this shift away from psychotherapy as the primary mode of treatment, Drs. Bowers and Greenfeld have wisely underscored the fact that the therapeutic alliance remains basic to all effective therapeutic efforts, be they chemical or psychological. These authors also offer a commendable note of realism to this assemblage of avowed clinical optimists, namely, that our expectations regarding the treatment of schizophrenia should be both modest, and properly respectful of the fact that many schizophrenics will require long-term care and therapeutic maintenance. Furthermore, many treated patients will continue to be limited by persistent "trait deficits and residual vulnerabilities to psychosis." Bowers and Greenfeld conclude that such patients may continue to require at least intermittent use of prophylactic medication.

On the other side of the psychological versus pharmacological treatment issue is the increasing evidence for a thesis long suggested by Dr. Lidz, namely, that the role of the family in the treatment of schizophrenia is critical. Research concerning the role of the family as reflected in the dimension of "Expressed Emotion" has been developed by British investigators. They have demonstrated that low-EE families appear to provide an environment for recovered patients in which it matters little whether the patient continues to take medication or not. Attempts to replicate these findings are actively being pursued in this country.

CHANGES IN RESEARCH ON SCHIZOPHRENIA

Lidz and others offer a rather wistful and perhaps ambivalent recognition that the opportunities for the clinician–researcher to use the long-term psychotherapy setting as a laboratory for the study of schizophrenia have been sharply curtailed over the years. This change appears to be due in large measure to the early and sometimes enforced diaspora of the medicated patient from the hospital to the as yet ill-prepared community. Some, like Carpenter, also appear to lament the possibility of lost opportunities for patients to gain and grow from their psychotic episodes, because of the "premature" artificial (chemical) interruption of their schizophrenic crisis. However, the fact remains in sharp memory that many backward patients, even after years of opportunity, routinely failed to achieve maximum benefit from their psychoses.

As we have heard today, each speaker has placed special emphasis on the researchers' need to identify relevant dimensions for assessing the effects of psychotherapy in the treatment of schizophrenia. Most striking is the fact that the constructs and criteria offered seem to represent a narrowing of focus, since attention to symptoms by psychotherapists has been reduced. It appears that psychotherapists are now prepared to concede that antipsychotic drugs can control the symptomatology of schizophrenia—particularly the most florid symptoms—more quickly and perhaps more effectively than can psychosocial interventions. As a consequence, clinicians have deemphasized the assessment of symptom reduction, and renewed their interest in the enhancement of social skills and in improving interpersonal relationships.

Strauss and his colleagues focus on the goals of improving social relations, work, and education, coping with life stresses, and improving psychological organization. Bowers and Greenfeld have proposed the study of developmental goals, such as autonomy, increased capacity for intimacy, realistic vocational objectives, and increased ability to tolerate changes in emotional experiences. Lidz has focused on improving social relations, cognitive skills, adaptive skills, and interpersonal skills. Drs. Carpenter and Gunderson have also identified goals, but, in addition, propose instruments for their assessment. Carpenter has developed a "Quality of Life Scale" which assesses social networks, occupational roles, and the treatment of other residual symptoms. Gunderson and his associates have constructed a "Psychotherapy Outcome Interview" to assess "longitudinal awareness," "insightfulness," "object-relatedness," and "subjective experience."

In short, there seems to be a high degree of consensus among the participants concerning the dimensions relevant to assessment of change in the treatment of schizophrenia; however, there may be less agreement with the narrower, psychodynamically based dimensions presented by Gunderson. While it is possible to cavil about the specifics of the measures proposed, I prefer simply to express my satisfaction with the fact that efforts are being made to develop measures of areas of putative clinical significance. The willingness to specify measures is in itself a relatively new development for clinicians, and is to be applauded. In the past, the clinician was content merely to specify concepts and constructs, without undertaking to objectify their measurement. It seemed to be an accepted rule of thumb that basic clinical concepts could not be adequately measured. Indeed, whatever was caught in the researcher's measurement net would automatically be dismissed as essentially trivial.

I do not wish to appear unappreciative of the developments in specification of goals and their measurement, but the point needs to be stressed that in the field of treatment research it is necessary to do far more. In addition to defining measures, we must now specify with great clarify what and who is being treated, the nature of the patient–therapist relationship, and the specific elements of the treatment intervention that is being offered. If research findings are to be replicable and generalizable, information on each of these essential treatment variables must be provided.

Perhaps the greatest single problem facing the researcher in the field of psychotherapy is the absence of adequate descriptions, let alone "standardization" of the form of psychotherapy being treated. It cannot be assumed that psychotherapy provided by a particular therapist or set of therapists in a given setting bears a close relationship to the psychological interventions provided comparable patients by other psychotherapists. I take great encouragement from the fact that some few clinician–researchers are beginning to develop detailed descriptions—manuals, if you will—of the psychological interventions they use in the treatment of specific categories of patients. For example, Dr. Aaron T. Beck and his colleagues have written an elaborate manual specifying their cognitive/behavioral approach to the treatment of patients suffering from a major depressive disorder. Similarly, Dr. Gerald Klerman and Dr. Myrna Weissman and their associates have prepared a treatment manual describing "Interpersonal Therapy" for use with seriously clinically depressed patients. Dr. Lester Luborsky has also developed a manual for short-term psychotherapy with anxiety disorders.

I believe that in the writings of Dr. Lidz we may discern the core of a treatment manual describing his approach to the psychotherapy of schizophrenics. Aspects of the paper presented today further encourage me to make this inference.

I wish strongly to underline Dr. Carpenter's point that, though research has not provided strong evidence to support the notion that psychotherapy has a powerful contribution to make to the treatment of schizophrenia, the research available does not permit us to determine whether this finding results primarily from the weak effects of psychotherapy, or from the weaknesses of research methodology. The recent report[1] of the President's Com-

---

[1] Task panel reports submitted to the President's Commission on Mental Health, Volume IV, Appendix, 1978. Superintendent of Documents, U.S. Government Printing Office, Washington D.C. Stock No. 040–000–00393–2.

mission on Mental Health surveyed the available studies, and offered the following conclusions: "Treatment (of schizophrenia) by various types of psychotherapy is as yet of unestablished efficacy" (p. 1684). The report further states that the foremost contribution of psychosocial treatment has been shown to be improvement in social adjustment, which occurs only when these treatments are combined with maintenance chemotherapy. The benefits of the additional psychosocial treatment seem to take many months to emerge. The report also cautions that some chronic schizophrenics respond adversely to psychological treatments (p. 1766).

I am concerned that these sorts of "negative findings" regarding psychotherapy may, indeed, inhere in the limitations of the research. Group-comparison studies which fail to describe, at a minimum, such salient variables as the nature and amount of treatment, the characteristics of the patients, the nature of the therapeutic relationship, and the reliability and validity of the measures, make it extremely difficult to reject the null hypothesis, or to assess the generalizability of the findings. Measurement error, coupled with the variance due to differences among patients, therapists, techniques, etc., will produce estimated population variances of such great size as to reduce substantially the possibility that statistically significant differences between group means can be found. Such negative findings impact differentially on the practitioner and the policymaker. The practitioner will dismiss negative findings as being unrepresentative of their own experience with patients they treat, and the policymaker may seize upon a "no difference" finding as scientific justification for unfortunate policy decisions. It is incumbent on the researcher, therefore, to devise research which does not, for artifactual reasons, make the rejection of the null hypothesis inappropriately difficult.

Perhaps the most exciting change which has occurred in the field of psychotherapy research is that researchers now appear more willing to abandon what has come to be known as the "horse race" style of psychotherapy research: "My form of therapy can beat your form of therapy." Increasingly, research is designed to answer, not simply the question of whether one form of treatment is globally more effective than another, but rather the more useful scientific question of what kinds of changes are produced by what kinds of interventions, applied to what kinds of patients, by what kinds of therapists, under what kinds of conditions.

Chapter 26

General Discussion

OPEN DISCUSSION

QUESTION TO DR. BOWERS: About your treatment model, two questions. One, do you inform your patients of their prognosis and diagnosis? And two, how do you define for your patients the primary effects that you expect the medications will have?

DR. BOWERS: The way Dr. Greenfeld and I went about looking at this is that we knew we had been doing something for a while, we wondered what we had been doing, and we looked back to define these suggested phases. Since we don't feel very secure about making prognoses, and certainly are hoping to influence them in a positive way, we would play that, I think, as we feel it—very soft. Regarding the second question, how to describe for patients the primary effects that you expect the medications will have, most of the patients have had some experience with medication. We try to get in a conversation with them about what that experience has been like and usually it has been mixed. If we know, for instance, that the dosage has been perhaps too high, or that side effects that are preventable have been present, we may be able to identify that as part of the story. So we attempt essentially to start a conversation about patients' experience with medication, and about our experience with medication, and to tell them what we think we know. In that way, they can identify feelings that they may have which are either troublesome or perhaps enjoyable, and we can make some comment about our experience regarding whether or not the medication is likely to affect those symptoms if they take it regularly. The emphasis is upon interaction, interchange.

QUESTION TO DR. LIDZ: How do you help the schizophrenic patient who has no parent alive or available, and no significant person in their life now living?

DR. LIDZ: Well, that, of course, is apt to be their problem, that there is no significant person, and here the question would be to some extent what has happened that prevents this person from ever making satisfactory relationships. I would like to make one comment, because of something that Dr. Ruth (Lidz) said to me after my paper. I want to make it clear that I do not blame parents, or feel that in any way they are villains in the situation. I know I don't blame the patient for being ill, and I don't blame their parents for being the way they are. It is a question of understanding the interrelationships and the transactions that have gone on. For example, in one instance I am quite empathetic with the mother in her situation, and this was what we tried to modify. It wasn't that she was being such a rejecting mother, it was that she was a rejected figure in the family, and therefore, in turn, was more or less rejecting of the daughter; and so we could work with how the parental relationship had rebounded to the daughter's disadvantage.

QUESTION FOR THE PANEL: In light of the importance of object-relatedness and the need to learn socializing skills, is group therapy not a potentially crucial modality in the treatment of schizophrenics?

DR. GUNDERSON: The literature suggests that the group treatment of schizophrenia is useful, especially during aftercare, when you can get patients to be engaged in it. There is a high dropout initially, but, once in, they profit from it, and largely in the areas of their social relations and comfort in social situations. There is no reason to think that group therapy is particularly good for sign and symptom remissions, or the kinds of changes which I talked about in my paper.

DR. LIDZ: I think that group therapy, at least in hospitalized patients, has been quite useful and effective for a number of reasons. First, patients will tell one another things about themselves that the therapist and the hospital personnel do not feel so free to tell them, and often bring very salient aspects of their behavior to the foreground for discussion, and perhaps for discussion in individual therapy. There is also, as was said, the socializing effect of interacting with other patients.

QUESTION FOR DR. PARLOFF: Do negative findings ever have nay contribution in research? Can you ever prove the null hypothesis, or are only positive findings meaningful?

DR. PARLOFF: That's the point that I was hoping to make. Obviously, you cannot prove the null hypothesis, but the credibility of a negative findind does not seem to be very great if there is considerable room to elude it; that is, if you say it is not my form of therapy because I don't know what form of therapy they were doing, or these measures are particularly inappropriate, or actually I see quite different patients.

QUESTION TO THE ENTIRE PANEL: Does anyone see value in the psychotherapy of acute psychosis without medications, as Laing and Carl Whittaker have advocated?

DR. CARPENTER: The answer may be yes. The work of Goldstein reported some years ago, to some extent replicated on our research ward at National Institutes of Health (NIH), suggests that at least good-prognosis, nonparanoid patients may do better on a number of dimensions, including time spent in the hospital and discharge symptom status, if treated without medication.

In the short run, there are several other important benefits that can accrue. I think a brief period off medication provides better diagnostic data. To the extent that this prevents erroneous diagnosis of schizophrenia, a whole course of pharmacologic mistreatment may be avoided. Another direct benefit of delaying pharmacotherapy until a therapeutic relationship is established is that some time is provided for environmentally induced or spontaneous remission of symptoms. I think a patient is more satisfied when experiencing some mastery over the psychotic experience, and we at least avoid the mistake of making a judgment that it is a drug-responsive psychosis, if it is actually a form of psychosis that may remit very rapidly, whether on drugs or not. Short- and long-term pharmacotherapy decisions can also be more sophisticated under these conditions.

DR. STRAUSS: There are two other related issues. One is the question of subtype, and not necessarily in terms of DSM III subtypes. There is at least the suggestion that there are certain types of patients, for instance from certain socio-cultural groups, whose psychoses will remit spontaneously and quite rapidly, or others that may remit with certain social supports where medication may not be necessary. Such subtypes would not be revealed in the current methods of diagnosis we have, but may be important.

Another issue reflected in the work of Will (Carpenter) and others is the type of recovery being sought. For example, sealing over may possibly be a less complete recovery than an integrative recovery. Use of medications could make a difference in influencing such recovery types. One of the issues that comes up repeatedly is that our research methods are in many ways trying to catch up with our clinical judgment, and in considering patient and recovery subtypes, we still have a way to go.

QUESTION FOR PANEL: What is an appropriate relationship between therapies that "reduce or eliminate" bizarre behavior, and those that seek to regard the patient's behavior as meaningful communication?

DR. CARPENTER: The judgment about when to reduce symptomatology rapidly should come from the same clinical data base as judgments about the use of exploratory psychotherapy aimed at insight and understanding. These are not mutually exclusive, but sequence and context are critical. At times, phenomenologic exploration for a few hours or several days before inducing symptom change with medication provides an entirely different basis for the therapeutic relationship to develop, so there is at least an opportunity for the patient to understand our rationale for interfering with his experience. This is quite contrary to usual practice, where there is an attempt to eradicate experiences rapidly, without any shared understanding of the basis for such a decision. Furthermore, modification of psychopathology with medication can facilitate an exploration of behavior as meaningful communication by enhancing ego functions, such as the capacity for introspection. One treatment should not preempt the other.

QUESTION FOR THE PANEL: The general theme through the conference seems to be that multimodality of intervention is good, for example, combining individual and family psychotherapy, medications, sociotherapy, and skill training. Is there any disagreement with this general principle, that is, are there times when the multimodal approaches can be antagonistic, rather than synergistic?

DR. GUNDERSON: I think they can be antagonistic most of the time, depending on the coordination between them. There is nothing inherent about multimodal approaches which would make them synergistic. It depends on whether there is communication among those using the various parts of a mulitmodal approach. it could be destructive if there isn't.

DR. LIDZ: In older patients who have a relatively effective life style, and then have broken and relapsed or regressed, I would probably frequently want to treat them only with individual therapy, depending, of course, on the circumstances. There is a question of restoring levels of previous functioning, and then going on to get a better understanding of what has worked and not worked, and straightening out their relationships. I think that this can often be done in individual therapy alone. Putting them in with groups, bringing in the family with adult patients, can be difficult.

DR. STRAUSS: The multimodal approach often is good, but it is not good enough. What is needed is both an assessment of areas of difficulty, and a better theory of what is wrong, and how these various pieces fit together. I think we still have a long way to go in that area. But, while we are working on that, it seems that, if there are deficits in certain areas, or several kinds of problems all going on at once, perhaps the multimodal approach really is the most effective.

DR. CARPENTER: I agree with Dr. Strauss, but wish to be sure that the distinction between multimodal and shotgun is made. When a number of modalities are available, the clinician must be discriminating about temporal priorities for each patient at a given time. A common example relevant to stimulus overload occurs in treating acute psychotic patients. In hospitals where staff endorse multiple therapeutic modalities, we tend to use medication, group activities, and individual psychotherapeutic work immediately. Indeed, we forget the difficulty that acutely ill patients have in simply functioning communicatively. We expect them to move too rapidly into coherent group activity, and we fail to provide a respite. In a sense, particularly now with emphasis on avoiding long-term hospital stay, therapeutic modalities are combined perforce, rather than integrated into a coherent treatment plan.

Index

"Abolitionists," denial by, 93
Acute schizophrenia, fluphenazine therapy in, 79–80. *See also* Schizophrenia
Adolescence, identity formation in, 161–162
Aftercare treatment
    antipsychotic drugs in, 77–80
    in Camarillo/UCLA program, 45
    deliverability and compliance in, 80–82
    emotional blunting and, 88
    expressed emotion in, 87–88
    family therapy in, 77–89
    patient selection in, 79
    phenothiazine in, 78–80
    relapse rate in, 81
    results in, 80
    symptomatic status following, 82
    thought disorder and, 86
"Alarmists," psychotherapy viewed by, 93–94
All-or-none phenomenon. *See also* Splitting
    developmental origin of, 186–189
    ego functions and, 206–207
    in psychiatric and psychoanalytic
        literature, 184–186
    psychotherapy in, 188–189, 204–205
    in sex, 185
    versus integrated personality, 184
Ambiguity tolerance, 186
Ambivalence, in schizophrenic patient, 183, 224–225. *See also* Splitting
American Psychiatric Association *Diagnostic and Statistical Manual*, 38
Analyst–patient dyadic system, 191–192. *See also* Therapist
Annihilation, fear of, 105
Antiparkinsonian medication, 80

Antipsychotic drugs, in aftercare treatment, 77–80. *See also* Neuroleptic drugs
Anxiety, in aftercare period, 88
Anxious depression, family therapy in, 82

Behavior
    bizarre. *See* Bizarre behavior
    Time–Sample Behavioral Checklist for, 169–171
Behavioral Assertiveness Test, 35
"Betrayal" delusion, 207–208
Biological determinants, theory of, 279
Biologic sphere, versus psychoanalytic, 250
Biologic systems, self-regulating properties of, 194–195
Biologic therapy, versus psychoanalytic, 248
Bizarre behavior
    incidence of, 171
    paradoxical intervention in, 197–202
    reduction or elimination of, 169
    Social Learning Program and, 176
Borderline patient
    regressive transference model for, 193
    splitting in, 181
    superego of, 186
Brief Psychiatric Rating Scale, 82–86

Camarillo Dynamic Assessment Scale, 258, 266
Camarillo Mental Health Clinic Research Center/UCLA training program, 37–46
    aftercare planning in, 45
    cognitive skills training in, 41–42

297

Camarillo Mental Health Clinic Research
    Center/UCLA training program
    (*cont.*)
  community homework assignments in,
    42–43
  community survival skills in, 43–44
  evaluation of, 45–46
  family therapy in, 44–45
  in vivo training methods, 48
  outcome measures used in, 46
  social skills training at, 39–40
Camarillo State Hospital Clinical Research
    Unit, 38
Camberwell Family Interview, 24, 38–39, 45,
    50
Caring Team, in community psychotherapy,
    125–126
Central nervous system arousal, genetic
    factors in, 250
CFRS. *See* Clinical Frequencies Recording
    System
Chemical intervention, Freud on, 94. *See also*
    Drug therapy
Chestnut Lodge Sanitarium, 5
Childhood schizophrenia, family interactions
    in, 7
Clinical approach, versus research approach,
    151–152
Clinical data, biologic versus psychoanalytic
    spheres in, 250
Clinical Frequencies Recording System, 173
Clinical invervention, 26–27
Cognitive Distribution Index, 170–171, 176,
    178
Cognitive problem-solving skills, 29
  training in, 41–42, 47
Communication styles, 8–9
Community homework assignments, in
    Camarillo/UCLA program, 42–43
Community Psychiatric Action Research
    Study, 115–127
Community psychiatry
  Caring Team in, 125–126
  individual psychotherapy in, 121
  psychiatric follow-up examination in, 126
Community survival skills, 43–44
Comprehensive psychosocial treatment,
    167–179
  outcomes in, 175–179
  programs in, 174–175
Conjoint couple therapy, 122

Conjoint family therapy, 122
Consensual validation, 8
Crisis-oriented family therapy, 80

Death, fear of, 183
Deficits, in maladaptation, 8
Dementia praecox, 3
Depression, 223
Depressive position, Kleinian concept of, 187
Developmental schizophrenic patient, 220.
    See also Schizophrenic patient
Divorce, of schizophrenic's parents, 222–223
Dread, 164
Drug therapy
  psychotherapy and, 98, 240, 293
  side effects of, 231
  therapeutic alliance in, 230–231
Dynamics of Psychiatric Drug Therapy, The
    (Sarwer–Foner), 228

Eating disorders, 73
EE. *See* Expressed emotion
Ego functions
  all-or-none approach in, 228–229
  disturbed, 5
Emotion, expressed. *See* Expressed emotion
Emotional blunting, following aftercare
    treatment, 88
Emotional disorder, explanation and
    interpretation in, 142
Emotional level, as predictor of relapse,
    23–24
Emotional overinvolvement, in family
    relationships, 25
Environmental change, schizophrenic
    symptoms and, 28
Environmental stress, in schizophrenic
    breakdowns, 146
Equilibrium, in paradoxical psychotherapy,
    195–196
Etiologic information, in psychotherapy,
    71–74
Explanation, understanding and, 141–144
Expressed emotion
  depression and, 73
  family attitudes and, 25, 50
  in psychodynamic psychiatry, 253
  research in, 288
  in schizophrenic evaluation, 24
  schizophrenic relapse and, 25–26, 87
  social competence and, 27

Family, paradoxical invervention of, 194
Family care, patient selection and, 79
Family Conflict Inventory, 45
Family dialogue, facilitation of, 17–19
Family factors
  emotional overinvolvement in, 25
  in problem-solving therapy, 21–51
Family interaction, human development and,
  6–8, 145–146
Family intervention, 191–202
Family systems, paradoxical interventions in,
  191–192
Family theory, seduction theory and, 16–17
Family therapist, intervention by, 18
Family therapy
  achievement of objectives in, 84–85
  in aftercare treatment, 77–89
  analysis of, 83–84
  anxious depression and, 82
  behavioral coordinates of, 87
  in Camarillo/UCLA program, 44–45
  conjoint, 122
  crisis-oriented, 80
  effects of, 82–83
  family as unit in, 209
  hostility and, 85
  measures in, 84–88
  mental health education and, 51
  objectives of, 84–88
  parental image and, 225
  psychodynamic psychiatry and, 252–253
  psychotherapy and, 98
  results in, 80–88
  suspiciousness and, 85
  withdrawal and, 82–83
Fantasies, positive aspects of, 106–110
Fluphenazine
  in aftercare treatment, 79–80
  and "psychotherapeutic nihilism," 49
Folie à deux, 7
Freiburg Psychiatric Clinic, 4

Garden of Eden fantasy, 107
General-purpose psychotherapy, 97. See also
  Psychotherapy
Global Assessment Scale, 84–86
Good–bad self, splitting and, 181, 184, 187
Group therapy, efficacy of, 294. See also
  Family therapy

Hallucinations, as "splitting," 183–184
Hostile–Belligerence Index, 170–171

Hostility, following family therapy, 85
Human development, family intervention
  and, 6–8

Identity problems, 158–161
Id psychology, 5
Idyllic fantasies
  reality and, 111
  therapeutic role of, 106–110
Indecision, "degradation" of, 183
Individual therapy, in community
  psychology, 223
Insight
  cognitive attitude and, 137
  "confession" and, 136–137
  in etiology of illness, 131–144
  kinds of, 134–135
  knowledge expansion and, 140–141
  patient's use of, 136
  as psychoanalytic goal, 134
Insightfulness dimension, 258–260
Instincts, theory of, 6–7
Institutionalized mental patient, monitoring
  of, 169
Instrumental role performance, 168
Interpersonal Skills Index, 174
Interpretation, understanding and, 141–144
Intervening variables
  functional aspects of, 254
  integration of with mental states, 249–251
Intervention
  chemical forms of, 94
  family. See Family intervention; Family
    therapy
Intrapsychic restructuring, as psychoanalytic
  goal, 192
Irrationality, transmission of, 8

Johns Hopkins Hospital, 5

Knowledge, insight in expansion of, 140–141

Legalists, psychotherapy of, 93
London Institute of Psychiatry, 23
Loneliness, psychotic states in, 163–164
Longitudinal Awareness dimension, 258–259
LSD psychosis, 224

Magic Mountain, The (Mann), 95
Maldevelopment trauma, concept of, 8
Manpower problem, in psychotherapy
  research, 148–149

Maternal figure, idyllic fantasy of, 110
Medical Research Council Social Psychiatry
    Unit, 23
Mental Health Clinic Research Center
    (UCLA), 26, 29, 32–33, 37–38. *See
    also* Camarillo Mental Health Clinic
    Research Center/UCLA
Mental states, intervening variables in,
    249–251
Method–method approach, 119–122
MHCRC. *See* Mental Health Clinic
    Research Center (UCLA)
Milieu Therapy Program, 176–177
Milieu treatment, versus drug treatment,
    152–153, 160–161
Minnesota Multiphasic Personality
    Inventory, 35
Motivation, understanding and, 141
Multimodal approach, in psychopathology of
    schizophrenia, 295–296

National Institute of Mental Health, 7, 23,
    38, 149
    Research Diagnostic Criteria of, 38
Neuroleptic drugs. *See also* Drug therapy
    efficacy of, 248
    limitations of disadvantages of, 21–23,
        49–50, 218
    psychotherapy and, 229–230
    side effects of, 23
Neuroses, seduction theory of, 13
Normal behavior, incidence of, 172

Object redefinition, fantasy and, 108
Object relatedness dimension, 258–261, 267
Object–relationship theory, 5
Oedipus complex, 13–14
Oedipal myth, 14, 16
Oedipus theory, Freud's abandonment of,
    14–15
Overlearning, use of, 47

PACT. *See* Program for Assertive
    Community Training
Painful experience, profit from, 94–95
Paradoxical intervention, 19, 191–202
    case example of, 197–202
    defined, 192–194
    and susceptibility to illness, 212
Parental image, family therapy and, 225

Parent–child relationship
    in developmental schizophrenia, 220–221
    divorce and, 222–223
Patient
    psychotic. *See* Psychotic patient
    schizophrenic. *See* Schizophrenic patient
Personality theory, 161
    schizophrenic patient and, 162
Phenothiazine
    maintenance doses of, 78–80
    in tardive dyskinesia, 154
Phipps Clinic, 5
Placebos, versus neuroleptic drugs, 22
"Positive connotation" concept, 19
Present State Examination, 35, 38
Preverbal phenomenon, operationalizing of,
    152
Problem solving
    cognitive, 29, 47
    social inadequacy and, 28
Problem-solving therapy, social and family
    factors in, 21–51
Professional nonconformists, psychotherapy
    of, 94
Program for Assertive Community Training,
    27
PSE. *See* Present State Examination
"Pseudo mutuality" pattern, 7
Psychiatrist, theoretical attitude of, 8. *See
    also* Therapist
Psychiatry
    infectious disease model in, 278
    19th century view of, 4
    psychodynamic. *See* Psychodynamic
        psychiatry
    psychotherapy as prestige form of, 242
Psychoanalysis
    family interactions and, 7
    insight as goal of, 134
    intrapsychic restructuring in, 192
    overdependence on, 219
    psychodynamics and, 240
    role of, 5–6
    in schizophrenia, 9–10, 132
Psychoanalytic therapy, versus biologic
        therapy, 248
Psychoanalytic methods, familiarity with,
    132–133
Psychodynamic psychiatry
    family theory and, 252–253
    history of, 239–240

Psychodynamic psychiatry (*cont.*)
  intervening variables in, 249–251, 254
  for schizophrenic patients, 239–255
  theory application in, 246–253
  treatment range in, 254
Psychological constructs, use of, 247
Psychological systems, self-regulating
      properties of, 195
Psychopathology
  model for, 280
  theories of, 278
Psychosis
  assessment of vulnerability to, 232–233
  outpatient vulnerability to, 227–236
  psychotherapy of. *See* Psychotherapy of
      psychosis
  "trait" deficits in, 233–235
Psychosocial approach, 66
Psychosocial orientation, "psycho-"
      component of, 167
Psychosocial stress, role of, 145
Psychosocial treatment, comprehensive. *See*
      Comprehensive psychosocial
      treatment
Psychotherapeutic community, 122
Psychotherapists, research classification of,
      96
Psychotherapy. *See also* Treatment
  absence of adequate descriptions in, 290
  in acute psychosis, 294–295
  all-or-none phenomenon in, 181–189
  case histories in, 57–58
  central task of, 13–20
  challenge to, 146
  defined, 156
  developmental goals in, 233–235
  different modes of approach in, 122–123
  doctor–patient relationship in, 229
  drug therapy and, 92–93, 98, 228
  "elements" of, 157–166
  equilibrium in, 195–196
  etiological knowledge and, 71–74
  as facilitation of family-wide dialogue,
      17–19
  family-centered approach in, 125
  family therapy and, 98
  future studies in, 235–236
  general discussion of, 71–74
  "general purpose," 97
  group therapy and, 294
  individual differences in, 97

Psychotherapy (*cont.*)
  individual planning in, 120
  intensive explorative, 257–275
  left-brain and right-brain therapy in, 99
  monitoring in, 95
  multimodal approach in, 295–296
  nature and value of in schizophrenia, 55–62
  outcome versus process in, 96–97
  of outpatients vulnerable to psychosis,
      227–236
  outpatient therapy in, 98
  paradoxical, 195–196
  prestige of, 242
  psychosocial approach in, 66
  psychotic experience and, 101–112
  research classification and nomenclature
      in, 96
  research diagnostic criteria and, 96
  Rorschach cards in, 102–112
  of schizophrenia. *See* Psychotherapy of
      schizophrenia
  of severe disorders, 181–189
  simplified concept of, 165
  specific focused techniques in, 97–98
  therapeutic alliance in, 230–232
  therapeutic relatedness in, 57–58
  therapist factors in, 99
  "toxic effects" of, 98–99
  "understanding" in, 143
  and vulnerability to psychosis, 232–233
Psychotherapy of psychoses, problems in
      study of, 115–127
Psychotherapy of schizophrenia, 203–208.
      See also Drug therapy; Psychotherapy
  clinical science and, 241–242
  decreasing emphasis on, 241–245
  developing guidelines to, 217–226
  future of, 91–100
  intensive versus nonintensive treatment
      groups in, 263
  interdisciplinary communication in,
      242–243
  length of treatment analysis in, 264
  multimodal approach in, 295–296
  "negative findings" in, 291
  partial eclipse of, 218
  primacy of, 287–288
  psychoanalysis and, 219
  quality of outcome for, 257–275
  rationale for, 65–69
  research issues in, 244–245

Psychotherapy of schizophrenia (*cont.*)
  theory application in, 246–253
  treatment goals in, 244
Psychotherapy Outcome Interview, 258–261, 289
  detailed outline of, 270–275
  reliability ratings for, 261–262
  validity and usefulness of, 266
Psychotherapy research
  advantages and problems of, 124–125
  manpower problem in, 148–149
  method orientation versus problem
    orientation in, 119–123
  procedures in, 133
  time requirements in, 153
Psychotic adolescent patient, 107
Psychotic experience
  major divisions of, 103
  nature of, 101–112
Psychotic patient
  annihilation fears in, 105
  disorganized reality of, 105
  psychotherapeutic orientation in treatment
    of, 123–124
  regressive transference model for, 193
  subjective experience of, 143–144
Psychotic states, loneliness and, 163–164

Reality, relational, 15–16
Regressive transference
  in schizophrenic and borderline patients,
    193, 220–221
  stability and, 191, 205
Rehospitalization, resocialization in, 168
Relapse
  emotional level as predictor of, 24
  expressed emotion and, 25–26
  family factors in, 23–30
  social competence and, 27–29
Relapsing schizophrenic, Camarillo/UCLA
    training program for, 37–42
Relational reality
  defined, 15
  Oedipus complex and, 15
  psychoanalytic situation and, 16
Relative autonomy, attainment of, 235
Research
  changes in direction of, 288–291
  in psychotherapy. *See* Psychotherapy
    research
  in schizophrenia treatment, 245–246

Research classification, versus research
    diagnostic criteria, 96
Research Diagnostic Criteria, 229
Residual populations, disability severity in,
    169–174
Residential treatment, minimum goals in,
    168–169
Resocialization, in hospitalization or
    rehospitalization, 168
Restitution fantasies, 106–107
Role playing, in social skills training, 31
Roommate, supportive, 167
Rorschach cards, in psychotherapy, 102–112

"Schizoid position," 187
Schizophrenia
  admissions for, 22
  adolescent, 161–162, 224
  advances in knowledge of, 219–220
  aftercare treatment and family therapy in,
    77–89
  biological determinants of, 279
  as biological illness, 21
  biologic versus psychoanalytic therapy in,
    248
  chemical measures in symptomatology of,
    56
  childhood, 7
  clinical versus research approaches in,
    151–152
  comprehensive understanding and
    treatment in, 277–284
  defined, 156, 220
  denial of by "Abolitionists," 93
  depression in, 187, 223
  dread in, 164
  eating disorders in, 73
  "elements" of, 157–166
  environmental stress in, 146
  historical perspectives in, 3–11, 159–160
  identity in, 159–161
  infectious-disease model of, 278
  insight and self-observation in, 131–144
  loneliness in, 163–164
  neuroleptic drugs in, 21–23, 49–50, 218,
    229–230
  "nonexistence" of, 93, 160
  origin of name, 4
  Present State Examination for, 35, 38
  psychoanalysis and, 5–6, 9–10
  psychological versus organic nature of, 3

Schizophrenia (*cont.*)
  psychosocial approach to, 66
  psychotherapy of. *See* Psychotherapy of
    schizophrenia
  recovery in, 11
  relapse and rehospitalization in, 22, 168
  "remission" in, 4, 11
  representation development in, 103–104
  research in. *See* Research
  social and family factors in, 21–51
  social relationships dysfunction theory in,
    279
  stimulus modulation in, 284
  stressful events and, 279
  suffering in, 131
  theories of, 278–280
  thought disorder in, 86, 90–91
  treatment of. *See* Treatment
  treatment principles in, 283
  treatment research in, 245–246
  understanding of, 277–284
  variables contributing to, 280
  viewpoints in, 160
  work function and, 279–280
Schizophrenic. *See also* Schizophrenic patient
  cognitive problem-solving skills in, 29,
    46–47
  communication in, 8–9
  "elements" of, 157–166
  feelings and attitudes of, 9, 24
  number of, 133
  problem-solving model of, 29, 46–47
  regressive, 220–221
  "revolving door" policy for, 49
  therapeutic relationship for, 9–11
  worsening of symptomatology in, 30
Schizophrenic adolescent, 161–162, 224
Schizophrenic Disorganization Index,
    170–171
Schizophrenic families, siblings in, 72. *See
    also* Family therapy
Schizophrenic language, 8–9
Schizophrenic patient. *See also*
    Schizophrenia; Schizophrenic
  ambivalence of, 224–225
  anaclitic or symbolic needs of, 223
  classical analytical treatment of, 192
  controlled study of, 152
  cost of treating, 62
  destructive behavior in, 59
  developmental, 220

Schizophrenic patient (*cont.*)
  early health care systems for, 240
  ego activity of, 260
  and external reality, 105–106
  fear and emptiness of, 223
  follow-up studies of, 60–61
  grandiose fantasies of, 106
  identity of, 161–162
  intensive exploratory psychotherapy for,
    257–275
  milieu treatment for, 152
  monitoring of, 169
  orality of, 106
  parentless, 294
  personal and simplified concept of,
    164–165
  personality theory and, 161–162
  psychoanalysis of, 132, 134, 192, 219
  psychodynamic psychiatry for, 239–255
  psychotherapy for, 55–62. *See also*
    Psychotherapy of schizophrenia
  psychotic experience in, 101–112
  regressive, 220–221
  representation of boundaries by, 103–104
  restitution fantasies of, 106–107
  reticence of, 60
  sadness and helplessness of, 58
  self-awareness of, 260
  self-observation in, 138–139
  "splitting" in. *See* Splitting
  suffering of, 131–132
  superficial "processing" by, 243–244
  therapist "matching" with, 99
  typical predicaments of, 222
  vulnerability of in "unstable world," 104
  "willingness to change" in, 191
Schizophrenic relapse, 22. *See also* Relapse;
    Relapsing schizophrenia
  in aftercare treatment, 81
  expressed emotion and, 87
  family factors in, 23–30
Schizophrenic symptoms
  environmental change and, 28
  situational challenges and, 27
Schizophrenogenic mother, 7
Schizo-present family, 18, 74. *See also*
    Family therapy
"Secret garden" fantasy, 107–108
Seduction theory
  family theory and, 16–17
  versus Oedipus theory, 13–14

Self-Care Index, 70
Self-esteem, development of, 284
Self-observation
    defined, 138
    in etiology of illness, 131–144
Self-representation, 138–140
Sex, all-or-none attitude in, 185
Sheppard and Pratt Hospital, 5
Siblings, in schizophrenic families, 72
Single-subject approach, in social skills
        training, 33
Situational challenges, schizophrenic
        symptoms and, 27
Social competence, schizophrenic relapse
        and, 27–30
Social factors, in problem-solving therapy,
        21–51
Social inadequacy, 28
Social Learning Program, bizarre behavior
        and, 176–178
Social performance, in role-playing
        situations, 29
Social relationships dysfunction theory, 279
Social skills training, 30–32
    behavioral alternations or response options
        in, 40
    behavior changes in, 34
    at Camarillo State Hospital, 39–40
    group comparison studies in, 35–37
    hours per week in, 51
    multiple baseline analysis in, 36
    objectives of, 30, 51
    results in, 37
    role-playing in, 31
    single-subject studies in, 33–35
    training procedure outcome in, 33
Splitting
    affective aspects of, 183
    all-or-none phenomenon and, 186–189, 205
    in borderline and schizophrenic patients, 181
    former therapist and, 184
    hallucinations in, 183–184
Stimulus modulation, need for, 284
Stress
    environmental, 146
    as unifying concept, 249
Stressful life events, studies of, 279
Subjective experience dimension, 258,
        260–261, 267
Superego, of borderline patient, 186

Supportive roommate, 169
Suspiciousness, following family therapy, 85
Tardive dyskinesia, phenothiazine in, 154
Thematic Apperception Test, 182
Theory application, new directions in,
        246–253
Therapeutic alliance, primacy of, 288
Therapeutic relationship, 9–11
Therapist. See also Psychiatrist
    "disciplined subjectivity" of, 143
    essential requirements for, 165
    identity of, 162–163
    "matching" of to patient, 99
    patient's self-observation and, 139
    "stronger reality" of, 19
    tools of, 11
Therapy. See Psychotherapy
Thought disorder
    drugs and, 92
    following family therapy and aftercare
        treatment, 86
    improvement in, 88–89
Time–Sample Behavioral Checklist, 169–171
"Tooting horns" technique, 210
Total Inappropriate Behavior Index, 171
"Trait" deficits, mastery of, 233–235
"Transmission of irrationality" concept, 8
Treatment. See also Psychotherapy;
        Therapist
    changes in, 287–288
    combined with understanding, 277–284
    history of, 159–160
    milieu versus drug, 152–153, 160–161
    principles of, 282–283
Treatment research, new directions in,
        245–246
TSBC. See Time–Sample Behavioral
        Checklist
Turku Community Psychiatric Schizophrenia
        Project, 116–119
    overall design of, 123
Turku University (Finland), 116–117

Unconscious, reality and, 13
Understanding
    search for, 141–144
    treatment combined with, 277–284

VA-Alcoholic ward
    bizarre behavior in, 171–172
    improvement in, 177

"Vapor spray" technique, 210
Vomiting, in paradoxical intervention case
    study, 198–201
Vulnerability to psychosis
  future studies in, 235–236
  in outpatients, 227–236

Wechsler Adult Intelligence Scale, 182
Whitaker Index of Schizophrenic Thinking,
    35

Withdrawal
  emotional blunting and, 88
  family therapy and, 82
Withdrawal factor, in Brief Psychiatric
    Rating Scale, 83
World Health Organization, 23, 38

Yale Psychiatric Institute, 60
Yale University, 115